Together
We Will Win

What Happens

When We Don't

Talk About

Testicular Cancer

A Young Man's Story

Together
We Will Win

What Happens

When We Don't

Talk About

Testicular Cancer

A Young Man's Story

Karen A. McWhirt

Outskirts Press, Inc.
Denver, Colorado

Together We Will Win
What Happens When We Don't Talk About Testicular Cancer: A Young Man's Story
All Rights Reserved.
Copyright © 2010 Karen A. McWhirt
v5.0 r1.0

Cover photograph by Jeff Kirchhoff, Copyright © 2005, courtesy of the Lee's Summit Journal
Medical Illustration Copyright © 2009 Nucleus Medical Art. All Rights Reserved. www.nucleusinc.com

Visit Ian's website at www.IansStory.org
Visit the authors' website at www.Togetherwewillwin.net

Outskirts Press, Inc.
http://www.outskirtspress.com

ISBN: 978-1-4327-4867-8

Library of Congress Control Number: 2010929074

Outskirts Press and the "OP" logo are trademarks belonging to Outskirts Press, Inc.

PRINTED IN THE UNITED STATES OF AMERICA

This book is for my son, Ian,
in loving memory and deepest gratitude for all the
love, joy, humor, affection, and adventure that you brought into my life
and into this world, just by being who you are.
And in deepest reverence for your amazing spirit, Ian,
and the tremendous courage and grace with which you
faced your suffering and your fate.
I love you forever, Ian, Wonderful You. - Mom

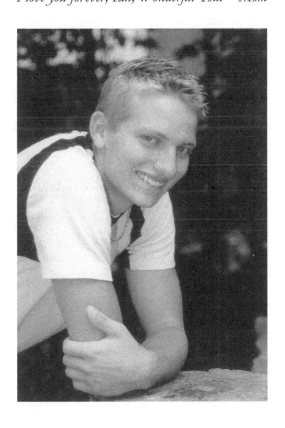

"This powerful narrative of a young man's fight to survive an advanced cancer provides the reader a vivid understanding of the fear, the anguish, the frustration, the anger, and the suffering involved in such a battle. Moments of little victories are overwhelmed by disappointment as disease progresses despite all efforts. The reader becomes painfully aware of the fact that such a disease is not experienced by the patient on an intermittent basis but is always present, physically and emotionally challenging the patient and frustrating his efforts to have even a little normal life. One also feels the struggle of parents attempting to relieve some of the burden thrust on such young shoulders and their pain and disappointment over the inability to protect their child or find an escape for him. The loyalty and courage of his mother and the benevolence of family and friends is compelling to witness. This story may have meaning to many people, but it is particularly revealing to those who care for cancer patients and provides invaluable insight into the aspects of this disease and what it means to the patient and those who love the patient that are often so private, so hidden."

— Allan R. Fleming, M.D.

"A mothers poignant memoir of disease and loss is also a moving call-to-arms in the fight to prevent a curable form of cancer.

Perhaps the most valuable part of Together We Will Win is a brief, appendix-like last chapter that lists the early-warning signs for testicular cancer, the most common cancer among men ages 14 to 45. The chapter also provides instructions for doing a testicular self-exam, the best means of detecting the disease in its earliest stages. McWhirt gives readers this information because the book is the true-life story of her son Ian's struggle with testicular cancer. The vibrant young man is thrust into a battle for his life by one abnormal cell. That one cell— which will multiply into billions— is the beginning of a cancer that will ultimately take Ian's life. The book recounts the story of his painful descent. The author is a talented writer and tells her son's story in surprisingly measured prose, mostly by channeling Ian's voice in the first person. This is a risky gamble, but it pays off, and the account is personal, relatable and compelling. We are with Ian when he first notices but ignores the small lumps in his scrotum. Then, McWhirt takes us into the room when Ian is diagnosed, when he receives chemotherapy and, sadly, when he dies. These scenes are not meant to be bathetic or melodramatic. The author tells her wrenching story as a journalist would, and her main goal is not to pull heartstrings, though she does. Her purpose is to inform and to explain, in the hope that others can be spared her son's fate. Her prose is therefore the most powerful kind of writing— the kind that can save lives.

A powerful, educational cautionary tale."

— Kirkus Discoveries

"Well I've just finished *Together We Will Win*, and boy I have the utmost respect and admiration for yourself and Ian. It was very emotional reading Ian's words and quite a few tears flowed at times, yet the way Ian's words have been written made me want to read on more, even when I had other things to do...I couldn't put the book down and in my view this is a sure sign of the book being written beautifully and having something that the reader has become attached to. Reading Ian's words really made me feel like I had known him for years and he sounds like the kind of guy I would have got along with and had a laugh with....I really mean that Karen, he sounds a brilliant lad and it's so sad what happened to Ian. It was so hard for me personally as a survivor to take in what Ian went through, I just can't believe he went through all that pain at times, whereas I just had one shot of chemo and didn't suffer nearly as much as Ian......I really am so lucky.....but this is why people like yourself and me do what we do....to make sure that other men don't have to suffer like Ian did, and his words toward the end of the book, where he wanted you to write his story so that other men would be educated...... well that's bloody brave and admirable of Ian to think of others whilst he was going through such a terrible time."

— Darren One Ball Couchman,
TC survivor, author of *One Lump or Two*

"THE BOOK IS AWESOME! I can't tell you how difficult it was for me to put it down at any point. I found myself getting home and going immediately to the book and I finished it very quickly. Karen - I can imagine how difficult that had to be to write that in Ian's voice but it was incredible. You must have taken some incredible notes throughout Ian's experience. It was perfectly written. It not only described in detail to a testicular cancer patient what to expect from diagnosis through treatment but also gives the patient and care givers a first hand look at how cancer and its treatment affects everyday life, relationships, right down to how difficult it is to simply get dressed. I also enjoyed getting to learn more about Ian as a person, as your son and about you and your family. It simply was wonderfully written and I can't explain how grateful I am that you honored Ian and how proud he is of you. Simply Incredible! Powerful! And it brought me to tears many times over."

— John Nigra, TC survivor

"When I finished the book I was absolutely amazed and terrified at the same time. The first thing that came to my mind was what an awesome mom you are. Your relationship with Ian is inspirational. At times, I would see glimpses of my relationship with my own mother as well as see parts of my own story played out on the pages of the book. As a matter of fact, I called my mom the evening I finished the book because I felt I needed to chat a bit with her. The struggle through highs and lows it must have taken to put together such an incredible book seems Herculean. However, I know your efforts are not only going to save many young men along the way but every expectation that Ian had to educate and enlighten others about testicular cancer will have been met. Your work is timeless."

— Mike Craycraft, TC survivor and
founder of the Testicular Cancer Society

Acknowledgments

I would like to thank God for the gift of Ian as my son, for Ian's grace, courage, wisdom, and strength in his most difficult months, and for providing the will, emotional strength and perseverance needed to write and publish this book. Thank you to Ian, for being the wonderful son that he is, for staying close to me, and helping with this book in many ways. To my husband, Mark, for his love and undying support in life, and in the process of writing this book. To my sister, Denise, for her caring heart, her gift of laughter, and constant support in trying times. To the hundreds of extended family and friends, for their aid, love, and caring encouragement, throughout Ian's treatment and during the writing of his book. To Ian's boss, Gina, and all of his friends for loving him, and remembering him always. And to Ian's friends—Carrie, Gina, Pat, Jess, David, Kyle, Karl, Jason, Jared, and Jesse—who have contributed details to portions of this book.

To the staff in every department of the University of Kansas Hospital and Cancer Center that guided Ian's treatment, for their attentive, compassionate, and professional care, and for their willing and gracious assistance with research and medical details, and sharing personal memories of Ian for this book:

- Dr. Peter J. Van Veldhuisen, M.D.
- Dr. Allan R. Fleming, M.D.

- Dr. Alvaro R. Alvarez-Ferrinetti, M.D.
- Dr. Darren Klish, M.D., MPH
- Margo Sweany, RN, OCN
- Angela Rueter, RN, BSN, OCN
- Tracy Sarin, RN, MSN, NP-C, OCN
- Mark Winkler, RN
- Carol Bomberger, RN, OCN
- Shari Thomasson, RN, OCN
- Michelle Bragg, RT
- Leslie Niehues, RT, CMD
- Beth Haines, RN, BSN, OCN
- Jo Babaren, RN, BSN
- Vici Liston, RN, BSN, OCN
- Kristy Delaney, RN, BSN, CCRN
- Michael Blomquist, RN, CCRN
- Lori Barham, RN, BSN, CCRN
- Andrew Chang, RRT
- Kimberly Clark, RN, OCN
- Cyndy Steen, RN, MSN
- Mary Moody, LMSW
- Erika James
- Carol A. Koski, RHIA, CTR
- Alberta Jadali
- Sam Sweeten, RHIA

And to countless other physicians, nurses, technicians, therapists, aides, transport techs, and housekeepers, for all that they did for Ian in a day's work. Every day they make a difference in the lives of cancer patients and their families.

Thank you to the owner and hair stylists at Salon Par, Veronica, Sheryl, and Kim for donating use of the salon, their time, and their talents for Ian's head shaving party.

Thank you to the hundreds of people who personally prayed for Ian, and to all the churches who prayed for him during his treatment and his transition: The Sisters of Saint Joseph of Carondelet in Kirkwood, Missouri; Saint Mark's Catholic Church in Independence, Missouri; Our Lady of the Presentation Catholic Church in Lee's Summit, Missouri; Our Lady of the Coronation Catholic Church in Grandview, Missouri; Redemptorist Catholic Church, and Our Lady of Sorrows Catholic Church in Kansas City, Missouri; Saint Paul Catholic Church in Nebraska City, Nebraska; Mother of God Catholic Church in Denver, Colorado; Lee's Summit Community Church, Deer Brook Covenant Church, and Lee's Summit Bible Church in Lee's Summit, Missouri; Pleasant Grove Primitive Baptist Church in Independence, Missouri; First Christian Church in Princeton, Kentucky; Open Door Church in Padukah, Kentucky; the Sikh Community Ashram in Kansas City, Missouri; Unity Village Chapel and the Silent Unity Prayer Ministry in Unity Village, Missouri; Unity Church of Lee's Summit, Christ Church Unity and Unity Temple in Kansas City, Missouri; and Unity Church of Maui, Hawaii.

Thank you to all who purchased Ian's music CD or contributed funds to *Ian's Story Fund for Testicular Cancer Awareness*, in honor and memory of Ian.

Contents

Introduction

Almost everyone knows someone who has had cancer. You may hear that they have cancer, are going through chemotherapy, radiation or both, in their fight against cancer. Then you hear that they have either survived the cancer, or they have died. But if you haven't been the caretaker, you didn't know what happened in between. Most people never hear the rest of the story. Even young men who have survived testicular cancer do not often talk openly about that experience. There are those brave souls who are out there in our world telling people about this disease every day, and I praise them for their continuous efforts. I pray that others are listening to these survivors. They know how bad it can get. They know what it feels like to have to give up one of their testicles to save their own life, and they are making every effort to help other young men learn how to detect this cancer in the earliest stage, a lump in a testicle, in order to increase the chances of survivorship.

Maybe you've heard of testicular cancer. And hopefully you are aware that it is the most common cancer in young men, and that early detection increases the chance of survival to around 90 percent. It's easy for a person, especially a young man, to shrug his shoulders and think this kind of thing only happens to other people, or older people. But consider the fact that testicular cancer is one of the more aggressive and faster-growing cancers, and think about the fact that testicular cancer begins as just one cancer cell in a testicle, and soon multiplies into billions of cancer cells inside that testicle. As embarrassing as that sounds, keep thinking about it, and imagine what would happen if nothing is done to stop the cancer from growing inside that testicle. Do you know how bad it can get? Do you realize how horrible cancer treatment will be, the longer a guy waits to get it checked out?

Together We Will Win is Ian's story, and is being told to increase awareness of testicular cancer, and with hope that young men will know more about what will happen to them if they find a lump in a testicle and do nothing about it. Ian's story illustrates the life of a cancer patient that most people never see. Probably you've heard how sick people become with chemotherapy. But have you ever thought about what it must be like, hour after hour? Do you understand what chemotherapy actually is, or how it works? Have you ever wondered what a radiation treatment looks like, or what it does to the body? Ian's story will tell you.

The life of a cancer patient may not be all that you think it is. Or it may be everything you think it is, and worse. No one can have the same experience as another person, yet my sitting beside my son for four months and observing the horrible suffering he went through cannot compare to the very real and frightening experience it was for Ian. His experience was sometimes so torturous that he could not put it into words. But as his mom, as every loving mom knows, there are always little things you notice that tell you how your loved one is truly feeling. Ian's suffering showed not only in his face, but also in the tender ways he so often spoke to me.

Ian, throughout his life, was a very affectionate, loving person. Our relationship was solid, built on trust and unconditional love. As Ian grew older, he didn't need his mom as much. He was strong, willful, and confident. But when cancer became the lonely reality of his every day, Ian showed fear in many ways. His eyes no longer sparkled with happiness when he spoke, and he never wanted to be alone for any length of time. His constant expression of gratitude to me was the most sure sign that he was suffering more deeply than even I could understand. All of our lives, we had never parted company without first saying "I love you," and every now and then, he thanked me for being his mom. After his diagnosis, Ian told me he loved me many times a day, and thanked me for being his mom almost every day, sometimes two or three times in one day, even though I never left his side. This expression of love alone told me that Ian was suffering more profoundly than he let anyone know. There was nothing I could do for him, there was no kiss to make it all better. My presence was all I could offer, and Ian appreciated it more and more each day.

Throughout Ian's treatment, I kept a detailed, chronological journal and calendar of every day and night during our hospital stays, every treatment, things that were said to us, things we said to others, and to one another. I lived at his side for days, weeks, months, watching him suffer, praying for him, and doing anything I could do to help him feel more comfortable. At the time, I thought this record keeping was helpful to Ian. I thought it mattered. But looking back, I think it gave me a sense of some control over the outcome. I never expected, though, that I would be using that information in writing about Ian's experiences. I read meticulously through Ian's medical records to expand the details and verify the events, treatments, times, and dates. I researched his chemotherapy drugs more extensively, and learned more about radiation. I spoke with his doctors, therapists, and nurses to gain a clearer understanding of things I wasn't sure of, and to hear their personal memories of Ian.

Ian had a comedic personality, and I loved listening to him tell a story, so I decided to let Ian tell this story, too. After all, it's his story. And even though in the end he was too sedated to talk, I believe Ian's spirit was very much present, and aware of all that was going on around him. It felt natural to me, that Ian should narrate this book to the very last word.

You'll get a taste of Ian's humor every now and then as you read through his four-month treatment. He didn't laugh out loud as much, or seek to entertain with funny stories as he used to, but his natural comedic look on life was still with him all the way. His casual one-liner style always earned a quick chuckle, but as funny as his comments were, he was simply expressing his honest, yet comical observation at the time. There were funny things he said and did so frequently that none of it got written down, but I remember sharing in his amusement, and chuckling at his humorous nature many times while sitting in the hospital with him, or talking with him at home. Ian often had a wise and philosophical take on life situations, too. We were talking once, about life, people, and those painful events and memories that each person holds inside of himself... the personal pain that no one talks about.

Ian looked at me as he was thinking, and then he said, "You know... you think you know people, but the truth is, you never *really* know a person until you know their story, and everyone has a story."

Ian's story is one of hope, struggle, and uncertainty. A story of the fragility of life, and what happens to a young man if testicular cancer gets overlooked for too long.

Please read this book with those you love in mind. It's not just about Ian. It's about creating awareness in our society of the most common, yet curable cancer in young men. Read it and learn how bad testicular cancer can get if not caught and treated early. Read it and remember how important it is to talk about testicular cancer with those you care about. Read it and remember how important your presence will be to someone you love who has cancer. Teach others what you learn from reading Ian's story. Create Testicular Cancer Awareness in your family, in your neighborhood, in your world. It is curable, and together, we will win.

1

Is It Bronchitis, Acid Reflux, Gynecomastia ...or the Most Common Cancer in Young Men?

I think that none of us ever fully understood just how sick I really was... how much cancer had continued to consume my body day by day... how strong the cancerous cells were. I didn't want to give that thought any power at all. I put my focus on my affirmations that I was going to be healthy again. In my prayers, I visualized myself as healthy and living my life again. I practiced knowing that God was going to make everything turn out okay, and that by next spring, I would be pronounced cancer-free. And Mom prayed for me day and night. She told me she was always praying, while sitting quietly beside me.

It's hard to believe that testicular cancer had started in my body, as one—just one—abnormal cell, inside my right nut. It lived there, abnormally, for—no one can know how long. It had secretly grown strong enough to multiply into two abnormal cells, and then three, then eventually millions, and then billions. Eventually the cancer cells worked their way into either my bloodstream or my lymph system, and from there were able to travel to and multiply in the rest of my organs. Freaky, isn't it? Just abnormal cells, growing in their own destructive path, starving off the good ones, and silently killing my living body.

By the time we learned I had cancer, the cancer cells had already grown into multiple lesions in my lungs, my stomach, and my liver. Why? Why had no one ever told me? The doctors say testicular cancer is the most common cancer in guys my age—so why isn't anyone talking about it? How come I had never heard about it until now—now that it's taking over my whole life? If only I had known about it. I just thought one of my balls was lumpier than the other. I was still growing, and so was one of my balls, a little bigger and a little heavier than the other one. It didn't hurt, it just grew a little tender. Hell no, I didn't tell my parents, or anybody. A guy doesn't say, "Hey Mom, do you think there could be something wrong with one of my nuts?!"

I had seen my doctor six months before my actual diagnosis, about a lump I noticed near my left nipple. I was really embarrassed about it, and I didn't tell my mom. It was a little tender, though it didn't hurt, but I was afraid people might notice it if I took off my shirt. The doctor didn't look at it much, but told me not to worry, said it was called gynecomastia, and that many young men my age have the same problem. He didn't ask me if I had any other symptoms at all. He just said to come back and see him again if it got larger or more painful. That breast lump never did go away, but it did not get larger or more painful, so I never went back. This doctor did not seem concerned at all that something else might be wrong.

Several months later, I developed a cough that flared up every time I ate something. I went to a different doctor for that. I told this new doctor that eating made me start coughing, and that I felt like the food was getting stuck in my throat. I had difficulty swallowing, and many times some green junk came up when I coughed. I wasn't nauseous, but I told him that I had what I thought was frequent heartburn. An x-ray was taken, but nothing abnormal was reported, not even in my lungs. I was diagnosed with chronic bronchitis, due to what they call peribronchial cuffing. The doctor gave me a nasal steroid and antibiotics to treat these symptoms.

When these medications didn't help after a week, he thought maybe

I had been suffering with acid reflux, and sent me to a gastroenterologist. Well, they thought I had some obstruction in my esophagus, and scheduled a procedure called an EGD to go down into my esophagus through my mouth. They tried it twice, without success. The nurse didn't give me enough anesthesia the second time and I apparently freaked out and tried to pull the apparatus from my throat. That sucked, and I was beginning to wonder if anyone knew anything about what they were doing. I never went back, and the coughing continued to get worse. I couldn't sleep at night. Mom kept on me to go see the doctor again, but I didn't want another episode of what had happened a few weeks earlier.

After a minor car accident in which a woman slammed into the back of my car, I began having some back pain. I had been to the emergency room just after the accident, where a doctor had viewed an x-ray of my spine and found no fractures, but the pain kept getting worse. Within a couple weeks, the pain in my back grew more intense and more constant. My stomach had started to hurt, and after a couple days, I started throwing up occasionally. I didn't tell Mom about that at first, but my boss at the shipping company where I worked part time had said I didn't look well at all on Friday, and kept on me to tell my mom and get to a doctor. A few days later, the nausea and stomach pain were too much, and I ended up calling in sick from work that Monday. That's when I finally told Mom. She thought I might have some kind of stomach flu, and gave me some stuff to calm my nausea. But by the next evening, the pain was so severe, I couldn't stand it. I woke my mom up at two o'clock in the morning to ask her what to do. I told her I had taken more of that pink stuff, but it wasn't doing any good. She wanted to take me to the emergency room, but I refused. She made a space for me to sleep near her until morning, and at about 6:30 Wednesday morning, I asked her if she would drive me to the clinic. My back and stomach hurt so bad I felt I could not drive myself. I couldn't even stand up. I told the doctor about the intense pain, the vomiting, and that I felt overall, very sick. He felt around on my abdomen and we noticed that it was very tender to the touch, especially around the pit center of my navel, or what he called the umbilicus. He didn't ask me if I had any other symptoms, and I didn't tell him about the still-existing breast lump, or my lumpy, heavy testicle. But he was concerned that I might have gallstones, or some kind of duct obstruction, so he arranged for me to have an ultrasound on my abdomen. He also had the nurse take some of my blood to analyze the enzymes in it. He was still looking for some type of gastrointestinal trouble.

The earliest appointment we could get for the ultrasound was later that afternoon. So I was forced to go home and wait it out. Mom tried all kinds of things to ease my pain—ice, heat, massage, music, laying her hands on my stomach and back—and even guided relaxation meditation. Nothing worked. The pain was too intense. I took some of the pain reliever that I had from the car accident, and that helped me to sleep for a little while. Mom woke me at four o'clock to go in for the ultrasound. During the ride there, my stomach started hurting worse. We didn't have to wait long, though, and they took me right in. Mom wanted to come in with me, but I thought I'd be okay on my own. I left her pacing in the waiting room. Having the ultrasound done wasn't too bad at first, and it only took a few minutes. I was watching the technician's face as she rolled the cold steel cylinder across my stomach and the rest of my abdomen. Her eyes looked serious—and for a moment, shocked, even, and her reaction got me feeling a little scared. I asked her what she saw, and she just darted her eyes away and said she needed to talk to the nurse. The nurse came in and I asked again what the ultrasound was showing. They both looked at each other and the nurse said they couldn't say for sure, but they wanted to do a CT scan. I was getting really worried, and I wished my mom was in the room with me, so she could help me find out what was going on. I asked the nurse if she would please go and get my mom, if she could come in my room with me. When Mom came in, she asked the same questions, and got the same answers—no answers. I told Mom that I was scared because no one was telling me anything, and I was afraid something was seriously wrong. Mom said it was too soon to worry, and to just be patient and let them do their job. She said that probably they are not allowed to discuss with the patient what they think, and that it's their job to do what the doctor has ordered for me, and report back to him.

The nurse brought in a delicious formula for me to drink that looked like a pink-orange milkshake, and tasted like something I described as "ass." It was bitter and chalky, with a metal-tasting film that covered my tongue, and made me want to throw up, but the nurse said I needed to drink the entire eight ounces. I lay on the ultrasound treatment table with the large Styrofoam cup next to me, drinking it out of a straw. Mom had pulled a chair up close to me. I showed her on my stomach where the ultrasound had been done. It looked like a normal stomach, but it hurt like hell on the inside. We talked about our concerns for tomorrow, my pain, and the delectable locker room-flavored nectar that I had to force down with a grimace at every sip. The purpose was to fill my body cavity with this substance called contrast, which I was told enhances the visualization of my organs and tissues during the CT scan. By absorbing the x-rays, the rest of my organs and blood vessels are highlighted, thus creating a "contrast." In the meantime, the nurse was getting the okay from my doctor to do the CT scan, and I had to wait a while for the contrast solution to work its way through my body.

I asked Mom if she wanted to come with me, but I already knew she wanted to. I was feeling a little freaked out, and I wanted her to be there. The CT technician escorted me and Mom to the lab, and told us all about what was going to happen in the scan. I had to lay flat on a table that moved slowly through a donut-shaped machine, as if going back and forth through a four-foot-wide donut hole. I was to stay as still as possible. There would be times when I had to hold my breath in, or out, and not even move to breathe while the scanning took place from my shoulders to my hips as the table I was on glided me through the process. The technician said he would be instructing me through a microphone in his observation room as we went along, telling me what to do, and assured me that if I had anything to say, he would be able to hear me as well.

Mom was scared, I could tell, because she kept asking all kinds of questions about this procedure. He helped us both to understand that nothing weird was going to happen, it's just like getting an x-ray, and he let Mom join him in the adjacent room and watch me through the large window. Mom later told me that this room was full of computer screens, and that every one of them was showing a different image of the scan that was taking place on me. She didn't understand what she was looking at, although she tried. She said she could tell by the look on his face that the technician was very concerned and was thorough in his work. She knew that he knew exactly what he was looking at, but he would not talk about it with her. With growing anxiety, she stood quietly behind him, closely watching me through the process. The scanning procedure I think took only about 20 or 30 minutes to complete. It was so hard to lie still—my gut was hurting so bad I just wanted to curl up in the fetal position—so even though all I had to do was lay there and breathe, or not breathe, I was relieved when the procedure was over. Although no one would tell us anything, I sensed the news was not good. The technician told us to call our doctor in the morning to learn the results.

By the time we left there, it was after 5:30 in the afternoon, and I was starving. I hadn't eaten all day because of the pain. I didn't feel I could eat any solid food, so Mom stopped at the health food store on the way home and bought some organic vegetable broth for me. She was in the store only a few minutes, but that time I spent waiting for her in the car was shear agony. My stomach had started to feel as if it was a big burning, gripping, stabbing, twisting muscle inside of me. All I could do was twist and writhe around in the seat, holding my stomach. I cursed and screamed at the pain. I couldn't stand it, and when Mom got back in the car I yelled at her, too. "Mom what took you so long? I can't sit still and feel this pain anymore!" I slammed my fist into the dashboard of the car. "GODDAMMIT I CAN'T STAND THIS PAIN! IT'S KILLING ME! I CAN'T TAKE IT!" My eyes were watering because it all hurt so bad. My mom had never seen me this way, and I could tell by the look on her face that I scared her. But she didn't get mad, she just told me never to punch the dashboard like that or I might set off the air bag to blow up in my face. Then she said in a very calm voice, that she was very sorry that I was suffering so much pain, and that she knew the pain was worse than anything she could understand, and that she was doing her best to help me. Then she added that yelling and cussing so loud and getting mad wasn't going to make the pain go away, it would just hurt the people around me. I took a deep breath and dropped my head back into the seat headrest.

"I'm sorry, Mom." I looked over at her, "I'm not mad at you... you know... it's just that this pain is so fucking bad..." My eyes were still watering. My arms were wrapped around my stomach.

Tears formed in her eyes, and she lifted a hand to touch my shoulder. "I'm sorry Ian. I'm so very sorry."

"Can you please hurry and get me home... I just want to lie down in my bed." I sat up and doubled over, still holding my gut.

She started the car. "You can yell now, if you want to. I can take it, if you just need to get it out. I'm prepared for it now," she said in a hopeful voice.

I shook my head. "I was just going crazy sitting there by myself. You're right, it doesn't make the pain go away, it just makes it hurt worse, getting all worked up like that."

I quietly suffered and she quietly worried, as we sped down the highway trying to get me home in hopes I'd be more comfortable there.

I couldn't eat anything when we got home, even though I hadn't eaten in over a day. That entire night, I just rolled around in hell, holding my stomach, trying to find a position to ease the pain. I couldn't stay still, I raised my legs up, then put them down straight, raised up one leg, then both, as I rolled from side to side. Even the pain medication I had didn't help. Mom sat on the floor right by me through the night. I know she wished she could do something to help me. I started feeling sleepy around two o'clock in the morning, and she had drifted off to sleep beside my bed. We would call the doctor first thing in the morning.

☽☽☽☽

2

Defense Can Win the Game, but First We Have to Take Your Nut

Mom woke me gently from a sound morning sleep at about 8:30. "Ian... wake up, honey. It's 8:30."

I opened my eyes and looked at her.

"How are you feeling this morning?" she asked.

"Okay..." I muffled in a cracked voice.

She waited for my face to show signs of comprehension, then she spoke with a kind, soft but nervous voice, "Ian, I just talked to your doctor. He wants us to meet him at the hospital."

"What?"... I rubbed my eyes, "Why?"

"He wants to talk to us about the CT scan..."

My stomach wasn't hurting too bad at the moment, so I wondered about the urgency. "Now? We have to go now?"

"Yes, we have to go now. Just get up and dressed, and we'll go as soon as you're ready. He wants us to go this morning. How's your stomach? Do you want something to eat?"

"No... thanks... maybe, could you get me a little milk?"

I rolled out of bed and went into the bathroom while Mom went for the milk. I threw on a t-shirt and jeans, and grabbed a baseball cap. Mom came in with a small glass of milk, and I took a few swallows as

I slid my feet into my white leather sneakers. I sat on my bed finishing the milk, and thought to myself... why the hospital?

As we were driving, I asked Mom what else the doctor said. She said that he told her I needed to have more tests done. "But why at the hospital?" I asked. "I don't understand why we have to go to the hospital."

I could tell Mom was nervous and scared, though she tried to look calm. "Honey, let's just get there, okay? We'll find out everything when we get there."

When we arrived in the hospital lobby, I claimed a chair nearest the door, and Mom went to the admissions desk to find out what we were supposed to do. I sat there still wondering why we had to meet the doctor at the hospital. Something must be wrong, I thought. I gazed around at the lobby, as if looking for clues, and Mom came back to tell me I needed to be with her at the desk, to answer some questions.

When we sat down, I asked Mom why we were there, at the admitting desk. "The doctor wants you to be admitted, Ian," she said with apprehension.

"Admitted?!... into the hospital?! I'm not that sick! I feel fine! Why do I have to be admitted?! What's going on!?"

She looked at me, and her eyes were sad and afraid. Her mouth opened slightly as if she was going to say something, but then she pressed her lips together as if something stopped her. "Please, Ian... we'll see the doctor soon, and he'll tell you," she pleaded.

"This is bad, Mom, I can feel it, and I want to know what's going on." I could still see fear in her eyes, and I could tell that she had words in her that she was afraid to speak, and that scared me even more.

"Let's just do what the doctor says, Ian, and we'll see, okay?" I didn't know it at the time, but she was praying the doctor was wrong, that it was all a mistake.

"But I want to know why he wants me to be admitted into the hospital, Mom, when I'm not even sick! I'm not going to be admitted into the hospital unless I know why, Mom..." In my mind, a hospital was a place only for people so sick they needed surgery, or those with a terrible disease, or dying. I wasn't any of those things. I just had a bad stomach ache and some nausea, maybe the flu.

She looked straight at me and in a barely audible voice said, "He thinks you have cancer, Ian."

"What!? That's bullshit..." I shook my head and raised my hands in the air, showing my disbelief. "I'm going to call him." I grabbed my cell phone out of my front pocket and opened it up, my thumb at the keypad, ready to dial. I looked at her, "What's his number?"

Mom looked nervously at the admitting representative, and asked her to give me the doctor's number. The clerk dialed the number for me on her desk phone, and told him that I was sitting in front of her at the admissions desk and wanted to talk to him, then she handed the receiver to me.

"This is Ian. I want to know why I have to be admitted into the hospital, why did you tell my mom I have cancer? Why did you tell her to bring me here?" I then listened as the doctor started to speak, and I felt my breathing stop. I felt my whole body change from a tense concern, to an almost numb, vulnerable feeling of alarm and dread. I felt my eyes redden and fill with tears as I looked over at my mom, who was biting her lower lip, and already had tears streaming down her cheeks. I felt a sense of hopelessness coming over both of us, as Mom leaned in closer to me. I had to look down, to keep from crying, and when I looked back at Mom, I could tell she knew what I was being told. She had heard the same words only minutes before she woke me up. The doctor was telling me there was a large cancerous tumor in my stomach. He said there were numerous lesions in my liver, and many in my lungs, which are also cancer, and that my spleen was enlarged. He continued that it was suspected and most likely that my right testicle was enlarged with cancerous tumors also, and that I must be admitted into the hospital for more testing and immediate treatment. He spoke with a kind of stern, impatient voice. He stated the hard evidence in no uncertain terms, that my situation was one of emergency treatment or death. He said he would be at the hospital to see me once I was admitted, and that he had already contacted other doctors, a urologist and an oncologist, to meet me there. I didn't even know what those words meant, but the idea that I had three doctors coming to see me brought a cold, weakening chill all over my body. I had never felt so much fear and instant dread in my whole life. I didn't even know what to think. I suddenly couldn't feel my legs or my hands. My mouth got dry, and I couldn't swallow. I felt dizzy, and sick to my stomach, as I laid the receiver down on the desk. I looked to my mom for that strength she often gave me, and when I saw her tears, it all just spilled out of me. Mom reached to hold me, and I wrapped my arms around her as we cried about the news we now shared.

"I'm so sorry, Ian," she cried, "I'm so sorry I couldn't tell you those things, Ian, I couldn't say it...I just couldn't look into your eyes and say those things to you! I keep praying it isn't true!"

I loosened my hug and sat back to wipe the tears off my face. "It's okay, Mom..." I sat looking at her, hoping she could tell me it's not as bad as it sounds.

She dried her tears, and suddenly had that assured expression that I was looking for. "We'll do what we have to do, Ian," she said, looking at me with the promise of strength I needed at that moment. "We'll do what we have to do, and we'll get through it. We will get through it, together."

I nodded and took a deep breath, my hands on my wet face.

She motioned to the clerk that we were ready to continue the admitting process.

I wiped my wet hands on my jeans as I looked back at Mom. "Does Mark know?"

"Yeah..." she nodded, "he's on his way here now."

Just then, I looked up and saw Mark coming through the door. He stood looking for us for a moment, then came straight over to us. He gave me a hug, and Mom, too, then he stood behind us like a support beam with one hand resting on my shoulder, while the admitting forms were completed. The pain in my gut grew more intense as we sat there waiting.

Mark and Mom had been together since I was four and a half years old. I sometimes called him Dad, but with others usually referred to him as Mark. When I was alone with him, I most often called him

Mook or Mooky, a nickname I gave him when I was about five. Mark is the strongest person I know, but I could feel his fear, too, and knowing I had them both with me made me feel protected and comforted, but at the same time, even more scared just knowing I needed them. It seemed like we had to answer a million questions before I could be admitted, but finally someone came with a wheelchair to take me to my assigned room. I felt like throwing up, and I guess I was kind of in shock, because everything started to look not real, like I was being wheeled through some kind of fake movie scene. Everyone seemed to be moving in a kind of surreal slow motion, and the sounds of everything around me were muffled. It felt very strange to be in my body, looking out at all of it. That morning only my stomach hurt, but now I felt like my whole body, my whole life was giving up on me.

As soon as I got to my hospital room, the nurses and aides started streaming in, hooking things up, bringing in supplies, taking my temperature, checking my blood pressure, asking me dozens of questions. My stomach had started to hurt so bad I could not lie still, and all I cared about was getting rid of that pain. Mom stayed very close to me, and Mark stood by the foot of my bed, pacing back and forth occasionally. A nurse came in and put an IV in my arm, which scared me. I'd never had an IV before, and it hurt like hell when she stuck it in my forearm. Pretty soon there were three bags hanging from the IV pole. One was fluid, the others contained drugs for pain and nausea.

The oncologist, who I only knew as the cancer doctor, came in and examined me, felt around on my abdomen a lot, then Mom and Mark left the room so he could examine my testicles. That was a really strange feeling, and I felt embarrassed as I lay there helplessly while he felt around on my balls, inspecting them and asking questions about them. He asked me how long ago I had noticed a lump in my testicle. I couldn't remember, and I was feeling embarrassed to say so. I told him it had been painful for the last couple of months.

As he stepped out of the room to get Mom and Mark, I laid there mentally kicking myself for not knowing that the lump meant something was very wrong. He then explained to all three of us everything that would take place in the next few hours, and the coming days. He didn't talk much about the cancer treatment, but he did say I would be treated at the new cancer center located about a 15-minute drive from our house. That seemed convenient enough.

My regular doctor came in to see me while the oncologist was there, and he gave me a very grim picture of my not-so-certain future. He was a young guy, a little over-zealous about it all, and what he said scared the shit out of me.

He knelt down on one knee at the foot of my bed, and propped his arms on the footboard. I raised the head of my bed a little to see him. He held my medical file in his hands, and looked at me very directly with his dark brown eyes.

"Ian, do you understand you are here because you have been diagnosed with cancer?"

I nodded. I figured my fear showed on my face and in my eyes. It was still shocking news to hear.

"I want to make sure you understand the seriousness of your situation that has put you in the hospital today."

I looked blankly at him. How much more seriously could I take it? This was the third time I had been told this news, and I was scared for my life!

"There is a very large mass in the duodenum of your stomach, do you understand?" He set my medical records at my feet, and used his hands to show me it was about the size and shape of a large potato.

"Yeah." I tried not to show my emotions, but I felt very nauseous and frightened at the thought of a huge cancerous mass growing in my stomach.

He continued in his urgent tone of voice, "There are numerous masses scattered in both lobes of your lungs, and multiple masses scattered throughout all lobes of your liver. Your spleen is enlarged as a result of the cancer. There is also a large mass in your right scrotum. You are in very critical condition, Ian, and it is very important that you get treatment immediately. That is why I've had you admitted today."

I imagined the cancer growing faster by the minute. "What would happen if I can't get treated soon enough?"

He paused briefly, taking a breath. "You will die. If you don't get this cancer treated, you'll die."

I couldn't help feeling that he actually enjoyed delivering such grave news. The fact that cancer can kill a person wasn't news to us, but Mark, Mom, and I all looked shocked to hear him say it so bluntly. While I did appreciate that he was very clear about the seriousness of my health status, I did not like the way he made it seem as if death was waiting at my door.

It was all too much, and I couldn't even take it in, I couldn't make any sense of any of it, except that my body was full of cancer, and I could die. That's all I could hear, and it was so hard to believe. My gut and my back hurt so bad I wanted to scream, and my thoughts were swirling together with disbelief, fear, helplessness.... My life had been going along just fine, and now all of a sudden, I could be dying. I thought this could not really be happening. This is too horrible.

Finally the doctors had gone, the nurses and aides were gone, and the room was quiet. Mark, Mom, and I just looked at each other. It all seemed like a nightmare I couldn't wake up from. I adjusted the head of my bed to sit up a little more. Mom and Mark talked to me about how everything was going to be okay, and that they would be right with me every step of the way, just like they've always been. While I knew that was true, I still felt so alone, just me and cancer. I can't even describe that fear.

Someone called Mark on his cell phone, so he left the room to talk. Mom came to sit beside me on my bed, and we sat quiet for a minute, just looking at each other.

"Mom... am I going to die?" I felt the whole room was full of dismay and uncertainty.

Mom took hold of my hand in both of hers. Looking right into my eyes, she said with complete confidence, "No, Ian, you are not going to die. You are going to fight this cancer and you are going to win. You are going to live. This is just a life challenge for you, and you are going to see how strong you really are."

I felt my fear ease a little, and feelings of hope rose up in me. "Will you pray with me, Mom?" I always trusted Mom's prayers. She seemed to pray with a kind of faith and power that I didn't think I had, and I felt like Heaven heard her. It seemed my prayers were always answered when she prayed with me.

She adjusted herself, sitting a little closer to me, and again took both my hands in hers, resting them on my legs. We looked at each other to kind of connect, as we always did for special prayer. Mom bowed her head and prayed the sign of the cross, and I closed my eyes, lying still to feel the prayer around us. We prayed the Our Father, and she asked Jesus, Mary, and Joseph to help us and pray for us. Then she continued in this way as she often prayed, where her words seemed to flow from some place within her heart and I felt a growing strength inside of me with every word. She said stuff that helped me to know and trust that God was strengthening us in that very moment, giving me the courage, and perseverance that I needed to overcome this health challenge and live in perfect health again.

We were still for a moment, then we both opened our eyes, and I looked up at Mom. I felt a peaceful new hope, and a slight smile came to my face. "Thank you, Mom." I pulled her close and she leaned in for a long hug. I kissed her a few times on her cheek. She laid her head on my chest, and just held me for a minute.

"I love you, Ian."

"I love you too, Mom."

She sat up and took a deep breath, and we sat looking at each other again.

"Mom? I'm afraid to be alone...will you stay with me? I mean... all the time... until this is over?"

She said that she absolutely would, that she would never leave me. "You are not in this alone," she said. She would be with me all the way through it. And she said that just like a football team wins the game together, that I would have a whole team of doctors, nurses, family, and friends who would be with me, supporting me to help me fight this cancer and win. "Together we will win," became my new motto.

My fears were not completely gone, but I didn't feel alone anymore, and the pain didn't hurt as bad.

I shifted around a little in my bed. "I'm going to rest a little, okay? I'm so tired."

"I'll be sitting right here when you wake up," she said.

She stayed there on my bed next to me, and told me later that when I had drifted off into a light sleep, she looked at my face and remembered the day a few weeks ago when she had thought I looked very sick. I remembered our conversation. I had come home one afternoon to change clothes for an evening out, and she came into my room to visit with me. She saw in me a thin, pale, sallow face, with dark circles under my tired-looking eyes. She had put her hand on my chest to stop and look closely at me. She had never seen me look so sick before.

"Ian, you don't look well at all," she had said. "Do you feel okay?"

"Yeah... I just haven't had much sleep in the last few days." I had turned away and wrote off her concern. I hated it when she made a fuss over anything. I just wanted to get on with my evening.

"Too much partying?" she had asked as I checked my hair in the bathroom mirror.

"Yeah, I guess so," I had said, smiling. "Well, you know I've been practicing with the band almost every night after work, and then the last two nights I played those open mic nights until close, and then with the band last night, and working all day today..." I had paused to look at her, and she looked worried at my appearance.

"I'll come home and get some sleep tonight, I promise." I reassured her with a quick hug. "But I have to change clothes now, so can you go?"

She had reluctantly dropped the subject. In the days that followed, I hadn't looked as ill as I had that afternoon, so she had let go of her concerns. But her memory of that afternoon conversation brought a heavy sadness to her heart as she realized it was probably the cancer that had made me look so sick that day.

The urologist, Dr. Teitjen, came into the room, and Mom woke me from my nap. She and Mark stood up to greet him. The doctor wanted to examine my nuts, so they had to step out briefly for that. He asked a lot of the same questions as the cancer doctor. My right testicle was enlarged a little, and it was very firm but tender to the touch. He asked me how long it had been swollen and hurting me like that. Just as I'd told the oncologist, I thought it had been about two months.

He had arranged for an ultrasound to be done on my right testicle right away. He told me what would happen after that, that the cancer in my right testicle would have to be removed, and that meant removing my entire testicle. He said it would be sent to the lab to see if it actually was testicular cancer that had spread into my body, or if there was some other type of cancer that had spread into my testicle. He was reasonably sure that it was testicular cancer.

So a transport came to whisk me and my IV unit off in a wheelchair to get the ultrasound, and when I came back, I was so exhausted that lying down in that stiff hospital bed actually felt good. It was dinner time, and a woman with a cart brought a tray of food in for me. The smell of it made me want to hurl, so I told Mom she could have it. I just wanted to sleep. She and Mark descended on that food like a couple of starved animals. I hadn't even realized that we had been there since nine o'clock that morning, and no one had taken the time to eat anything. It had all been about me.

I didn't get much rest, because at some point my IV unit started beeping, so someone came in to check that. Then just when I started to doze off again, an aide came in to check my vitals. I had become so used to those interruptions that as soon as I saw the aide coming toward my bed, I held out both arms, one for the blood pressure check, one with a finger extended for the blood oxygen level check, and I held my mouth open for the thermometer. Soon everyone around me got a kick out of my quiet little joke each time an aide came around, and even though I didn't feel like laughing, I was doing it to be funny.

It seemed like I had just drifted off into the quiet when Dr. Tietjen returned. He said that the ultrasound was successful and the report confirmed there was cancer in the testicle. He said I would be scheduled for surgery as soon as possible. The surgery is called a radical orchiectomy, aka, say goodbye to my right nut. The nut itself would be sent to the lab for a biopsy to find out exactly what type of cancer was in there. I was pretty freaked out by the thought of it, and Dr. Tietjen told me that what is removed is on the inside... they don't actually just whack it off, as I had pictured it in my head. They would make a small incision just to the right of my pubic bone, then take out the testicle inside of the scrotum, like an egg slipping out of a shell. Just a few stitches would sew up the small incision. He said there would be very little pain afterwards, and that I would notice just a little extra loose skin than what I was used to having down there. The whole idea of this surgery made me nauseous and weak, I mean, losing a nut! I told him I think I'd rather lose a finger!

Mom was writing everything down on the back of some papers I'd received when I was admitted. Dr. Tietjen said that the type of cancer he suspected they'd find in my testicle is called embryonal carcinoma, and choriocarcinoma, also known as testicular cancer. I looked at my Mom, and then at Dr. Tietjen. "Can she come with me?" I nodded my head toward Mom. I just wanted her to be there in case something went wrong... to know she was there with me... someone I know and trust watching over me, just in case. The doctor told me that no one could be in the operating area with me except for those operating on me, but he assured me that she could be just outside the door.

After he left the room, Mom, Mark, and I talked about my fears concerning the surgery. I was afraid the surgeon might remove the wrong testicle, or that the anesthesiologist might not administer enough drugs, and I might feel the pain during the operation. I was so afraid of losing a part of my body, a part of myself, especially that part... and even though the doctor told me that having only one testicle most likely would not affect my natural abilities where sex was concerned, I was still afraid it would ruin my chance for future relationships, my sexual ability, and even the possibility of fathering children later in my life. I was afraid of bleeding, especially from my nuts, and I feared being asleep while strangers surrounded me and cut on my body. Mom promised me that she would stay with me as long as possible, and that she and Mark would not be any farther away than the other side of the surgery room door.

The pain in my gut was hurting bad again, and the nurses said I had to wait a while before I could receive more medication. All I could do was try to sleep. Mom got an extra pillow and a warmed blanket for me from the nurse, which made me a little more comfortable. I managed to sleep off and on through the night. Mom got some extra blankets and pillows, and stayed with me in a chair next to my bed. She kept her hand on my bed near me the whole time, so I would know she was right there if I woke up. It's not that I felt scared like a little kid who is afraid of the dark or something like that... I felt scared for my life, and even for my sanity... I felt like I still didn't know what was going to happen. I didn't want to chance dying alone in the night. I felt helpless in the midst of all I'd been through in the last two days, and with the thought that cancer was quickly growing inside me in every moment. It's a whole different thing than being scared as a kid. Suddenly I was very doped up in a hospital, and everyone was making a fuss, sticking needles in me, taking my blood, testing me, poking me, asking what seemed like thousands of questions, and everything was so serious and urgent. I felt like I didn't know what was happening to me, and I felt like I didn't have any control at all, and it was so hard to keep up with everything that all these strangers were saying, or doing, or planning for me. But I knew Mom would keep track of things, and understand things for me, and explain it to me when I needed her to, and I knew that if she was with me, I would be okay. I could rest knowing she was right there watching over things.

The day starts early in a hospital, as the aide came in to check my vitals at 5:00 a.m. From then on, it was all I could do to get a little bit of rest in between the constant pain in my back and my stomach, and everything else going on. My body was stiff from lying in bed for so long, but the pain wouldn't let me stand or walk, and the drugs made me weak and tired. I felt a little hungry, but I couldn't eat or drink anything. I could have nothing but ice chips before my surgery, and as the day wore on, that alone made me all the more miserable. My thirst made it hard to swallow sometimes, and I got pretty cranky. My stomach felt so nervous that I puked in the wastebasket next to my bed. That made my stomach hurt twice as bad. Mom kept me supplied with fresh cool damp washcloths. She'd fold one in half and place it on my forehead, and I'd lay back and close my eyes.

Mark had taken the day off from work to be with me and Mom. He had worked at the same construction company for almost a decade. A lot of the other guys in the company including his bosses were like family to him, and made arrangements to cover for him for as long as he needed. Mark had calls coming in on his cell phone all day it seemed, family and friends who had learned of my news overnight or early that morning. Lots of people wanted to come and visit, or wanted to know how to help in some way. Mark was taking care of all the information that needed to be passed along to everyone. I was so grateful that he was doing that. I didn't want a lot of people rushing in to look at me, asking me all kinds of questions... and I didn't even want to tell people that I had cancer. It was enough just having my family around me. I appreciated the support. My grandpa sat with me for a long time, just holding my hand and being with me, quietly. Other family members came for brief visits throughout the day, but I wasn't much in the spirit of having any conversation at all.

Mom and I had talked earlier about how I was going to tell all of my friends, especially my best friends, Jared and Keaton. We three were like brothers. I had known Jared since we were in sixth grade class together, and the three of us started hanging out around eighth grade, when Keaton was new to our school. We all joined the football team in high school, and by eleventh grade, our bond of friendship was unbreakable. Everyone knew us as best friends, because we were nearly always together. Man, we sure had some good times... some crazy times.

One of my favorite memories with them was what we came to jokingly call by our code name, "midnight panda runs." The word panda in itself was a joke code of ours that we used to describe any comical situation of trouble or pandemonium. Jared's dad owned a couple four wheelers, and we'd sneak them out in the early morning hours and drive them to a wildlife reserve a couple miles away. In pitch blackness with only the moon and a small headlight on each four-wheeler, we'd get those puppies sailing at what seemed like 40 miles per hour over shadowed dirt hills, and across the grassy open fields, screaming and laughing like a bunch of wild monkeys. Oh, my God we had some good laughs, the three of us... good times.

I didn't know how I was going to tell them now that I had cancer, and how bad it was. There had been so many friends calling me on my cell phone leaving voice mail and text messages, wanting to know what was wrong, but I didn't want to let it out that way—over the phone— to be spread like a virus through casual friends. I wanted to tell my close friends in person, before anyone else knew. I planned to call or text Jared and Keaton and ask them to visit as soon as they could.

Mom, Mark, and I sat quietly for a minute. I had been thinking about how we had to tell people, and how hard it felt to have to do that. "Hey Mom? When Jared and Keaton get here, will you let me tell them alone? Can you and Mark go for a walk or something? This is going to be hard, and I think it might be easier for them if it's just us." I looked at her. How was I going to say it? What would be my first words? I felt sadness as I thought about what I might see in the face of my friends as I told them the news.

Kristen and Tracey, my stepsisters, both walked in. Mark had filled them in with the details, so I didn't have to explain anything. We exchanged hellos and comments about how my situation sucked. I got a sense that they didn't know what to say, and being a brother, I didn't want them to feel sad, so I started in with my typical humor. I told them about all the things that had been done to me in the last day and a half, and about the nurses, trying to keep our conversation light. We were all about the same age, within about nine months of each other, Tracey being the youngest, and Kristen the oldest. But I still felt like the older brother to both of them. We sat as a family just visiting, as they told me all about their different lives and times of campus life. We hadn't seen each other as much since we'd all been in college. And as we talked, I actually thought for the first time that someone needed to call student administration for me and let them know why I'd be drop-ping my classes for maybe the rest of the semester. Kristen was taking a couple of classes at the same college, so she said she'd stop in and make sure they had all the information on me. We talked about people spreading the news around campus that I had cancer. Mom told them that Jared would be coming sometime soon, and that they would all leave the room so I could talk to him.

Jared had left work to come and see me. He worked for his dad, who understood how close our relationship was. Jared's dad had been like another dad to me, since I spent so much time at their house. When Jared walked into my hospital room, his face looked nervous and tense with concern. He looked at me, and then at Mom, Mark, and the girls as he greeted us. Mom stood up and gave him a hug, and he and Mark shook hands and hugged each other, too.

"We'll be just down the hall, okay? I'll let the nurse know you have a visitor and don't want to be disturbed." She kissed my cheek, they filed out, and closed the door.

Jared stood at my feet as I used the button to raise the head of my bed to more of a sitting position. He pulled a chair up close to my bed. He sat down, then he stood up again as he saw me trying to adjust my pillows and the IV lines in my arm to get comfortable. He looked wor-ried, "Do you need some help?"

"No, sorry, it's just that it takes a little effort to get adjusted..." I faked a chuckle. I had given a lot of thought about how I wanted to start, but now I was feeling tense by the thought of it. Jared sat down again on the edge of the chair, with his hands together, his elbows leaning on his legs. He waited for me to talk.

I tried to say something, but I couldn't... just like Mom couldn't say the words to my face, I couldn't bring myself to say it to him. I just looked at him.

"What's up, man? Are you going to be okay?"

Just spit it out, I thought to myself. I took a deep breath... "Well... the doctors say I have cancer." I forced the words out, and Jared's eyes just locked on to my face. He said nothing, but his eyes filled with tears. He didn't move.

I tried to make it sound not so bad and not let my fear show, "I'm going to get through it, though. But I have to have chemo and all that shit."

He frowned and swallowed hard, to be able to speak. "Are you serious?...cancer? where?...how?"

I explained as well as I could all the things that the doctors had told me, including how far the cancer had spread. He couldn't believe it, just like we couldn't, and tears forced their way into our conversation, no matter how we tried not to cry. I told him that I would need his support, his friendship to help me stay strong, and he said he would do whatever he could to help me, whatever I needed, he'd be there for me. I added my own optimism that everything was going to be okay. I asked him not to tell anyone until I had the chance to tell Keaton, and he gave me his word. He agreed that Keaton shouldn't hear it from the chain of gossip that would start up as soon as the word got out. He said friends were already buzzing with the question, what's happened to Ian? I actually wanted everyone to hear it from me. I knew there was no way I could tell every single person, but I was working on an idea for a way to tell as many people as possible at the same time, and trying to figure out how to do that.

Mom knocked on the door and opened it slowly, peeking in. "Can we come in?" she whispered.

"Yeah... come in." I motioned to her.

Jared stood up as she walked slowly in. I knew Mom noticed our eyes were red from tears. She smiled softly at us, the way moms do sometimes. Mark and the girls followed her in. Jared offered his chair to her, and she insisted he stay and visit with us if he wanted. He stayed for a little while, but then Dr. Tietjen came in, so Jared said his good-byes, with his promise of silence until he learned that Keaton knew.

Dr. Tietjen asked me a few questions, checked me out with his stethoscope, thumped and poked around on my abdomen a little, and chatted with me for a while. I liked him okay. I felt confident that he seemed to really care about me. He asked if I had any more questions about the surgery, and confirmed that I knew it was scheduled for two o'clock that afternoon. He wanted to mark my testicle and incision site for surgery, so he pulled the curtain closed around me, as Mark and Mom stepped out of the room for a minute. After that, he wished us a good day, and he was gone.

I asked Mom if she had any ideas about how I could gather my friends all together in one place, so I could tell everyone at once, and I wouldn't have to keep telling the same story over and over again. Mark said there was a conference room just down the hall. She could check with the nurses' station and ask if I could use it, maybe to-morrow. Mom could take me there in a wheelchair to see everyone. I wouldn't be walking much after my surgery. I thought that would work out great.

We talked about how I would tell Carrie, the girl I loved for four years now. She'd want to know. I hoped she still cared about me. Carrie was living on the other side of the state, going to college. I wanted to hear her voice. We hadn't gone out in over a year, and we often fought when we were together. I had screwed up bad by being unfaithful to her, and lost her trust in me, but I never had loved anyone like I loved my Carrie. We went out for two and a half years, and we had talked often of marriage. I was always hopeful that someday, she and I could work things out.

We talked of another of my close friends, Aaron. He was away at trade school, and I would have to call him. Aaron and I had been friends since sixth grade, also. He was an amazing drummer, a lot better than me. We had some great times through the years, jamming together at his house and mine. And while sports, music, and girls had taken us into different social circles through high school, we had always kept in touch and partied together often.

I was so tired from all of that thinking and feeling. I tried to sleep until time for my surgery. It came sooner than I wanted, and fear slammed into me as I realized it was about to happen. As if the whole two-day event hadn't been frightening enough, now I had to go alone, wearing nothing but a hospital gown, into a cold operating room with several people I'd never met, while a stranger gave me enough drugs to knock me out, so this new doctor in my life could remove a part of my manhood forever. I told Mom and Mark how scared I was. Mark tried to break the stress by saying funny things, and helping me to crack a few jokes about it myself.

A couple of people came with a different bed to transport me to the operating room. Mom and Mark walked beside my bed as we traveled the hallways and elevators. The stress of the event, the idea of what was about to happen, and the feeling of my bed being swung and turned and bumped around, made me feel like I was going to throw up. I felt the fear squeezing at me. Mom held my hand, and prayed aloud with me as I kept my eyes on the hallway ahead. She affirmed that God was present, in every doctor, every nurse, and every moment, taking care of everything, and I nodded in acknowledgment. Mark stayed in the waiting room, while Mom went with me to the pre-op room. She asked Dr. Tietjen if he would briefly tell me the entire surgical procedure, so that I could feel more secure about everything that was going to take place. He was really cool about it, and as he talked, I started to feel a little more relaxed. He showed me all the instruments that would be used, and told me who would be using them. He let Mom and me glance around the operating room, as he explained each area. He introduced us to the anesthesiologist, and the other nurses who would be present, and described to me what each of them would be doing during the operation. I felt my anxiety lift away a little bit. Dr. Tietjen then lifted the covering from my lower half. I shifted my eyes to look at Mom. She knew what I was thinking, and smiled as she made sure her body and head were facing toward my head, to make sure I knew she wasn't going to see that part of me. The doctor asked me a few times, to make positively sure which testicle is the one to be removed. He knew my fears of losing the only good nut I had.

"Do you know which testicle we're going to remove today?" he asked, looking at my face for an answer.

"The right one." The corners of my mouth turned up, as I heard the humor in my answer. "I mean, the one on the right side... but of course, the right one..." I couldn't help but grin at the doctor when I looked at him. I knew he understood the all of it. Mom smiled, chuckled, and shook her head slightly, as she looked at me. She looked proud of me, for some reason.

Dr. Tietjen chuckled, "And which one do you consider to be the one on the right, meaning the right one?" He smiled, continuing the humor. "Please reach down and show me which one you understand as being the right one."

He was just so cool about it. He knew I was scared to death. He had a diagram, all my medical records, the CT scan image and reports, and the ultrasound results, which showed him which of my balls had the cancer in it. And he knew that I knew which one was bigger than the other, which one had the lump, which one all the doctors had been looking at, and which testicle he put the black marker writing on, marking it for surgery. This was the good doctor's way of helping to get rid of my fears, by making absolutely sure without question what was to be done. So, we both agreed on which one would be removed, and Dr. Tietjen gave Mom the word that they were ready to start preparing me for the surgery. Mom held my hand close to her heart with both of hers. She leaned in and kissed my cheek, and I hugged her with my other arm around her neck. We exchanged I love you's quietly, then she stood up, kissed the back of my hand, and held it in both of hers.

"I'll be right outside that door, okay? I'll be right here waiting for you when you come out."

"I nodded, trying to keep the fear and apprehension out of my throat.

"Everything is going to be okay…" she said "I'll see you very soon." She backed away toward the door, moving her lips to say "I love you," one more time.

I tightened a gratuitous smile and signed to her "I love you" with my thumb, first and last finger extended. The door closed behind her, and everyone around me started preparing for my surgery.

The next thing I remember was looking up and seeing Mom. She was holding my hand, and I could feel her rosary intertwined in her fingers. She told me that the doctor said everything went fine. She added that there was a whole waiting room full of people waiting for me and praying for me. She had contacted the ministers at our church that morning, and a prayer circle had been started for me. They, and all my family were together for me, now. I was embarrassed to think that so many people knew that I now had only one nut, but I was also grateful that they all cared so much that they would be there waiting for me. Dr. Tietjen told us that we would have the results from the biopsy within a day or two. I was happy to see Mark waiting at the door, as I was wheeled out of the recovery room to head back to my room. People cheered, clapped, and reached out for me as we passed the waiting room, and I felt loved and embarrassed at the same time. But I was so glad to have the stress of the surgery behind me.

I was still really groggy while in my room, and slept most of the night. Mom and Mark stayed with me. The nurse had come in and told them that she had checked on the conference room, and it was available for me if I wanted to use it to talk to my friends during the weekend.

The following morning was Saturday, and after I woke to the morning hospital ritual, I contacted Jared to ask him if he'd help spread the word that I was asking anyone who wanted to know about my situation to meet me at the hospital in the conference room on the second floor at twelve o'clock noon that day. He was relieved to hear the news. He said he had heard that people were saying all kinds of untrue things…

that I had died, I was dying, that I'd been in an accident. This made me feel anxious to tell people what was really going on with me. Keaton had been told, and I would call Carrie before the meeting.

The oncologist came to visit me that morning, to let me know that I would be released to go home later that afternoon. I was to call his office and we would meet in the coming week to start my outpatient chemotherapy treatment. He said he'd give me a prescription of Vicodin to take for pain during the rest of the weekend. None of us felt comfortable with this waiting until next week, but what did we know? We would do as the doctor said.

My stomach and back were hurting with mild pain, and my surgery site was pretty sore. That made it hard to move around in any way. Mom kept me supplied with a fresh ice pack to keep on my swollen incision, and that helped. It was about 11:45 as she was going to the nurses' station to freshen my pitcher of ice water. As she walked down the hall, she saw a large crowd of about 25 people rounding the corner at the nurses' station, looking for the conference room. She didn't even recognize them at first, but then someone called out, "Hey, there's Ian's mom!" Her eyes flushed with tears as she smiled with awe, that so many friends had gathered at the hospital to see her son. A few of them hugged her as she guided them to the conference room. She told them I was feeling okay, and asked them to wait. She would bring me in to see them. She returned to my room with fresh water and a wheelchair. She and Mark both helped me out of bed and into the chair. Moving made my nether region hurt like hell. Mark unplugged my IV machine and draped the cords over it so the wheels wouldn't catch on them. Mom pushed me in the chair, while I held my IV pole rolling along at my side. When Mark opened the door to the conference room, I couldn't believe my eyes. It was full of my friends, sitting and standing there waiting for me. I had to stop as soon as we entered. My throat felt a lump in it, and I couldn't see for the tears in my eyes. I was amazed that so many of my friends were that concerned about me that they would take the time to be there. Mom handed me a tissue and a cup of water. Everyone waited patiently while I took a few swallows and wiped my eyes and dripping nose. Some of them looked shocked at my appearance. The last time they'd seen me, I was partying with them, laughing and making jokes, playing my guitar and singing. I was aware I now looked pale, thin, and unshaven. The wheelchair and IV pump made me look all the more pathetic. I thanked them for coming and told them how much it meant to me that they all cared so much. I said I had to keep it short, because I was really tired, but that I would say what I could, and if they had any questions, I'd try to answer them, or Mom or Mark would. I asked them to squelch the gossip that I had died, or that I was dying, and to tell people that my doctors were saying that testicular cancer is curable, and that I was being released from the hospital to go home, and would be going through chemo treatment for a while. They all hung around and visited, shaking my hand and hugging me. After about 20 minutes, I started feeling very tired, kind of nauseous, and the pain from the surgery was driving me crazy, so I had to say my goodbyes. I thanked everyone for coming again, and Mom and Mark wheeled me back to my room. When we got there, I just wanted to crash into my bed and rest quietly for the rest of the afternoon, until I'd received my discharge papers.

My room had been pretty quiet for a while, when my nurse came in and said I had a visitor. I asked Mom to go and see who it was. When she came back into my room, she was smiling. "Ian, it's Jeff!"

I looked at her blankly for a moment... 'Jeff...' I thought, '...how did he know?'

"Jeffy Lube!" Mom said, cheerfully reminding me of the playful nickname I'd given him more than ten years before.

I felt a big smile come over me. My good old friend Jeff! Wow, I hadn't seen him since high school! Jeff and I had been best friends all through grade school. He'd lived behind us, and we'd played together every day since we were six years old. We'd not been hanging out in the same social circles since the sixth grade, but Jeff was always like a brother to me, even still. He had been in college about five hours away, and had made the trip home just to visit me. We visited for a good long time, catching up on each other's news.

The time finally came for me to go home, and I was so exhausted once we arrived. It felt incredibly good to be in my own room, in my own bed. I was able to eat a little bit without feeling sick, which was a welcome change. But as the night wore on, my pain started getting worse. Mom stayed with me, and tried massaging my back to help ease the pain, and I took the Vicodin every four hours as the doctor prescribed, but nothing helped. By one o'clock in the morning, the pain was so bad I couldn't lay still. Mark had come to my room, and together he and Mom and I discussed whether or not to take me back to the hospital. I really didn't want to do that, so Mom called the oncologist to ask if there was something else he could do to help me, if he could call in a prescription for extra pain reliever at a 24-hour pharmacy. She told him how bad I was hurting, her voice cracking a little from trying not to cry. He had seen me writhing in this kind of pain when I first went into the hospital three days ago. He had seen the CT scan of the four-inch tumor in my gut. Surely he could help. He told Mom that there was nothing he could do, that I would just have to wait it out and deal with the pain until Monday.

Mom looked mad and sad, as she slowly hung up the phone. She looked up at me and Mark, "Tomorrow, we're going to find a better doctor for you, Ian. That doctor doesn't care enough."

Mark suggested I go back to the hospital, but I couldn't bring myself to agree. Nobody realized how awful I felt lying in that place. "I'll try to get through the night," I said. "Maybe I'll feel better in the morning."

I didn't sleep very well, but I did sleep a little bit. I kept taking the Vicodin every four hours, but the doctor had told Mom that if I took more than prescribed, it could damage my liver... my liver which was already loaded with cancer. Mom wouldn't let me have over the prescribed amount, even though once I begged her. But she stayed with me through the night, waking up to sit with me when I could not lie still from the pain.

She got on the computer early the next morning, to look for a new oncologist for me. She brought me some oatmeal, which I tried to eat, but the pain in my stomach was just too much. By mid-morning, the pain was more than I could stand, and I agreed to go to the emergency room. They admitted me on the spot, but being a Sunday, there were no oncologists in the hospital who could prescribe more drugs for pain. The charge nurse took control, and immediately called the hospital's pain management team, as she referred to it, to get permission to begin administering morphine to control my pain. Mom later told me that she had no idea just how horrible the pain was for me, until she saw how much morphine I had to have before the pain started to go away. It took several hours for the pain to ease enough that I could actually rest.

The nurses were so compassionate and kind to us. They were very professional, and did everything they could to help me feel better as quickly as possible, and I was very thankful for them. But they told us there was nothing they could do except help manage the pain. They knew how bad the cancer was, and saw throughout the day, how intense the pain could get. Mom and Mark had still been busy trying to find another oncologist for me, and by that evening, decided to take me to Kansas University Medical Center, a local hospital renowned for progressive cancer treatment. The charge nurse offered to arrange transportation for me, so I could have constant medical care along the way. She gave Mom all my medical records to take with us, and called ahead to introduce me as a patient being transported there. Mom rode with me in back of the EMT unit, and Mark followed us in the car. The EMT in back with us was cool, and he made conversation and told some funny stories to try to help me feel better.

It was about nine o'clock Sunday evening when I was officially admitted to the University of Kansas Hospital, Oncology/Hematology Critical Care Unit 42. The feel of the place was entirely different from the other hospital. I was in the presence of cancer treatment specialists, whose conversations with each other surrounded us with the realization that I was in serious, critical condition. Several people were taking care of me, while Mom and Mark stood by watching every detail, feeling helpless, and hopeful. I felt like the desperate case that I was, having been wheeled in and out of places, hooked up, doped up, unable to walk, and still suffering that incredibly intense pain in my stomach and my back. The nurse had to replace my old IV with a new one, and of course go through all the routine of checking vitals and asking questions all over again. I was so wiped out by the pain and the whole experience that I didn't even feel like myself anymore.

Margo, the charge nurse, was doing everything necessary to get me settled into my new room, and took on the responsibility herself to care for me through the night. I also met three other nurses, and two aides when they came in to see this seriously ill young guy admitted to the cancer ward so late at night. Word had spread that I was there. Margo explained the priority over the course of the evening and into the morning was, first and foremost, to get my pain under control so I would be more comfortable. She would be keeping a close check on me. She explained all the oral medications I would be receiving, and why. To get me started feeling better, I got Zofran for nausea, and a constant IV drip of two milligrams of morphine, with a self-administer button called a PCA, that afforded me an extra milligram every six minutes if I needed it, and, when both of these were still not enough, an additional one milligram kick of the same stuff to add to the rest of what I was getting, called a bolus dose, given to me as an injection directly into the IV in my arm. I was allowed a bolus dose only a couple of times a day. The total morphine I was to receive was not to exceed ten milligrams per hour. In that first midnight to morning at KU Med Center, I needed all I could get.

I was pretty out of it from the pain and the medication, when a doctor came in to see me. He introduced himself as Dr. Van Veldhuisen, and said he would be my primary oncologist. He extended his hand and I gave him a drugged handshake. Mark and Mom stood and introduced themselves, then he stepped closer to me and stood looking. He asked more detailed questions than the usual, inquiring where the pain was most intense, had I been coughing blood, stuff like that. He listened with his stethoscope to my lungs and abdomen, and felt around on my stomach, finding the large tumor that was causing the pain. He explained that I would be meeting an additional oncologist,

Dr. Fleming, in the morning, and we would talk more about my upcoming treatment. His visit was brief, then he nodded good night to us, and made a quiet exit.

Mom, Mark, and I became increasingly freaked out by the entire unpleasant new experience. The reality had begun to sink in, that I had cancer all inside my body, and that I was suffering this immense, horrible pain because of it, in a cancer hospital, with cancer treatment professionals, people that I now desperately needed to take care of me and stop the cancer from killing me. The whole experience felt like a nightmare happening to all of us.

Margo brought some extra pillows and blankets for Mom and Mark, and they started settling into the chairs on each side of me. The room was quiet, so quiet. Everything was still. There was no sound except the clicking of my IV machine and the clock on the wall, and no sound beyond my hospital room door. Mom kept the light on over the sink near the bathroom. It was enough light that we could see each other, but it wasn't bright near my bed. I drifted off into a drugged, light sleep, with the comfort that both my parents would be right beside me through the night.

My slumber was ended instantly, when I was suddenly filled with feelings of fright and panic, and a sense that I was completely alone and falling backwards into nothing but darkness. My eyes were wide open, but I couldn't see where I was, and I didn't know where I was.

"MOM!...MOM!...MOM!" I called out to her. She was right next to me, but I couldn't see her. "Mom...what's happening, Mom?!" The expression on my face was one of complete terror.

She was holding both my hands and sitting on my bed, talking to me. "Ian, I'm right here with you. What's the matter?"

"Mom! I'm scared! What's happening!? Mom, help me!"

"Ian, I'm right here, honey, I'm right here. Look at me, I'm right here," she said, still holding my hands.

Mark was standing beside me too, calmly telling me that everything was all right.

My eyes wouldn't focus on Mom. I couldn't see anything but myself falling. "Mom! What's happening to me? What's happening?!" I cried out in fear. I was afraid that even she couldn't see where I was.

She moved closer to me, her face right in front of mine, "I'm here, Ian... I'm here, holding your hands. Look at me, Ian, I'm right here. Feel me holding your hands. We're here together, in your hospital room, in your bed, and everything is okay, you're having a bad dream... Ian, I'm right here with you..."

As she continued talking to me, I started to feel my hands gripping hers, as if I was holding on to save my life. Slowly her face came into focus, and her voice sounded more clear.

"Mom...Mom...oh my God, Mom...oh my God." I whispered as I came slowly out of the hallucination. I took in a deep breath, and she leaned in to hold me. I wrapped my arms around her neck and squeezed her, feeling intense gratitude that what ever had happened, was over, and for the rest of the night, she slept with her head next to me on my bed, and her hand holding mine, resting on my stomach. That hallucination was the scariest moment of my life, and as I laid there almost afraid to go back to sleep, I wondered if that was what cancer treatment was going to be all about.

3

DNA, Cancer, and Chemo: The Loser's Lottery

My vitals were being checked every thirty minutes in my first night at KU, so we didn't get a lot of sleep. When I did sleep, I had these horrible nightmares, and woke up terrified. Suddenly I wouldn't know where I was or what was happening around me. I always reached out for Mom's hand, and looked for her face. She was always right there next to me, and immediately took my hand in hers, and spoke a few words to help me wake up. I got so tired of this happening that I asked her if she would just keep holding my hand while I slept, so that as soon as I woke up from a bad dream, I could feel her right there. I wanted the security of someone holding on to me in that first moment between dreaming and waking, when my eyes were still closed and my fearful body jolted out of a dream. For the rest of my hospital stay, she was always sitting at my side, with her hand resting on mine, and I felt more secure with that constant contact. Her presence made it easier to fall asleep, if only for a short while. Yes, those nightmares sucked that bad and came that often.

By morning I was feeling pretty cranky because both the evening and morning staff had been buzzing in and out of my room since 5:00 a.m. Margo came in to check on me, and said that my in-patient doctor, chief oncologist Dr. Fleming, would be in to see me around 7:00. The pain was still with me, but not quite as intense, and I tried my best to just deal with it in between doses of morphine.

We heard a rap on my door, then it slowly opened as Dr. Van Veldhuisen and Dr. Fleming arrived accompanied by Margo and six other people wearing white coats. It freaked me out when I saw eight doctors walking into my room. In the beginning of my stay, I didn't know that KU is a university hospital, a teaching hospital, so seeing that many doctors at once was like a vision of doom for me.

Dr. Fleming first introduced Dr. Van Veldhuisen as the head of the oncology department and Cancer Center, acknowledging that we'd met him last night. He then introduced himself, the doctors each shook my hand, then turned to Mom and Mark and did the same. The resident also introduced himself, and Dr. Fleming explained that the others in white coats were students who would be only observing our interactions as they stood at a distance. Dr. Fleming knew that Margo had been taking care of me through the night, but he formally introduced her as well, stating her full title as a registered nurse, oncology-certified, and telling us that I couldn't be in better hands, that she was one of the finest oncological nurses he'd ever worked with. That made me feel good, that I had been assigned one of the best to care for me.

Dr. Van Veldhuisen stood to one side near Margo, listening and watching me. The resident doctor stood nearby, as Dr. Fleming did all the things that doctors do, examining my stomach, feeling around on me, listening to my lungs, heart, and gut with his stethoscope, and asking me dozens of questions. Dr. Fleming talked to the resident and the students, teaching as he went along. Margo was taking notes, and Mom was listening and writing stuff down, too. She was trying to learn all that she could, so we could better understand this new cancer world we were now living in.

Dr. Fleming asked me to recall the first time I noticed something different in my right testicle. I told him that it had been kind of swollen and tender in the last two or three months. He asked me to think back even farther, to the very first time I remembered feeling even a small lump. I wasn't sure, but I thought it was late sometime in my senior year in high school. I told him that I didn't think it was anything to worry about, because it didn't hurt. That would have been about a year and a half ago. I sat quietly grieving the fact that I hadn't done something about it back then.

Dr. Fleming nodded. He had seen all my medical records that we brought with us, and began to talk to us about the types of cancer cells that were growing in me. He called it a nonseminomatous germ cell tumor, or NGCT, composed mostly of embryonal carcinoma, with amounts of choriocarcinoma, a very highly malignant germ cell, and both of which are very aggressive and fast-growing. He also talked about the kinds of chemotherapy I would soon be receiving, explaining that treatment would be given to me intravenously every day for five days, and then they wanted to keep me in the hospital for a few days afterwards to make sure I was tolerating it okay. I would most likely be receiving the highest doses possible. He told me about what is called a "port," a catheter with a sort of porthole opening that would be surgically placed under my skin just below my right collar bone, so the needle could be easily inserted into it, and the chemical drugs could be infused directly into a major artery through the catheter attached to the port. A catheter is a plastic tube, like an IV line that is placed inside the body. This catheter would be threaded a few inches into my artery. I could be wearing this Port-a-cath under my skin for as long as I needed chemotherapy treatments. He would order the surgery to be done on Monday or Tuesday.

I asked why I needed that.

He answered that the drugs were very strong and would irritate and burn my smaller veins, and also that the port was a simpler means of tapping into the artery for each treatment.

I wanted to understand everything that was happening to me, but sometimes the answers just made me feel more scared.

He said that he would be working together with Dr. Van Veldhuisen, who would oversee all my treatment and outpatient care. He explained to us about what is called staging, a process they use to figure out how much of each type of cancer cells I have, and how much the growth of these cells had spread into the rest of my body, and the rate at which they were growing, in order to put together a perfectly suited treatment plan. The schedule of chemotherapy is set based on the type of cells, the rate they divide, and the time a chemo drug is most likely to be effective. Some chemotherapy drugs have to be given when the cells are actively dividing, and others work better when the cells are at rest, or between growing cycles. This, he explained, is one of the reasons my chemotherapy regimen would go in cycles, as he mentioned before, which also allowed my body time to strengthen itself between treatments.

I was going to have to get an MRI done on my head to see if there was any cancer in my brain. Dr. Fleming suspected there was after reading my CT scan reports. He wanted to see all the actual images of my CT scan and the images from the ultrasound taken on my right scrotum, and he wanted the lab at KU to run a biopsy test of their own on the cancerous testicle tissue. The images and slides containing my precious right nut tissue would be transported to KU on Monday or Tuesday. All these things we had to wait on. Dr. Fleming said it would be Wednesday or Thursday before treatment would be started. I asked him if we could go ahead and get started with some of the treatment in the meantime, while we were waiting for this staging process to get finished. It was only Monday, and I was more than ready to start killing this cancer. I still didn't have a good grip on everything he had been telling me.

He looked straight at me, and at Mom and Mark. His voice was very sure. "Now, there's no question, Ian, that you are a very sick young man. But it is extremely important that we know precisely the type and stage of cancer growth before proceeding. It would be irresponsible— and even dangerous—to start treatment before we have a complete report of the stage and growth cycle of these germ cells. But be assured, your treatment will be started within the next few days."

Dr. Fleming sometimes used medical terms that I didn't understand, but he was very clear and thorough when he wanted to get his point across. He was a tall man, a lot taller than all the others who followed him around. He was friendly yet serious, dedicated, and seemed to be well experienced at treating cancer. I felt good about that, and so did Mom and Mark. He was strict with me about my responsibilities as the patient, like eating right, getting exercise, and following doctors' orders. He shook my hand again, patted me on the leg, and said he would check in on me later. Dr. Van Veldhuisen shook my hand to say good bye, and nodded to Mom and Mark. The team of white coats filed out. The heavy wooden door of my room closed, and the thick metal latch handle clicked, as we heard Dr. Fleming's voice trail off down the hall.

My head was spinning with information overload. I was scared, confused, I didn't understand why, or how... I was bewildered, frustrated, terrified, in shock... I was in disbelief... I felt empty, nervous... and horrified.

Mark, Mom, and I looked back and forth at each other, and after a moment our eyes just naturally turned their gaze downward at the blankets on my bed or the white linoleum tile floor, as if to be letting all that information sink into our thoughts. I heard Mom take a deep breath as she reached to touch my hand. She hadn't moved from the chair next to my bed. Mark leaned against the covered air register, a long solid wooden bench-like shelf that stretched the length of the window of room 4211.

None of us said anything, and the silence in the room was like a loud ringing in my ears. The ticking of the large wall clock in front of me seemed to be saying this was going to be a long, hard, and frightening lonely road. I was just sitting there in my bed, staring off into the space around us. "I'm so scared." The words just came out of my mouth, as I looked over at Mom and Mark.

Mark paused to look at me, then stood up and walked over to the other side of my bed and sat in the chair, pulling it up close to me. He leaned toward me, resting his arms on my bed. I looked over at him, and he looked straight at me with his coach's game face, then said, "You're going to beat this, Stretch. You know that. We're going to beat it together."

I just nodded. I felt like crying, but I was too depressed and numb to have tears.

Mark had supported me 100 percent in everything I'd ever done. He had been my coach in year-round sports since I was six years old. It was during one of our Junior League Baseball seasons that he'd started calling me Stretch. I'd grown pretty tall for my age, and as a left-hander, I could make any catch with my foot still on first base or home plate. We had a few different nicknames for each other, and a playful affection that was equal to any father and son. He never lied to me, he never broke a promise. He was always there for me, and he took good care of me and Mom... good care of everything. He was the best step-dad ever, and he earned his nickname, Mook, because he was so loveable and funny. And I knew he loved me, and I knew he meant what he said.

"Together we can win..." I quoted my new motto as I looked back at him.

"We will win," he assured.

Mark grasped my right hand, and I raised my left hand, still holding on to Mom. I gave him a weak, yet hopeful smile. We all looked at each other, and Mom smiled and kissed the back of my hand.

"I love you, Ian," she whispered.

"I love you too, Mom..." I laid my head back on my pillow. "Could you lay the head of my bed down for me? I'm too tired... I'm just so tired."

She pressed the button on the bedrail and the head of my bed moved slowly down flat. "We'll be quiet and let you rest," she said.

"You won't leave, will you?" I didn't feel sure of anything, and I didn't want to be sleeping there alone.... My eyes fell closed. I was feeling very drowsy.

"No, honey, we'll be right here. We won't go anywhere." She put her other hand on top of mine.

I squeezed her hand that I was holding on to. "Thank you, Mom..." I shifted my head on the pillow.

I had just drifted off to sleep when the pain woke me. I tried to let it go, but it just kept squeezing at my gut, and my back. I reached for the PCA button and gave myself a dose. Just then the nurse came in. She had a needle and some vials, and said she needed to take some more blood. I had confided to her earlier that I was afraid of needles. There had been dozens stuck in my arms over the past few days, and I wasn't getting used to it. As I squirmed in my bed, I suddenly felt nauseous, and told her I needed the trash can right away. She reached for it near the sink and pulled it over to me, and immediately I threw up in it. I grabbed a tissue from my bed table and wiped my mouth. I apologized for being such a baby, trying to keep a humorous tone in spite of my embarrassment. She was very compassionate and patient with me, and when she stuck the needle in my arm, I looked the other way, and hardly even felt it.

I told her the pain was getting bad again. She said I couldn't have more medication than I was already getting, so I would have to hold out for a while. She told me about the three different kinds of pain medication I was getting in my IV, morphine, fentanyl, and hydromorphone. I was kind of nervous about getting all this pumped into me, but at the same time, it was good to be getting some relief from the pain. She said she could come in and give me a bolus dose a little later, if the pain was still too much. After the aide came to check my vitals, Mark went to the hospital cafeteria to get some lunch for him and Mom. The room was finally quiet again, and I lay with my eyes closed, trying to get some rest.

The frightening feeling came on me like a silent hidden shadow, and suddenly I felt I was falling completely alone again, into an abyss of darkness. Instantly my whole being was tense with horror. "MOM! What's happening!? MOM!" I gripped my bed blanket in my fists, "MOM!" I didn't know where I was. I didn't know what was happening. I could hear her voice, but I couldn't see. I felt like I was trapped in a void.

"Ian," I heard her say. "Ian... Ian... I'm here with you, I'm right here. You're okay. Ian. Look at me, Ian... look at me. You're safe, everything is okay, you're okay. I'm right here, Ian. I'm right here with you..."

Her face came into focus, and I kept my eyes locked on her.

She kept talking to me, and finally I felt myself being eased out of the horrible place I thought I was, and I could feel her hands holding mine. "Oh my God...." I looked at her face looking back at me, "Why is this happening to me, Mom? What's happening to me?"

"I don't know, Ian," she said sadly. "Maybe your fear of the unknown is making you have these bad dreams or hallucinations...you know, just being afraid of what the chemo is going to be like, and not knowing what's going to happen next."

"But it seems so real." I looked at her, and thought about it for a minute, "I'm awake, and my eyes are open, aren't they? I can hear you, but I can't stop falling, and I feel like there's nothing around me to hold on to. I can't stop it from happening, and it scares the shit out of me, Mom. It's like I have no control at all. I just don't understand." I heaved a sigh and closed my eyes.

"I'm sorry, Ian," Mom said, sympathetically.

I looked at her. "Stay right here, okay, Mom?"

She kissed the back of my hand. "Yes."

I closed my eyes and hoped it would never happen again.

Mark had come in quietly with food for both of them, and they ate quietly while I dozed lightly. I woke when I smelled the lunch cart being brought around, and someone brought a tray of food in for me. The smell of my food made me feel nauseous at first. I didn't have any appetite, but Mom urged me to try to eat something. I had a few bites of a pear and a couple of french fries, but I was too tired and nauseous to eat the rest. My stomach still hurt, like someone had jabbed their fist into me, so I just laid back and closed my eyes to rest again.

After lunch, we learned that I would have to start peeing in a bottle so they could keep track of the electrolytes and stuff in my urine, and I was going to have the opportunity sometime on Monday to bank some sperm, in case chemotherapy destroyed my chance for future fatherhood. The doctors and my nurse said this could be a very likely situation, what with all the intense chemotherapy I was going to be receiving. Great. As if I didn't feel bad enough about myself, now I had to worry that for the rest of my life, I could be shooting blanks. This was embarrassing, nerve-wracking, and very depressing. I had one or two chances to save some of my little guys, or I might never have kids. No pressure there. I had to produce sperm at my appointed time in the reproductive clinic on the fifth floor. Everyone would know why I was there, everyone would know what I was doing in that little room, with all the magazines in it. And with all those pain medications in my veins, the chance that I could even get it up was looking pretty grim.

Well, Monday came, but I didn't. I gave it my best effort, but just ended up being wheeled back into my room, feeling more depressed than I had ever felt before. I'm telling you, I felt like I just wanted to crawl into a dark hole and hide, and never come out. The pain of that depression crushed me, my soul and my heart were so heavy. Mom couldn't hide her sadness. I knew her heart was hurting for me and my sorrow. But she kept her faith that everything was going to be all right and tried to help me keep my faith, too. We wouldn't need the saved specimen because God was in control, and by the miracle of living, I would still be able to father children later in my life, once this cancer journey was over.

Dr. Fleming checked in on me, along with the resident and the team of med students streaming into my room behind them. This is how it was going to be every day, a group of people coming in to stare at me, intruding on me, while Dr. Fleming did his job. It irritated me, being observed by a whispering group of onlookers, but I tried to ignore them and focus on what Dr. Fleming was saying or doing. Eventually, I grew to hope that they were learning something from watching me, and would go on to tell others about testicular cancer, and how bad it can get if a guy finds a lump and does nothing about it.

When Dr. Van Veldhuisen, came to see me, he was alone. I liked that. He was very kind, more soft-spoken than the other doctors I had seen, and he had a serious and gentle caring nature about him, an unassuming presence, I felt. He examined me as I was used to after the past few days, feeling for the tumors in my abdomen, listening to my lungs, heart, and digestive system, and asking me questions about how I felt.

He said the cancer was Stage III B, which meant it had spread into the lymph nodes, with numerous tumors in more than one organ. To me, it just meant there was a shit load of cancer growing in me. He spoke a little about the tumors seen in my organs, the general progression of this disease, and the chemotherapy plan that was being arranged. He asked if I had any questions. I had hundreds, but I could think of only one that mattered to me the most at the moment. How would the chemotherapy make me feel, and was all my hair going to fall out? He told me about all the common unpleasant symptoms, like nausea, vomiting, fatigue, and generally feeling sick. They sounded very bad, but I wasn't to understand the severity of bad and unpleasant until a week later.

Mom wanted to know, that in his experience with cases like mine, what was the most common outcome? She wasn't asking what my chances were, exactly, just what were the odds. She was looking for more hope. Dr. Van, as he was known and invited us to call him, told us there were several cases like mine where the outcome was very good, and that he felt confident that I had just as good a chance for a successful result. Dr. Fleming also had shared this confidence with us, that even though this cancer was far advanced, I was still an overall, healthy young male, with a very strong chance for survival. This comment made us all feel very good, and we thanked God for this news. I had medical confirmation that cancer was not the death sentence I had once thought it was. It was just a health challenge, a life challenge as Mom put it, that I had to overcome. I had to fight hard, with the help of my doctors, nurses, and also my family, but I would win. Together, we would win.

We built up our faith and team spirit after he left, talking about all the ways we would work together to help me win the fight. "Hey Mom, you know that picture of me making that great tackle in high school, when we played North?" I looked over at her as if she could see my idea.

"Can we get that blown up bigger, and hang it here on my wall? That's the way I'm going to tackle cancer...I'm going to keep looking at that picture to remind me what I have to do."

Mom said she would make sure it got done. And for the first time, I laid my head down on my pillow feeling some confidence, some fight in me. I think I even smiled, imagining that picture, that perfect tackle I made as a defensive back in my senior year, when I knocked that kid right out of his shoes. Then I used his chest to push myself back up, shoving him into the ground he laid on, looking him square in the eye, feeling like a total bad ass. Yeah. This is how I was going to treat cancer. I was going to kick its ass.

I lay quiet and thought about the attitude I needed in order to beat this cancer. I had been inspired by Lance Armstrong's LiveStrong bracelet given to me by one of my nurses in the other hospital. I wore that bracelet every day to help keep my spirits up. I had told Mom and Mark that I wanted to have my own bracelets made in a bright green color inscribed with my slogan, Together We Will Win. Once I had won my own fight with cancer, I would sell my bracelets to help raise money for testicular cancer awareness, just as Lance was doing. I thought about the bracelets and pictured myself in high school auditoriums talking to guys about this disease once I was healthier. I would do my best to make a difference.

A nurse came in again to draw my blood, as they had been doing each day for labs, as it was called, checking my complete blood count, and among other things, the tumor markers. Dr. Van had explained it to me simply, that as cancer grows in the body, proteins are produced that show up in the blood. By watching for the presence of tumor markers like certain peptide hormones and proteins, mainly beta hCG and alpha feta protein in testicular cancer patients, they can know how the cancer is advancing or responding to treatment. A high or rising number means the cancer is growing, while lowering numbers show the opposite, and obviously, the faster the count declines, the better the chemotherapy is working. He told us that currently, my tumor marker count of beta hCG was at about 200,000. That count had risen from 72,742 at my diagnosis just four days earlier. The hCG stands for Human Chorionic Gonadotropin, and yeah, beta hCG is also known as the pregnancy hormone, because it's produced by the woman's body after she conceives to protect the fetus from infection. In a healthy male without testicular cancer, the amount of beta hCG in the blood would be 0, or 3.0 at the most. That was painful news, but he expected the count to drop considerably after my first round of chemotherapy.

My oncology team would be consulting regularly with Dr. Lawrence Einhorn for my ongoing treatment. He's an oncologist in Indiana, recognized as the world's pioneer in testicular cancer treatment, the guy who came up with this successful chemo cocktail known to testicular cancer patients and oncologists as BEP (bleomycin, etoposide, and platinum), or CEB (cisplatin, etopiside, and bleomycin). This treatment dramatically and consistently raised the survival rate of testicular cancer patients to 95 percent, from 10 percent. Dr. Einhorn is also the doctor who treated Lance Armstrong. How could we go wrong with that? This information gave me great hope.

I was scheduled to have an MRI of my brain that afternoon, and the Port-a-cath implanted on Wednesday. Dr. Van Veldhuisen had ordered the first dose of chemotherapy to begin Wednesday evening around 11:00 p.m., starting with a small test dose of bleomycin. After that, I would receive the full dose through my Port-a-cath on the first day only.

Bleomycin is an antibiotic that is derived from a bacterium that grows in the dirt. It interferes with a cell's ability to divide and reproduce, causing it to die. After the first bleomycin dose, I'd start getting my doses of cisplatin and etoposide, one right after the other, for five nights in a row.

Cisplatin is basically platinum, a heavy metal. It prevents cell division also. The side effects are scarier, like hearing loss, nerve damage, kidney damage, and sterility, to name a few. But it's like the grandfather of cancer drugs, because it's the most used, and one of the first drugs to be effective in killing cancer cells.

Etoposide, also known as VP-16, is a plant alkaloid derived from the root of the Mayapple plant. The fruit is apparently edible, but the rest of the plant is very toxic. Etoposide screws up the process of cell division in a different way from the others, but with the same outcome, death to the cell.

The main problem with chemotherapy was that there wasn't any way to aim these drugs at only certain cells, like the abnormal ones known as cancer. They would have this effect on the normal cells, too, because the chemical compounds of the chemo would attach to all DNA. With chemotherapy, it's all or nothing.

Dr. Fleming helped me to understand chemotherapy a little better by trying to teach me what cancer actually is. I couldn't explain it myself in medical terms, but basically what I learned is that a cancer cell is just a mutated normal cell, and its DNA is jacked up. DNA holds the chemical code that tells the cell what to do, to divide and multiply, or to stop, like it does when a wound is healed. The damaged DNA of a cancer cell never tells the abnormal cell to stop dividing, so it keeps replicating its messed-up self and takes over territory of good cells. That's cancer in a nutshell.

Dr. Fleming explained that as chemotherapy drugs attach to the DNA, they work in different ways to interrupt the chemical code, so the cells will stop dividing and die. This is also what causes most side effects of chemotherapy.

There's really a lot more detail to the process, but basically that's how it works. The good news is that cancer cells often are not able to continue growing after a cancer drug has affected the DNA, but normal cells are strong enough to make a comeback. I was actually more worried about the side effects of chemotherapy than whether or not my normal cells were going to be able to keep up. I kind of trusted that they would. But the thought of feeling like shit every day, possible infertility, and losing all my hair and eyebrows had me feeling very afraid of the days ahead.

Wednesday morning came, and it was time for my surgery to get my Port-a-cath implanted in my chest. Here was another dark tunnel to get through. My fear and anxiety made me feel alone and helpless. Mom and Mark walked beside my transport bed all the way to the operating room. They stayed with me while the surgical nurse explained to us everything that would be done. She assured me that it was a very noninvasive surgery, just a simple implant under my skin and into a vein. She even showed the port and catheter to us, but I was still very nervous about it. Mom and Mark would wait for me by the door until the nurse wheeled me back out. We exchanged "I love you's" as always, then they wheeled me into the operating room.

I was scared of being operated on again, but I didn't have a choice. I figured, if this is what it takes to keep me alive, then I'll just have to surrender to it, fear and all. I was afraid of being under anesthesia, but after a few minutes, I didn't have any notion of what was happening to me, anyway. I was really tired when they wheeled me to my room. I hadn't ever thought I'd be glad to be back in that bed, but it felt good to be in my room, with no one doing anything to me.

My nurse came in and asked me if I wanted to try the sperm banking again. This would be my last chance before chemotherapy got started later that night. One more element of pressure, and three days more morphine in my system. I did try, reluctantly, dreading the likely outcome, or should I say, lack of outcome. Short story, no bank deposit. Severe depression again. I returned to my room in shame, and tried to escape in sleep.

I was too depressed to sleep, so Mom and Mark and I just sat and talked about everything that had been going on, all that we had learned about cancer in such a short time, and how we were going to deal with the coming days. I started to feel a little overwhelmed again, and wondered why this happened to me...why me?...and why had I never heard of this cancer that the doctors were saying is the most common cancer in guys my age...this cancer that has so far, fucked up my whole world? I heaved a big sigh. "You know..." I looked straight ahead thoughtfully as I spoke, "cancer is a loser's lottery, and you don't even have to buy a ticket to win." I looked at Mom and Mark, both sitting to my left, looking very sad for me. I continued my thought, "Yeah, it's like, Hey! Congratulations! You've been chosen... you've got the winning numbers...you get cancer! Let me shake your hand, you poor fucker..." I stuck my right hand out into the air in front of me, as if the person awarding me the cancer prize was shaking my hand. I felt a hint of a chuckle in my breath, and a slight smile came to my face, and I looked over at them, shaking my head in disbelief at my fortune. Mom nodded her head, in agreement and disappointment of it all, and Mark leaned back in his chair, clasped his hands behind his head, and sat gazing up at the ceiling in thought. He looked like he was trying not to cry.

Word had gotten around to my friends that I was going to be in the hospital for another week and a half, so I was getting a lot of calls and text messages on my cell. A lot of people were coming to visit me. I was grateful to Mark for having gone home earlier this week to bring us some clean clothes, toiletries, and my cell phone charger. Mom had drawn my name in big bold letters on an 8-by-10-inch piece of paper, and hung it on the outside of my door, so people could find my room easily. I liked it. It made me feel like I wasn't so invisible to the rest of the world, and now that the pain wasn't so bad, I felt like communicating again.

Mom made a comment about the ring tone that I had on my phone. It was a song from a band called Story of the Year. I put it on there because it reminded me of Carrie, the one girl who still had my heart, but Mom said that I might want to change it, because it kind of sounded like an affirmation of something we didn't want coming true. The song rang, "Until the day I die, I'll spill my heart for you..."

"Yeah, I guess you're right..." I agreed with her. I wanted something that sounded more positive, too. I changed it to a song titled "Dare You to Move," by a band called Switchfoot, because the lyrics to that song are more an affirmation of living life. But eventually, I just put the phone on vibrate, because I was getting so many calls that the ring tones were getting kind of annoying, and I was growing more irritated at being awakened from any amount of sleep that I was able to get, especially since I rarely slept more than an hour at a time. Sleep was such a welcome escape that I didn't want to be interrupted.

I lowered the head of my bed a little more, told Mom I wanted to sleep, and asked if she would please put my phone in the drawer of my night stand next to the bed. She kept the room phone near her also, with the ringer turned down low. I was still feeling a little afraid of sleeping, because of all the nightmares I was having, but I dozed off and on through the rest of the afternoon. Aides and nurses came in, and dinner came, and nightfall came, and at ten o'clock came the preparation for my first experience with chemotherapy.

I had to receive extra fluids and several medications to support my body and help it deal with the chemicals that would soon be flowing through my veins. I was really scared and nervous to get it started because I was so afraid of how it was going to make me feel. The thought of it haunted me, chemicals flushing into my body to kill the cancer... the cancer that I still couldn't believe was growing inside me. I didn't know which scared me more, the cancer or the treatment. The nurses had all been great, and I was glad that I already was acquainted with the one who would be hooking me up with chemo for my first time. Her name was Carol. She told us about the different "pre-meds," the drugs I had to take before receiving chemo, and how each one helped keep the possible side effects at a minimum. She joked around with me, and that helped me to relax a little bit. The treatment order was that I would receive the chemo starting at midnight each night, and it would take until about four o'clock in the morning to be finished. That way I could hopefully sleep through it, and all the better that my body would be at rest through the process. But we were wide awake the first night we got started. I couldn't sleep well through the night, and Mom didn't either, mostly because of the constant nightmares I was having. The dreams would wake me, then Mom would wake when she felt me move and look with wide eyes at her. But eventually the morning sun came, and the chemotherapy treatment was over, and I had to pee like crazy. Our fifth day in this hospital was getting started, and I felt even more crabby and irritable than the day before.

Overall, though, I didn't feel too bad that morning. The nurse said that I wouldn't notice symptoms of nadir for a few days. Nadir is when the body's white blood cell count is depleted, and the effects of the chemotherapy are evident. Basically it means I would feel like hell, but at that point, I had no idea how bad it was going to be.

I was receiving the prescribed 17 different kinds of drugs, counting the three chemotherapy drugs, but not including the pain relieving opiates on constant drip in my IV. Most of the others were to help counter the side effects of the chemotherapy, like nausea, poor digestion, constipation, diarrhea, acid reflux, kidney failure, itching, insomnia, depression, anxiety, nerve damage, and headaches, to name a few. As for nadir, all they can do for that is to make sure the blood count doesn't get too low. If it does, I would get a daily shot of neupogen to help my body build up its white blood cell count, or Epogen for anemia, to help my body build up its red blood cell count, or I could receive both.

The doctors told me that if I became too anemic, I would need a blood transfusion. I asked where the blood would come from, and was told it comes from anonymous donors, but I wasn't feeling too good about that. I mean, getting blood from another person's body injected into mine? Isn't that sort of like taking a bath in someone else's dirty water? It's used blood, isn't it, it's already been around inside some stranger's veins. Gross. I asked Margo if my mom could donate her blood if I needed any. The answer wasn't one I wanted to accept. But of course, they can't just take blood out of Mom's body and put it into mine, like syphoning gas from one car to another. The blood has to be tested, screened, and processed first, and that takes about 20 hours on average. If I needed blood, I would need it right away. Mom tried to tell me it was fine, and that if I needed it to save my life, then I'd better be okay with it. I asked her if she would please check to find out if she can donate some blood, then they can save it in case I need it.

When Mom came back from the blood bank on the second floor, she didn't have good news for me. What she learned was that an autologous donation, meaning a blood donation given for a specific person, yours truly, would be very expensive. They told her that it requires segregated processing, and special handling and storage, all costly for us, and that even with the added expense, the blood would still only keep for 42 days. So she could have been looking at over $800 to donate and store one unit of blood for me, and if I didn't need it within those 42 days, it would all be wasted. Then what? Donate more red blood cells, and spend another $800 just in case I might need it within the next 42 days? And what if I needed more than one unit? $1,600? $3,200? I knew we didn't have that much money, and insurance wouldn't pay for it. And how much could she spend to prepare for the off-chance that I might, in 42 days, need so much blood, when I could have all that I might need already waiting for me from a stranger, for only the cost of the blood and transfusion itself, mostly paid for by insurance. So I'd like to say I surrendered to the idea of an anonymous donor if I ever needed a blood transfusion, but to tell the truth, I was never comfortable with it, and I prayed I would never need it.

4

Nadir, Magic Bullets, and Cancer Mountain

It was Thanksgiving Day already, and I couldn't believe I'd been lying in the same hospital room for five straight days, except for my trips to labs in the hospital. My world did expand beyond my room from time to time. The pulmonary clinic was on the fourth floor of the Northwest wing. That was where I went for a complete pulmonary functions test for my lungs. I had to sit in a glass tubular booth, hold a tube-like mouthpiece in my mouth, and breathe in whatever way the therapist told me. He watched the results on a couple of computer screens, as he measured my lung capacity, how my lungs were able to move the air, and the amount of oxygen I was able to take in from the air. The test took about 30 minutes, and it was a long trip to get there. Two corridors to an elevator, down to the main floor, three more corridors to another elevator, up to the fourth floor, then two more corridors to the lab. I felt like they wheeled me to a different hospital. And when I needed an MRI on my brain or a CT scan, I traveled seven corridors zigzagging from the main lobby to the radiation oncology department. Mom and I learned our way around that hospital pretty fast.

I was getting used to my surroundings, and living in the hospital. Mom had settled us into my room earlier in the week by putting all our belongings in place. I hadn't had the energy to do any of the things she automatically took care of. She hung my clothes and coat in the closet;

put my shoes and duffle on the shelf; and lined up my toothpaste, razor, deodorant, and contact lens solution on the vanity by the sink for me. My soap and shampoo were in the shower, and my KU thermal water mug, and my cell phone charger were always within my reach on the rolling chest of drawers next to my bed. She kept my eating table at the foot of my bed, so it wouldn't be in the way of my IV unit and all its cords when I had to get up to go to the bathroom, and she arranged all my cards, gifts, and flowers on the other bed table in the room. She had gotten permission from the nurses to go into the nurses' kitchen in case I needed water or ice, or something to eat, or if she herself wanted some coffee or tea. It saved the nurses the trouble of doing it, and Mom was happy to be able to get me something if I suddenly got an appetite for a snack at any hour, which usually was in the later part of the night. They had a variety of cereal, milk, fruit juices, crackers, bread, Jello, and soups, stuff like that. They even had little packets of peanut butter and jelly available to make a sandwich.

Right around the corner from my room was a linen cart, and the nurses told Mom she could take what we needed from there, more blankets or linens, towels, extra pillows... they had realized that Mom was there to stay with me, and they were very nice to us. Mark stayed when he could, but he had to keep working to take care of everything. And when we had worn all our clothes, he brought clean ones and took the others home and washed them.

Mom adjusted everything in the way I liked to have the room, dark and quiet, with the blinds completely closed and pale green leaf print curtains drawn to cut the sunlight as much as possible. I liked the curtain drawn across the room in front of the door, and the door closed... always, the door closed, and no lights on in the room. At night, she left the bathroom light on and the door just cracked open, so we could easily see when we had to. It also prevented the nurses and aides from turning on a light when they came in during the night. But the silence was something I couldn't compromise on. I didn't want people talking around me, and I didn't want to hear anyone talking on their phone, or out in the hall. I didn't want people talking about me, and I didn't want to lie in my bed, wondering if they were. I was so tired, I didn't want to have to pay attention to a conversation, or have to think of things to say, myself. It was all stress to me. I didn't want the TV on ever in the daytime, but sometimes we'd watch at night. I just wanted silence, so I could sleep, and stay asleep as long as possible. Was it normal for me? No, it wasn't, but the people who loved me and cared about me didn't question it or try to change it. They just honored my requests, and I appreciated it so much.

I had a real problem with people coming into my room and not being quiet about it, and even the sound of the door bothered me. Mom was always careful to pull the metal latch slowly and gently so it wouldn't make a sound to disturb me, and when she returned, I barely heard the door open or close. I was so grateful to her for that, and if I saw her coming in, I always greeted her quietly, saying "hi Mom..." as she came around the bed to sit next to me. I wanted her to know I was awake, and that I appreciated the quiet way she moved in the room. She even mentioned to all my nurses that I appreciated low voices, low light, and minimal noise, if possible, and most of my nurses were very kind to me in that way. I really, really hated it when someone would let the door close hard in my room. I knew I was irritable, but I couldn't help it. There were times when it was so noisy out in the hallway that it irritated me even through my closed door... closets closing and doors slamming in the rooms near me, wheels rolling on the vitals carts and IV machines, dozens of people talking loudly.

I'd say, "Mom! What the hell is going on out there?! What are they doing?! Will you please go out there and tell them all to be quiet?"

She'd stick her head outside my door, and she'd tell me there were doctors talking, nurses and aides doing their jobs, housekeepers cleaning, the whole hospital staff doing what they are supposed to be doing, but in my own private misery, I couldn't understand why they were making all that noise in my space, in my world, just outside my door.

I'd say, "Mom, can you tell them to go down the hall? Tell them to shhhhh!...to be quiet! Don't they know I'm trying to sleep?"

Mom would assure me that they would be gone soon, that it

couldn't be helped. She tried in her soft-spoken way to tell me that the others weren't aware of me and my anguish, that it was their hospital, too, but in my personal hell, it drove me crazy. So Mom at some point, bought a package of earplugs for me, and kept them in her purse for whenever I wanted them.

My evening nurse, also named Mark, had given me a CD player and headphones as an early Christmas gift. He had felt sorry for me when I told him I'd dropped mine on the floor and broken it. He also gave me a couple of copies of his own CDs. He was a really cool guy. Mook brought my CD wallet I'd kept in my car so I'd have plenty to choose from. Hearing music helped a little, but a lot of the time I was too tired to hassle with it, and sometimes just wearing the headphones bothered me.

There really was no getting away from the noise sometimes, and the constant ticking and frequent beeping of my IV unit was always by my side. I even thought I could hear it at home, sometimes. Welcome to my cancer world.

I didn't know how Mom did it. She sat quietly next to me every day, hour after hour, while I slept or just lay still with my eyes closed. When I wanted to talk, she listened, and when I had a problem or complaint, she took care of it, or found someone who could. I thanked her every day for that, and told her often that she was the best mom in the world, and that I could never get through this without her. I meant it. I had heard lots of my friends complain about their parents, or their home life, and I had mentioned that to Mom once or twice through the years... reminding her that I felt so lucky that she's my mom. She was one of my favorite playmates when I was young. She'd get down on the floor with me and we'd play with all kinds of toys and games... we made up chase games, and hiding games, and when I grew older and bigger, I got a kick out of being stronger than her and hiding to jump out and scare her, or tackle her. She took me everywhere she could afford to, showing me the world, and creating adventures for us. She read to me every night until I was about 14, and sometimes we laid awake for hours into the night, laughing and talking about life. She was always at my school helping out through the years, and she never missed a program or sporting event. She even went to all my practices. She said she loved just watching me live and be who I am. Before every game, she said the same words to me— "I love you," and "Have fun." She'd always been right here for me. Whatever I was doing or wanted to do, she did her best to help me out. She taught me it was important to always pray and to trust God. I sure needed her and God to help me out now.

Mom would ask me a couple times a day, if I wanted to pray with her, or if she could help me visualize myself being healthy again, in an effort to keep my spirits up and build my will to get out of bed and go for a walk. The doctors had told us that I need to keep moving, and to at least get up and walk around as much as possible. It took all the energy and willpower I had just to go to the bathroom. I needed to build up my willpower first, just to get myself sitting up in bed. I'd swing my legs over to the side of the bed, then had to sit there for a minute to concentrate my energy on standing up, as if waiting for my brain to relay instructions to my legs. This rest also gave the room a chance to stop wobbling. Mom had learned this process, too. My IV unit needed to be unplugged, because the cord wouldn't reach to the bathroom. I was usually too weak to get that large square plug pulled out of the wall... that's right... me... a guy once able to lift 150 pounds from the ground, was now too weak to pull a plug out of a freaking waist-high wall outlet. So Mom walked around my bed and did that for me, while I grabbed hold of the IV unit to brace myself and pull up to stand and walk. After standing up, I had to wait another few seconds for my equilibrium to be restored before I could walk. I couldn't just get up and do something anymore; everything took time and effort, and everything caused more pain. Mom had to drape the cord and IV lines over the unit so they wouldn't get tangled in the wheels as I shuffled my way to the bathroom, rolling my IV unit in front of me. We had learned by experience that this was an important step, watching the cords. While I was away, Mom always straightened the covers on my bed and fluffed my pillows. When I came to lay down again, she plugged the unit back in and held the IV lines loose for me, so I could fall into bed without laying on them and pulling on the needles in my arm. When that happened the first time, it hurt enough to make me cuss and roll around in pain for a while. After that, Mom was there to help each time. Sometimes I was even too weak to pull the covers up over myself, so she would do that for me, too. I was 19 years old, and I hated needing her so much, but I was so grateful she was there.

Dr. Fleming visited usually around 11:30 each morning. This Thanksgiving morning he had some bad news. The MRI revealed two lesions in the left occipital lobe. That's the part of the brain at the lower back of the head that controls vision. He said I would need radiation to treat those lesions, because the chemotherapy would not get through because of the blood brain barrier, which is basically where the blood vessels are tighter to prevent toxic stuff from getting to the brain through the blood. My oncology team was discussing whether to begin the radiation treatments immediately, or wait until after I had finished the first couple of rounds of chemotherapy. Dr. Einhorn and Dr. Van Veldhuisen thought it was best to wait, trusting that the cancer in my organs would respond well to the chemo and I'd be physically stronger to handle radiation, but Dr. Fleming wanted to start radiation treatment right away. There was a slim chance that the large amount of chemotherapy I was receiving would cross the blood brain barrier enough to get through to the lesions seen in my brain, but there was also a chance that more lesions would grow if left untreated with radiation. It was possible that other tiny lesions not yet visible on the MRI images already existed. On the other hand, at this point in treatment, my body was very weak, my blood counts were very low, and being treated with both chemotherapy and radiation at once would weaken my body twice as bad, and risk permanent damage to my central nervous system. The decision was up to me, and Dr. Fleming suggested I take some time to think it over, talk to Dr. Van Veldhuisen and my parents about it, and let him know what I decide within the next couple of days. If I decided to wait, they would watch the lesions closely with MRI. He said a doctor from Radiation Oncology would also be in to talk with us about it.

A guy from the respiratory care unit came and hooked me up with an oxygen line in the wall behind my bed. I had to wear this in my nostrils for at least a day. The pulmonary test I'd done earlier showed that my vital lung capacity was reduced, and that the residual volume was increased, which means the air wasn't moving through my lungs well enough. I didn't feel short of breath, but that's one of the reasons

I had been feeling so tired.

My nurse came in to give me my first experience with an epo-etin injection, which is the generic form of Epogen, also known as Procrit. This injection was needed because my red blood cell count had dropped very low. This man-made protein would help my body to get the red blood cell count built back up again. If the injections helped to raise my count enough, then I wouldn't need a blood trans-fusion. Epoetin has to be injected into muscle tissue, not fat, and she said it usually stings a little more than your average injection. She gave me a choice of taking it in my upper arm or my outer thigh. I chose my thigh, and rolled to one side to raise the leg of my gym shorts to receive the shot. While the nurse was sterilizing the site, Mom asked if I wanted something to grip onto, like the bed rail, or Mark's hand. He stood and reached over to me, and as soon as we clasped hands, the nurse jabbed my leg with the thick needle.

There aren't enough cuss words to describe that pain. It started burning at the injection site, stabbing like a hot metal rod all the way into the bones in my leg and foot. I clenched my fist, grabbing the blanket on my bed. I cried out some really foul words, and I clenched Mark's hand with all the strength in my other hand, trying to squeeze the pain out. Tears were coming out of my eyes. My body tensed up and my leg drew upward, as if trying to stop the torment, and I slammed my foot back down into the bed, cussing and writhing some more. It took a couple minutes for all the pain to dissipate, and Mark and Mom stood beside me, looking very sad. I decided I would never have the injection in my leg again.

Mark's aunt and uncle were hosting the family Thanksgiving dinner that day, and that afternoon, his brother Curt and his wife Debbie brought a few plates of food up to my room for Mark and Mom, and me, if I was interested. I couldn't eat for feeling a little nauseous, but Mark and Mom appreciated the home cooking. The rest of the family came up to visit with us later that evening. It was nice to see everyone, but I was very tired.

Within two days, I had begun to feel the effects of chemotherapy on my body. In addition to feeling exhausted by all the other things going on and being done to me, I was feeling very lethargic and uncomfortable. The pain in my abdomen was still a major part of my total discomfort, my muscles were stiff and hurting, and all my bones ached from the inside out. I was constantly nauseous with no appetite at all, and even though I took the opportunity to sleep whenever I could, I couldn't manage to stay asleep. Imagine feeling completely uncomfortable and restless, but not having the energy to even stretch, or stand up and walk it off. I felt like absolute hell. Mark would help me out a couple of times a day, stretching my legs for me, lifting one leg at a time with one hand on my foot, and one hand on my knee, bending each leg and pulling it up close to my stomach, and then straightening it out to lay back down slowly. He offered calisthenics on my arms, too, putting his palm against mine and telling me to push and pull against him. Mom massaged my feet and my neck, shoulders and head sometimes, and that helped me feel a little better for a while, too. But as each afternoon came, I started feeling great anxiety about the coming chemotherapy treatment for the evening. The anxiety made me feel very nauseous and too nervous to sleep.

Saturday morning I heard the bad news that I was still anemic, even after having an epoetin shot every day since Thursday. This meant I was going to be receiving two units of blood. That made me feel more sick than I already was. Not only the fact that I needed two bags of blood hanging on my IV pole and dripping into my veins, but that I didn't know whose blood it was. Mom continued to try to help me with that, saying the kind of stuff she often did, trying to get me to trust that God provided the right person to give blood for someone they didn't know, either, and that they gave it out of love, and that it was all in divine order, sent here just for me. I did my best to get past the idea that it had already been through someone else's body. I had no choice but to buck up and take it, and try not to look at the maroon bag hanging there above me.

Later that day, I got a call from Carrie. She said she wanted to come visit me. I was more than excited to see her. Just knowing that she cared enough to come see me made me feel better. I wanted to take a quick shower, so I called Margo to come in and help me cover my Port-a-cath and the IV in my arm to keep the injection sites from getting wet. She took a couple of the large six-inch-square plastic sheets out of the drawer in the vanity, and peeled the tape off to expose the adhesive edges as I held them in place with one hand over each site. Then she sealed both sites with extra tape. I hated having to use that clear medical tape, because it left a sticky residue that was practically impossible to scrub off, even with alcohol. The lint from my clothing stuck to the leftover adhesive, and after a day or two, turned into fuzzy gray tape outlines on my chest and arm. After my shower, I put on some clean clothes and added a little cologne. I called Margo to come in and make sure both my injection sites looked okay. As she was helping me to remove the plastic coverings, I mentioned I was expecting a special visitor, and told her a little about Carrie while she helped me slip my arm into my shirt. Margo noted my uplifted spirit, and added that Carrie must be a very special girl.

I laid back to rest, wondering how I looked. I wanted to be as normal and attractive as possible, trying to ignore the thoughts in my head, telling me I was just a thin, cancer-filled shell. I raised the head of my bed up a little, and Mom helped fluff my pillows to help me sit up comfortably. When Carrie arrived, Mom and Mark left us alone for a good visit. Carrie made me feel like myself again, the old me, before cancer. I felt happy, and loved. Nobody ever made me feel as good as Carrie could. It was just like old times, the two of us, laughing and joking around. Her laugh was one of the many things I loved most about her, and it felt so good to be with her again. We even shared a long, romantic kiss. I so missed her, and who we were together. I hoped she'd come back to visit me again.

We had four years of history together, some bad, and a lot of very good fun and happy memories. I met Carrie in the summer before my junior year in high school, when I was working my first job as a cook with my good friend Karl, in a Sonic drive-in restaurant. Karl and I had met in the sixth grade. He lived only a block away from me and was my most trusted friend. He had introduced Carrie to me when she came to visit him there. It was heartthrob at first sight for me. She was the most beautiful girl I'd ever met. She was almost as tall as me, with a slender, hourglass figure, tanned satin skin, long brownish blond hair, sexy brown eyes, a gorgeous smile, and a voice that made my heart pound. She wore no makeup at all, and she was radiant as she talked and laughed with us. After she left, I asked Karl if he could hook us up, and he said he'd talk to her.

Several nights later, he told me she wanted to meet me again, and within a couple of weekends he had arranged for the two of them to meet up with me and some friends at a restaurant near the local movie theater. Carrie and I hit it off, and went out for two and a half years after that. Carrie was my other half, and together we were a playful, passionate, and comfortable perfect fit.

I loved doing fun things for her. Like once I invited her over for a romantic dinner, just the two of us. I bought a bunch of roses and sprinkled red rose petals from the doorway, up the stairs, and into the living room, which I had lit with candles on the floor, and on all the tables, including the one in the kitchen. I even sprinkled petals on the table, and had a vase of roses waiting there for her. I had planned to make lasagna, but when Carrie learned I was using a box mix, but had forgotten to buy the ground beef, we decided to send out for pizza. We had a good laugh about that. At 17, I hadn't trusted my culinary abilities to make anything more than a romantic cheese sandwich.

For her birthday one year, I planned a treasure hunt for her that took her around the city looking for different clues for a total of nine surprises. I told her to dress nice, and to ask her mom for the first clue. Mary was excited to be a part of it. She handed Carrie a cassette tape and told her to listen to it in the car. I had recorded the tape in a Mission Impossible sort of fashion, telling her that her mission, if she chose to accept it, was to follow my instructions exactly. The first tape had instructions on where she needed to go first, what to look for, who to talk to, and what to do. There was a tape waiting for her at each destination. She was to listen to each tape as soon as she received it, and follow directions on that tape. Each tape started with one of our favorite songs, and then I faded the music out and talked like a radio deejay, giving her the instructions on where to go for the next clue tape. I even gave her directions, and then recorded another of our favorite songs to play during her drive to the next stop. I had figured the length of each tape would play almost as long a time as it took her to drive to the next destination. At four of the stops, she also received a gift... flowers, sparkling cider, a nice watch, and a movie rental. I had arranged everything with store clerks a day in advance, and I had it all worked out in a two-hour-and-ten-minute time frame. I stayed two stops ahead of Carrie according to the time, and dropped off the clue tapes just before she arrived at each destination. Mom had helped me to orchestrate things on the afternoon of the event, calling the merchants to see what time Carrie arrived, then calling me with the updates to make sure I was staying ahead of Carrie. She dropped off a couple of the later clues and tapes for me so I'd have time to get in place at my last point, then she watched for Carrie to arrive at the last clue stop. When Mom called me on my cell, I had just a few minutes to make sure I was in place for Carrie's final stop at our church. There was a special place in the garden there, where she and I used to like to go once in a while. I parked my car at a distance so she wouldn't see it, and I stood waiting behind some trees in the garden and watched for her car. Her instructions were to park near the garden, get out of her car and walk toward the water fountain. On the stone wall of the fountain, in plain sight, I had set a silver matchbox car she had given me, with a note underneath it. The note said, "Say my name three times, and turn around."

The sun was just beginning to set behind the large buildings, and cast a glow down the lane of trees leading to the garden, and a very faint rainbow shown across the fountain in the middle of the garden. As she got out of her car, I could see Carrie's hair shining in the sun behind her, and I listened to her footsteps on the brick path as she came closer. When she stopped at the fountain as she'd been instructed, I saw her looking around. She picked up the car, read the note, and I could tell she was smiling as she said my name three times. While she was saying my name, I came out from hiding in the trees and walked toward her, and when she turned around, there I was. I couldn't help but smile a big smile at her. Her face was so beautiful it lit up the whole garden. We shared a long, happy embrace, and I asked her if she was having fun. She said she was having a great time, and thanked me for all the surprises. She had thought that was the end of it. I told her that I had one more surprise for her. We excitedly walked to my car, left her car there and I drove her to a place called the Country Club Plaza. I parked in a nearby parking garage, and we walked a short distance to the restaurant where I had made reservations. The host showed us to our table by the window where I had a vase of red roses waiting for her. Carrie was amazed to see I had planned anything that far in advance, and I told her I had been planning and scheming on it for weeks. We sat eating, talking and laughing about the night's events, and gazing out the window at the people walking past. A horse drawn carriage passed by, and Carrie made a comment about it.

"Who would ever want to ride in one of those things? I'd be so embarrassed to do that." She laughed.

I just looked at her. "Well..." I started, "We're going to do that after dinner. I have one reserved for us already."

She burst out laughing. She didn't believe me, but I swore to her, I really had.

"No you didn't! You would never be seen riding around in something like that."

"Okay, I swear I did, but if you don't believe me, just wait and see." I had a big grin on my face. Then I thought to myself as I took a drink of water, maybe she really wouldn't like it. I set my glass down and looked at her. "Well if you really don't want to, I guess I could cancel it."

She still had a skeptical look on her face. "You really did?"

I nodded my head and smiled.

"Okay." she said, a little embarrassed that she'd made fun of the carriage passing by.

After dinner, we walked to the carriage booth on the corner to wait for our carriage. She still didn't believe me. She thought I was playing the joke out, until our large round white pumpkin-shaped carriage arrived, and the man wearing a black coat and cap stood down and opened the gate for us to get in. He bowed to her and lent his hand to help her in. She looked at me with an enchanted smile, and an amazed look in her eyes. I thought I'd maybe made her feel like the princess she was to me. The carriage was lined on the inside with red velvet and two leather bench seats. The frame of it wasn't solid, it was more like an ornate cage wrapped and decorated with a shiny white Christmas garland, white ribbons and tiny white lights all around us. The man stepped up into his seat at the front and the horse began to take us on our tour of the plaza. Every building was outlined in brightly colored Christmas lights and music played through the air from speakers around the stores. The weather was a perfect chilly November evening, and the sidewalks and streets were full of people walking and shopping, seeing the sights and enjoying the season.

Carrie and I must have had a regal look about us as our carriage rolled us along the streets of the plaza, because people began to look at us, pointing and waving.

We heard a woman say to the crowd around her, "Hey, look! It's The Bachelor!" Then she started taking pictures of us.

I started waving just to be funny, and after a few minutes, people started gathering to watch us, snapping photos as we passed by them. Carrie started waving at everyone too, and we started playing the game that we were the famous people they thought we were, from that show.

Before long, a couple of guys came up to us and asked for our autograph on a bar napkin, so I gave them my signature as they rode with us, standing on the step of the carriage. When they jumped off, more people cheered and waved at us. Carrie and I laughed at how we started to feel like movie stars, and playing along with it was so much fun. It was one of the best times I ever had, and we laughed about that night every time we recalled the memory.

Yeah, Carrie and I had some amazing times together. That is, until I screwed things up with infidelity. She found out, and I thought I was going to die if I lost her. We fought and talked for days, and after a while she forgave me. I was so grateful that she was giving me another chance that I swore off even flirting at school when she wasn't around. Carrie had given me the silver matchbox car as a gift once, saying that someday I'd have the real thing. It was kind of a fun joke between us. I started carrying that toy car in the pocket of my jeans every day to school, and when I felt the urge to play the flirting game with some cutie, I'd reach into my pocket and feel the car that Carrie gave me. It made me think of the future we wanted together and how much I loved her, and it helped me to focus on being trustworthy to her. It worked for me for a long time, but then I had another weak moment and cheated on her again. She found out, we broke up, then she said she forgave me again, but lack of trust became our nemesis and tore us apart. She was deeply hurt and angry, and I couldn't handle the consequences. I was impatient, and mad that I couldn't earn her faith in me again, and by the summer of my first year in college, I'd lost her. She had given up on us, and so had I. We still remained friends, but never could work things out again, and I had spent the last year and a half wishing we could, and trying to stay in her life in any way she'd let me.

I was so glad she came to visit me in the hospital, but after she left my room, I felt completely exhausted. I hadn't even realized how much energy I had been using to sit up and visit with her, it had just felt so good to laugh with her. Mom and Mark understood, and sat quietly to let me sleep. The room was quiet for hours, with only the clicking of the IV machine, and the ticking of the wall clock.

Margo came in that afternoon, and told me I had several visitors. She wanted to know if I felt up to it. I wasn't sure I felt up to a whole group of people trying to talk to me at once.

"Could you find out who it is?" I asked.

Margo smiled, and nodded, and closed the door. A few seconds later she rapped on the door again and walked in. "There are six of them... they said they're from... Longan?"

I felt my face light up. "Are you serious?... oh, my God... yeah... send them in!" I raised the head of my bed so I could sit up. I felt overwhelmed and amazed, and cared about, knowing that so many of my childhood friends had gathered to see me. We'd been separated since middle school, because they all lived in the city, and I had been attending school in the suburbs since sixth grade, but I felt no apprehension in seeing all of them.

I couldn't believe it. Adrien, Eric, Nick, Libby, Jessica, and Shiva filed in, all smiling and gathering around me. Adrien was the first best friend I ever had. He and I were the only two suburban kids in the class, and for a couple years rode the 20-mile trip together to our inner city French magnet school, Longan Elementary. After fifth grade, we'd both ended up going to the same suburban schools all the way through our senior year in high school. We were like brothers and sisters, all of us. We'd grown together through grade school in the same class from kindergarten through fifth grade, and then sealed our graduation with a ten-day trip to Belgium and Paris together with some of our teachers. We'd had a couple of reunions through the years. I had a lot of great memories of playing around with my friends, and we talked and laughed about those good times.

We reminisced about the teachers we loved, Muriel, Odette, Magali, Veronique, and Mrs. Burr, and I had recently received calls and cards from Muriel and Odette. I'd kept in touch with them all through the years, visiting them once in a while. I had even invited them to my high school graduation party. Muriel came and hung out with me, we reminisced about the Longan days, and she even joined me and a few of my friends in a sandlot basketball game. She and Odette had been a big part of my early years, and I loved them both a lot.

We talked about our brother classmate, Rian. He lived in the not-so-good part of the neighborhood, several city blocks to the east of our other Longan classmates. At age 15, Rian took his own life, God rest his soul. Rian was everybody's friend. He was obnoxious and rude sometimes, but also a lovable, funny, and generous friend. He'd had a rough life, and didn't get to go to Belgium with the rest of us, because of his grades and his behavior. His passing was the last time our childhood family had gotten together. We gathered at Libby's house for a memorial to Rian. Muriel and Odette were there with us, and several of our parents. After a meal together in the dining room, we kids filtered into the living room and lounged on the floor and the furniture, chatting and laughing about old times. Everyone had a funny story about Rian, and once everyone had spoken, a hush came over all of us, as if it had something to say. It was a natural tribute, a moment of silence that came on all by itself. We each sat still in it, looking at one another, and I could feel it, the emptiness of grief in every one of us, realizing that our brother Rian was gone. None of us had seen him in a couple of years before he did that, but we all loved him and missed him, and felt sorrow for the life he must have been suffering.

It was fun to see how much everyone had changed since our last time together as kids in middle school, though, and I enjoyed the visit even though I could feel my energy draining away as we laughed together. Mom wrote down some of their phone numbers and e-mail addresses in hopes to keep in touch with them. They all wished me good luck in my treatment, and with hugs and handshakes, they left us in the quiet again.

I lay back and thought for a moment. It felt like they came from out of a different life that I'd lived, yet it felt so close to the present. I'd had such good times with them back in those days, no cares, just playing together, being kids. I looked over at Mom and Mark and remarked, "That was cool... all of them coming here... it was good to see them."

They both smiled and nodded. Mom looked kind of sad. "You're all grown up, all of you. I was looking at everyone's face, and I could still see them as they looked when you were all so young, as I watched them talking, and it's weird, to see how you've all grown and changed, but in some subtle ways, not changed."

"Yeah..." I closed my eyes.

"It all went by so fast," she sighed.

I drifted off quickly into a light sleep, until the aide came in to check my vitals, then I went right back into my nap.

A couple hours later, a few of my other high school friends dropped by for a short visit, and although I was still very tired, I managed to carry on a bit of conversation with them. I hated letting them see me this way, so weak and tired and pale. I didn't like it when people asked me how I felt, because I couldn't describe it except to say I felt like shit. They all stood around me and talked, making jokes once in a while, but I was so tired, I couldn't share a hearty laugh. I know they meant well, but I was grateful that they kept the visit short, because I really didn't have it in me to stay awake and keep up with the conversation. I was totally spent from all the visiting earlier in the day.

The days felt like months, but eventually the last day of chemotherapy was over. I had felt better on Sunday, much better, a little like my old self, emotionally. I even felt good enough to get out of my room for a wheelchair ride to the cafeteria for breakfast with Mom and Mark. Mom rolled my IV unit next to me as Mark pushed me along, down the long bustling corridors to the elevators that took us to the main floor.

As we entered the open doors of the double entryway, the smell of crisp hash browns, buttermilk biscuits, and smoked bacon filled my senses and made my mouth water for a plateful of biscuits and gravy. I told Mom what I wanted and she relayed my requests to the server. The bright yellow eggs were steaming as she fluffed a spoonful on my plate, and I could practically taste the creamy white gravy as she poured it over my biscuit. Mark carried my tray for me as Mom steered me toward the milk cooler. I opened the door and reached in for a bottle of skim for myself, and a small carton for Mom, then we caught up to Mark standing in line for the cashier.

We looked around the half-crowded eatery, and found a booth at one end, next to the wall of windows. Christmas wreaths hung in every window in the place. They were all different, and there was a sign below each one noting which department had donated or arranged it. They were being sold for charity. Mark set our trays down, and I maneuvered my IV machine to be near me so I could get out of the wheelchair and sit in the booth with them. I salted and peppered my food and took a big bite of bacon, followed by a forkful of hash browns and gravy. The gravy was rich, creamy, and salty, the biscuit was warm and soft, and the bacon was just the way I liked it, brown but not too crispy. Mom was looking around at all the wreaths, and asked Mark and me which ones we liked best. It got us both looking around and noticing the differences in the wreaths. I sat still for a moment, looking at them all, trying to recall the feeling of being excited about Christmas. By this time of the year at home, Mom would have had the whole house decorated, including my room. I would have already made my Christmas lists of what I wanted and what I planned to buy for everyone else, and been shopping with my friends. I'd been in the hospital for so long, I'd forgotten about that, and I wondered if I'd feel the Christmas spirit as it grew closer. I started to feel depressed with the knowledge that because of cancer, this Christmas would be very different.

I kept eating as I thought about it. I ate about six more bites, then my stomach started to hurt a little. It was churning and not feeling so good. I sat back and took a couple swallows of milk. Mom noticed the look on my face, and she knew I was done. She didn't say anything, but put down her fork and wiped her mouth. She waited for me to move. I wanted to eat that breakfast, it tasted so good. I picked up my fork and took a couple more small bites of hash browns. All I got was the sour taste of nausea covering my taste buds and bringing that tingling feeling to the sides of my throat. I knew it was time to quit. I reluctantly put my fork down and pushed my plate to the side. Mark was finished with his food already, even though he'd eaten more food than both me and Mom put together. Mom sometimes teased him about not even tasting his food for eating it so fast. His defense was that he'd grown up in a houseful of boys, and if you didn't eat fast, you didn't get seconds, and you left the table hungry.

Mom sighed and sadly looked at me. "You ready to go?" she asked.

"Yeah," I said, disappointed I couldn't eat more. Sitting among all the noise and people made me feel very tired, but it felt good to have gotten out and about anyway. It felt good to have wanted to get out and about.

When Dr. Fleming visited me a couple hours later, he noted the remarkable difference from how I looked when I was admitted, to the smiling young man he was talking to, just nine days later. I was actually able to sit up in my bed, move my limbs, and have a conversation with him, joke around, and laugh a little bit. I asked him if I could be released to go home, since my chemotherapy was finished, and he said I would probably be released on Monday. He and the nurse both told me, though, that I would probably continue to suffer the side effects of chemotherapy seven to ten days after my last treatment. Well, at least I was going home, and I felt good about that. I felt as if I had been enclosed and away from the outside world for a year, but it had only been a week. I looked forward to seeing the sky and the trees, my home, and my friends.

Dr. Alvarez, the radiation oncologist, came to talk to me on Monday, before I was released to go home. He spoke of the two small lesions seen in my brain, and shared his opinion concerning whether or not to proceed immediately with radiation. He was concerned about the long-term effects that chemo and radiation together might have on my central nervous system, due to my young age and potential for long-term survival. He had presented my case to the tumor board, and had also discussed my case with Dr. Einhorn personally. The tumor board was a group of doctors who met to help make treatment decisions like mine. The board included a neuro-oncologist, a neurologist, a neuropathologist, a neuroradiologist, and the chief radiation oncologist, Dr. Alvarez. It was the consensus of the tumor board and the recommendation of Dr. Einhorn, to hold off the radiation and continue with chemotherapy as long as there was tumor response and the tumor markers continued to decrease. He noted that Dr. Fleming still felt it would be best to start radiation right away.

A radiotherapist also came in to talk to me about radiation and the side effects. I was so worried about permanent hair loss. She assured me that the amount of radiation I needed would not be significant enough to cause permanent hair loss, or even total hair loss. She made sure we had plenty of reference information to take home and learn more about the side effects. I had not yet made a decision when I left the hospital for home, but I would be seeing Dr. Van Veldhuisen in a few days for a follow up, and another of those torturous epoetin injections. I could let him know then, what I had decided.

Every emotion I was feeling had a contradictory emotion to go with it. I was glad to be leaving the hospital for my home 45 minutes away, but I was afraid of leaving the medical staff that had kept a watchful eye on me for the last nine days. I dreaded the long ride home, but I felt excited to get there, to see my room, my car, and my cat. And as I walked up the steps to the front door of our house, I was filled with relief and the comfort of being home, but fearful of what the coming week would be like without the constant drip of pain meds into my arm, without a button to call the nurse. I wondered if we could handle it on our own, now.

After Mom made sure I was settled and comfortable in my room, she grabbed the checkbook and left for the corner drug store to fill my many prescriptions while Mark stayed at home with me. We had tried to fill them at the hospital before leaving, but our insurance had denied my coverage there. Mark figured it was just a glitch. We could get what we needed at the drug store that had been serving us for years near our house. The morphine, I needed as soon as possible, to keep it in my system before the pain got too bad. As it turned out, insurance still denied payment, so Mom charged the cost on her credit card, hoping Mark could straighten out the matter later.

Mom cleaned up my room and bathroom, put clean sheets on my bed, washed all my laundry, and brought a small bookshelf into my room to hold extra food for me to eat, and all the gifts that I had received in the last week. She put our land line phone next to my bed, and a small table to hold my water mug, my cell phone, and anything else I wanted to have nearby.

I talked to Mark about getting cable TV, so I would have more channels to choose from. We were probably the only people I knew who didn't have some kind of pay TV. Mark said he'd work it out in the budget for me. He also bought a universal box and hooked up everything in my entertainment system to one place, so I could easily switch from VCR or DVD, to stereo or any of my game systems, mainly Sony Playstation, and even hooked up my old Nintendo in case we felt nostalgic and wanted to play one of those games. They did everything they could think of, to make me more comfortable about being stuck in my room with barely enough energy to use the remote.

Mom prodded me often to get up and walk, and we tried walking around the block at least three times a week. I usually could only make it about a fourth of the way, then we had to turn back, but the idea was to keep moving and get some exercise each day. We had some exercise equipment at home, and Mom kept on me to use it, but I was feeling so weak that I didn't want to get out of bed to do it. I'd get frustrated with her for pushing me, even though I had asked her to do that. I was supposed to drink a couple of bottles of Ensure or Boost nutritional supplement each day, but it tasted so bad to me, I threw it up every time. Mom tried other nutritional shakes, mixing them with ice water, ice cream, juice, or cold milk, thin and thick, shaken or blended, but nothing worked. They all had the same effect on me, even when I tried just sipping them slowly. I grew so tired of throwing up after the first few days, that I didn't even want to try drinking or eating anything anymore. It seemed the anti-nausea meds weren't doing any good at all.

Nadir was setting in on me. The lethargy and weakness made me feel like the life in me was leaking out of every cell in my body, leaving me empty. I felt horrible, ten times worse than any flu I had ever had, and the nausea with dry heaves exhausted my patience and twisted my stomach in knots. Let me tell you, this was not just the ordinary dry heaves like you have with the flu. This was ten minutes bent over the toilet, with my stomach feeling as if it was trying to leap out of my mouth, causing a wretched pain from my lower intestines all the way up into my head. My eyes watered so bad, the tears streamed down my face and dripped off the end of my nose. My nostrils burned with the stomach acid that had worked its way up through my sinuses as I violently lurched, over and over. My legs weakened, and I crouched even lower to the floor, sometimes falling to one knee from the agony of it all. The only substance that came up out of my empty stomach was water, followed by a disgusting, burning, and bitter-tasting bile. When I could finally feel my stomach start to relax and my throat loosened up a bit, I didn't even have the strength to stand up again. I could hardly breathe. I usually just pulled myself toward the vanity and rested my head by the sink for a minute. Mom was always waiting for me to come out, ready to get me a cool washcloth and a fresh drink of water. As I'd open up the bathroom door and stumble to my bed, I couldn't even look up at her, but I knew, I could tell, that she was feeling so sad, she wanted so bad to make it all go away. But it was all I could do to fall back into my bed, close my eyes and try to wait out that feeling, the complete exhaustion of my body involuntarily heaving like that, and the intense headache, and stomach and back pain that followed.

I began to keep a trash basket next to me because a couple of times I hadn't made it to the bathroom quick enough, and threw up stomach acid on my bed and on the carpet. I was constipated from the pain meds, even though I had been taking stuff to prevent it, and that was causing me some excruciating abdominal pain that made me yell out loud. I had to take Milk of Magnesia for that, which of course, also made me throw up. In the hospital, I'd had to have an enema to get rid of the constipation. I was shamefully embarrassed that another person had to insert that little capsule into my anus, so I requested a female nurse that I wouldn't have to face later on, someone who wasn't regularly taking care of me. She gave me what they called a "Magic Bullet," and it was just that. It wasn't but about half an hour after she'd given it to me that I had to sprint to the bathroom, and everything in my intestines came shooting out of me. I had to admit, it was a relief. But I couldn't have that Magic Bullet at home, and constipation was a very painful, ongoing problem. I had become increasingly depressed, and didn't even have the energy to have a conversation or watch television. It was all I could do to lie in bed and breathe, taking the occasional sip of ice water from the straw in the mug next to me.

Friends dropped by to see me, but I was worthless, so tired and pale, and embarrassed that I could not even sit up to talk to them. They brought candy, snacks, and presents, but no one knew how to act or what to say, and even though I tried to be cordial and speak a few words, the eventual one-sided conversations usually kept the visits pretty short. I wasn't the Ian that people were used to.

I later wrote in a short cancer journal on my laptop about this period of nadir, which I had titled *The Cancer Mountain;* "Treatment 1: Complete and total hell. Too miserable to move, yet it hurts not to move. Everything's a chore."

This was why each day, I felt more and more thankful for my Mom. Neither one of us felt any discomfort in the silence, or the need for space-filling conversation. She never left my room to take care of other things unless I had visitors, or I was awake and she could tell me where she was going. At night, she slept on a bedroll on the floor next to me, and kept her hand on my bed near me. Sometimes I reached for her and held her hand, and sometimes I just needed to feel her hand on my arm or touching my side. I still had insane nightmares almost every time I fell asleep, and even though I was in my own room, I still would wake up feeling disoriented and alone. Insomnia was getting worse for me, too, and even when I was awake, hallucinations haunted me. Sometimes I would be lightly resting but not asleep, and a hallucination would snap me into a startling fear. My instant reaction was to squeeze Mom's hand and look at her, checking on my existence, validating where I was. I often quickly forgot what the vision was, and that was fine by me, but it happened so often, that I started getting paranoid about it. I was so glad she was willing to stay close by, so she'd be right there in those moments.

She had arranged all my medications on a tray in my room, to make it easier to take the right medicine at the right time of day. She labeled the top of each bottle with white tape and bold letters, to make everything easier to see at a glance, and she lined the meds up in grid fashion according to their purpose and time of day they needed to be taken. I had two pain meds, three for nausea, two for constipation, one to soften the stool if I had one, one to assist kidney function (or more to the point, to keep my kidneys from suffering the adverse effects of cisplatin), one for anxiety, one stomach acid reducer, and one for overall digestion assistance. Mom ended up dosing all my meds out for me, each morning, noon, and evening, so I didn't have to worry about it, or even think about it, but she showed me which ones were which when I took them, as the nurses did at KU, so I'd know if I had to dose them out myself at some point. Once in a while I threw up before all the medicines made it through the digestion stage. They tasted like shit and burned my throat coming back out.

I had a followup appointment with Dr. Van Veldhuisen on the Friday of my first week home. I was still so tired with extreme fatigue that I didn't want to have to make the trip, even though all I had to do was sit in the car while Mom drove. My stomach was hurting really bad, too. I was scheduled to have a treatment of bleomycin that day, and the thought of it made me feel sick and nervous. Mom packed her purse with some dried banana chips and a bottle of water for me, her notebook in which she was always keeping track of everything about me, and grabbed a pillow and an afghan for me to use in the car. We headed for the long highway drive to KU Cancer Center.

As we approached the hospital, I started feeling really sick to my stomach. I shifted around a little in my seat, trying to get the feeling to go away. I told Mom I thought I might throw up, and she said to just say the word and she would stop the car. We were about to enter the parking garage, so I tried to mentally push the feeling down as Mom found a close parking space. Getting out of the car and standing to walk helped to stave off the nausea a little bit, but the closer we got to the hospital entrance, the more sick I felt. The smell and sounds of the world going on around me had never seemed so intense before. Outside there was car exhaust, diesel fumes, and cigarette smoke, and the air smelled of a cold, stale, wintery day. Cars were parked with the engines running, dropping people off or loading them in, and voices came from every direction. Once we walked through the doors, people were moving around me every which way, coming and going, pushing wheelchairs with depressed-looking patients or strollers with fussy children, people talking on cell phones or to each other, walking fast, or lumbering slowly. Some people smelled like an old house, like mildew or moth balls, others reeked of body odor or cheap perfume, and it was all blanketed in the basic sterile hospital smell, with the hint of cinnamon.

When we walked through the door, the smells and the people, the activity, and atmosphere, it all just came rushing at me, and I told Mom I was going to throw up. Mom motioned me toward a men's room just around the corner from the main lobby, and I barely made it into the stall. When I came out, Mom was standing next to the door waiting for me, and asked if I wanted her to get a wheelchair for me. I felt I could walk, because the Cancer Center was just back through the main lobby from there. I felt drained of all energy, and we walked in a slow shuffle to the waiting room, where I was relieved to be able to lay down on a couch near the back wall. Mom had to go up to the desk and give them all the information about me and our insurance for their records before I would be seen. I just lay there in misery, my legs hanging off the couch as if I had fallen over from a sitting position onto my stomach. The lights, the noises, the stress, all made my stomach feel as if it was sitting in my throat. My body felt so fatigued that I didn't even care that my face was touching a couch where thousands of strangers had been sitting. Mom came over to me when she was finished at the desk, and knelt down on the floor beside me. She put her arm around me, and rubbed my back a little. Her face looked very sad as she told me how sorry she was, that I was suffering so much. She took her scarf off from around her neck, folded it and offered it to me to lay my head on. She kissed my shoulder and laid her head on her arm next to me while we waited.

The nurse called my name and took me directly to the lab where another nurse took all my vitals and weighed me. I was down to 174 pounds. I had lost ten pounds in the last ten days. She drew a few vials of my blood, then she escorted me to a treatment area with a reclining chair and privacy curtain, and a chair for Mom to sit next to me. Apparently I was dehydrated, even though I had been drinking lots of water. They hooked me up with IV fluids first thing, and I needed more than the prescribed amount that was to precede the bleomycin dose. We had to wait for the lab work to be done on my blood before anything else would happen, anyway. I just laid the chair back and tried to rest. After about an hour, we learned I was anemic, so I had to have another one of those epoetin injections in my arm. Since I didn't have Mark's hand this time, I chose to grip the arm of the chair. I was thinking Mom probably couldn't handle the pressure of my squeeze on her hand. I wouldn't have been surprised if I had left finger imprints indented in the leather and metal arm of the chair. I think for a moment, though, I had forgotten about my abdominal pain, which I had just rated a seven on a scale of one to ten, ten being unbearable.

Dr. Van came to visit me there in the treatment area. He said my white blood cell count was only slightly low, so I would be okay to receive the scheduled second dose of bleomycin before I left to go home. I figured I already felt like hell, so what did it matter now to have more chemotherapy in me, as long as it's killing the cancer! The nurse came and gave me an injection of morphine for the pain. That injection kind of sucked too, because at first, as the morphine got into my bloodstream, all my muscles tensed up, I mean every inch of fibrous tissue in my body burned like a light muscle cramp, and I hated it... but then after a few seconds, everything just let go, and I felt like I didn't even have any muscles in my body at all. It was so relaxing after that, and then I usually fell off to sleep a little. When the nurse came to access my port for the bleomycin dose, I told her my port site was sore, and that I hated the feeling of it being accessed. She said she could spray the site with a cold substance called ethyl chloride. This would numb the skin at the site a little, so it wouldn't hurt so bad when she stuck that big needle in. The bleomycin dose would take about an hour to drip into me, so Mom and I would be sitting for another hour and a half, or that is, Mom would be sitting, I would be sleeping.

When it was all over, the nurse removed the bleomycin bag. To keep my blood from clotting around the port, she flushed it with heparin before pulling the needle out, and I woke from my groggy semi-nap state. When that was finished, she sterilized the port site, and covered it with a sterile pad in case it bled a little afterwards. She pulled my IV needle out and did the same with it. Dr. Van came back in, and handed Mom instructions on what serious symptoms to watch for in the coming days, and reasons to call his nurse. He said if all went well, I would continue with more chemotherapy in a week.

5

Vertigo, Neutropenic Fever, Falling Hair, and Hallucinations

It was good to be home, but the bleomycin was having its effects on me. More friends came to visit over the weekend, but I was too sick to sit up and talk to them. All I could do was just lay in my bed and hope they understood. They'd try to keep a conversation going, but in the middle of a sentence, I'd have to leap out of my bed and stagger to the bathroom a few feet away to throw up, heaving and retching while they waited. So they sat on my couch, listening to me vomit, not knowing how to act or what to say when I came out of the bathroom pale and weak and falling into my bed again. I'd apologize, then they would apologize, and we'd all feel embarrassed in the following silence. After one or two visits, most people stopped coming around and sent me text messages instead. I felt very sad about that, but it was okay, really, because I hated throwing up before an audience, and I didn't want to be pitied. I just wanted to be normal again.

Mom checked my temperature twice a day, then asked the routine questions about any pain, blood in my urine or my poop, nausea, and stuff like that. She kept a record of all of it, including the exact time I took my medications, so she could accurately answer any questions the doctors might have, and so we could easily check her notes instead of relying only on memory. She was considering the idea of going to work on Monday. She cleaned homes for a living, and I knew we could use the money, and it would only take her about three hours. I did not want to stay at home by myself, because if I got seriously ill (which we'd learned I could do very unexpectedly), I wanted someone else to be able to call the doctor for me. We talked about finding someone to stay with me while she worked, and the only people I felt comfortable staying with me were my stepsisters. Tracey had a full class schedule an hour away, but it happened that Kristen had no classes on Monday, so Mark arranged with her to come over early that morning.

Mom gave her all my discharge instructions we'd received at the hospital, and the phone numbers listed in order of importance. She updated Kristen on how I'd been feeling over the last couple days, and what to expect as "normal," and what to consider an emergency. Mom gave me my morning medications before she left, so Kristen didn't have to deal with that. This would be the first time since my diagnosis that my Mom wouldn't be with me. Less than ten minutes away, she could rush home for any reason. We all knew everything would be fine, but we were also a little nervous about her return to work. I had become accustomed to her taking care of everything.

The morning went well, and I felt okay enough. Kristen and I watched a movie, I played a video game, and when I got hungry, she made some instant oatmeal for me. She asked me a couple of times if I was sure it wasn't too thin, and offered to make another bowl if that one wasn't just right. She seemed sure she had messed it all up, and that I didn't like it. I knew she didn't fully understand that I was glad to be able to eat anything at all. Thin or not, it had flavor and substance, and I told her it was fine, but I don't think she believed me. I rarely finished a meal, and the bowl of oatmeal was no exception. Nausea demanded I put the bowl down and tried to lay still and rest for a while.

Mom arrived home a little after noon, and I think Kristen was relieved that the responsibility shifted from her shoulders to Mom's. They talked about the possibility of Kristen relieving Mom from time to time so Mom could earn some money at least once a week. I was grateful that Kristen was willing to do that, if we needed her.

I started feeling more sick through the night, and Mom and Mark stayed close by. Mom settled in on the floor next to me, and Mark sat on my couch, and we talked as the night grew dark. We had all gotten a little quiet and sleepy, when all of a sudden I felt that I was falling, that everything around me was gone, and I was just falling...falling...and falling as the space around me seemed to speed past me from behind. I felt completely consumed with fright, and I tried to grab hold of the bed with each hand gripping the blankets in my fists.

"MOM!? What's happening?!! MOM!" I cried out to her. "MOM! Help me, Mom!" My eyes were wide with fear, trying to see what was going on, but I couldn't see any detail, only muted colors as I fell deeper and faster. My heart was racing, my whole being, my mind, my soul was clenched in terror. I couldn't feel anything around me, I just kept falling and falling, with a horrifying sense of being completely alone. I tried to find Mom's face, to see her, but I couldn't grasp onto the reality of my surroundings.

Mom was right there, I heard her voice, but I still could not see her. She saw the complete terror in my eyes. She took hold of my hand and was on her knees beside my bed, looking straight at me, and holding my gripping hand close to her heart. Softly she spoke to me, trying to coach me back to reality... "Ian...look at me...you're at home, in your room, in your bed, and me and Mark are right here with you... you're okay...just look at my face, Ian... look at me, I'm right here...look at my face...just keep looking at me, I'm right here with you, Ian, I'm right here and I won't let go of you, I promise, just keep looking at me... you're okay... everything is okay..."

"Mom... Mom... okay, Mom... help me, Mom... don't let go of me, Mom!..." is all I could hear myself say. Finally my eyes found her, I didn't dare look away. "Okay, Mom... okay, Mom..." I could see that Mark was right beside me, but I was afraid to look away from Mom's face. I could hear his voice softly telling me to hold on to Mom, and that they loved me, and that I was safe.

As the sensation started to subside, I was exhausted, but tense and afraid that it would happen again. I felt like I had been put back into my body after a horrible nightmare. It had been just as intense as the episodes I'd had in the hospital. They were the most terrifying experiences I'd ever had in my whole life. I didn't know what to think, and I know it made Mom and Mark both feel so sad and scared for me. We three talked about it, and I tried to describe how I felt. They said it only lasted a minute or two, but to me, it felt like a day had been taken off my life.

Mom sat down slowly on the floor next to my bed. She took my hand in hers and kissed the back of it, and held it close to her face. "I'm sorry, Ian..." she said in a soft voice.

Mark went to get me a cool damp washcloth to put on my sweating forehead, and when I laid it across my eyebrows, I began to feel a kind of peaceful relief, like I was home, safe again. He knelt down on one knee next to me, and I could feel his sorrow, and his concern.

"Thanks," I said in my tired, dry-sounding voice. I reached for my cooler mug of water, took a sip from the straw, and set it back on the floor next to me. I lay my head back onto my pillow. I felt so miserable, so helpless, even worthless. "Why is this happening?" I asked myself in a whisper. Mom said she would ask Dr. Van about it.

Mark sat back down on the couch, to stay and visit a while longer, and when he got up to say goodnight, I reached for his hand.

"Thanks, Mook." I looked up at him.

"You're welcome, brother," he said softly. He gave me what we called a "brother-brother-handshake," which sometimes ended up being kind of crazy or silly, but that time it was just us holding hands for a quick moment, a silent gesture of affection. He leaned over and gave me a one-armed hug, and then kissed Mom goodnight. "You sleep good, brother. I'll see you tomorrow," he said as he closed the blanket curtain I used for a door on my room.

Mom sat down on the floor next to me again, and looked at me with sad eyes.

I opened my palm, and she took hold of my hand.

"Mom..." I still could feel the fear as I thought about what happened, and I figured it showed on my face, "Please don't leave me..."

She looked sincere and assured me, "Of course I won't leave you, Ian. I will always be right here."

"I mean it, Mom... I mean right here, next to me. I couldn't handle it by myself if that happens again. I've never been scared like that... I thought I was dying... I don't ever want to be alone with that fear...and I don't think anybody but you or Mark could get me through it. And I don't want anyone else seeing me losing my shit like that."

Mom nodded, and her eyes leaked a couple of tears.

"Please say you'll always stay right by me... don't let go of me," I whispered.

"I will always stay right beside you, Ian. Hold my hand through the night if you need to, that way you'll know I'm right here, even when I'm sleeping."

That night as we laid awake and talked, Mom assured me she would not go back to work at all, no matter what. She and Mark would talk about the finances, and they would work it out, but I was not to worry that I would ever be left alone to go through that fear by myself. I didn't sleep very well that night, mostly because nightmares would scare me awake. I instinctively reached for Mom since the episode of vertigo earlier, and feeling her presence helped me to realize I was still alive, not alone, and safe enough to fall asleep again.

By morning, the nausea was getting worse though, and I was feeling more sick as the day wore on. Mom started taking my temperature four times a day. She watched my symptoms, and often asked me how I was feeling. She didn't want a generic answer, like, "okay," or "like shit." She wanted details. It irritated me a little bit, but I knew she needed to keep track of my symptoms just like they did in the hospital. She came up with a standard list of symptoms, and asked me to rate them on the scale of one to ten, like I rated my pain. That worked better, because I didn't have to give a lot of thought to putting my answers into words. Twice a day, she rated my upper and lower back pain, chest pain, head pain, stomach pain, nausea, fatigue, and depression. Of course, if some pain became worse in between her log times, I told her about it and she logged that, too.

I tried to have an appetite, and Mom tried fixing healthful food that she knew I liked, but I just couldn't eat. I'd have a few bites and then my stomach pain would get worse, the nausea would intensify, and I'd eventually throw up. I was having trouble keeping my medicines down, too. By Wednesday, I started feeling so horrible that I didn't think I could handle it. I had constant nausea with lingering dry heaves, stiffness, and I ached all over. That evening I had started having a really bad headache, and about seven o'clock, Mom found that I had a fever of almost 101 degrees F. She called Dr. Van's nurse to ask what she should do. The nurse told Mom she needed to bring me to the emergency room.

Mom called to Mark upstairs, and he went outside to warm the car. Mom helped me to get my shoes and coat on, and Mark helped me out through the garage to the car outside. I lay down in the back seat, and Mom covered me with the afghan. I wondered if this was what dying felt like.

Mark pulled up to the curb near the emergency entrance, and got out to help me out of the car. He parked the car while Mom and I walked toward the entrance, but I stopped suddenly to throw up on the walkway. I felt weak and dizzy, so I braced myself against the wall with both hands, and threw up some more. Mom stood by, waiting and worrying. Once I was finished, I had to stand there for a minute before we started walking slowly again, my hand resting on her shoulder for stability. We finally made it inside and saw the place was crowded with weary-looking people and crying children. Some were seated in chairs that lined the walls to the waiting room, and others paced back and forth. People looked up as we walked in and stood looking for someone to help us. Mark caught up to us as Mom helped me to the nearest chair, which was across from three admitting desks. I sat down and leaned over to hide my face in my hands. The smell of other people around me was making me nauseous, and closing my eyes to my surroundings made me feel dizzy. I just held my hands over my mouth and nose, and stared at the cold white linoleum tiled floor.

The atmosphere was cluttered with the chatter of nurses, admitting reps, and waiting patients. Mark walked up to the admitting rep at the nearest desk and told her that I was a cancer patient there and that I had a fever. The admitting rep called the triage nurse, and told Mark to take me right in to her office. I was sure I looked as bad as I felt as he and Mom walked beside me, shuffling my way to the small room. I sat down in the chair nearest the door, and heard the nurse already talking to another nurse on the phone about me. She checked all my vitals and asked the routine questions, and within about 15 minutes, another nurse came to take me to an exam room. I was glad to see there was a bed for me to lie down in. We were there for several hours, and I was feeling worse and worse by the hour, just laying there in that bed, helpless and depleted of life. They did a strep culture, a urinalysis, a chest x-ray, and accessed my port to draw more blood. Apparently I had a urinary tract infection, and I would be admitted as soon as a room was prepared for me upstairs in Unit 42.

As it turned out, my white blood cell count was extremely low, and I had what is called neutropenic fever. That is when I had almost no resistance to any kind of virus or bacterial infection, because of the low white blood cell count. The x-ray of my lungs looked good, and the masses appeared to be a little smaller, so that was pretty good news. But I still felt like crap, and I'd be staying there for a day or two so they could keep an eye on me. They gave me an antibiotic, and an injection of neupogen, the one to help build white blood cells. Those shots didn't burn as bad as the epoetin, because they could be injected into fat tissue, but they still hurt very bad and made my bones ache for days.

The next day, I met another nurse on the cancer ward who became one of my favorites. Tracy was very nice and took the time to explain everything to us. She said that the blood lab work done the night before showed that my hemoglobin was a little low, so she was to draw more blood again, and if it was still low, I might have to receive a unit of blood. She gave me all my regular medications, plus more antibiotics. I was already feeling a little better than I had the whole week before, and my temperature was back to normal.

Dr. Fleming came for his daily visit a couple of hours later. He said I would be receiving another dose of neupogen, and as it turned out, would not be needing the blood transfusion after all. That made me very happy. Also, I would be getting an antifungal medication in case there was a mild fungal infection in my mouth or throat, because even though the throat culture didn't show anything positive, I had been complaining of a sore throat. He was going to wait until later in the day to consider moving my third bleomycin dose, which was scheduled for the following day. Sometimes bleomycin can cause sweats and fever, which could interfere with the observation of the symptoms I had come in with.

By about one o'clock that afternoon, I actually was beginning to feel hungry. The cafeteria delivered a tray of food, but I wasn't able to eat much of it, though I tried. I still felt too nauseous, and I just wanted to rest. A couple of quiet, IV clicking hours went by, and Tracy came in to give me another neupogen shot and drew more blood for the lab.

Friday morning came, and Dr. Van Veldhuisen checked in on me around nine o'clock. He would be getting back to me about the bleomycin dose scheduled for that day, but suspected it would be changed, due to my low blood counts for the last couple of days. He said I would need another injection of both neupogen and epoetin, and this news bummed me out pretty bad. I was so tired of feeling the stress and the pain connected to those injections, and I told him of that.

My spirits were getting really low, being stuck in the hospital with all the testing and blood taking and pill swallowing, and daily shots that hurt like hell. I felt like I wasn't getting any real rest, for all the stuff going on and my continuing struggle with insomnia. When I did fall asleep, it seemed something always happened to wake me up... nightmares, nurses, aides, phones ringing, or my IV machine beeping for one reason or another. I became so fed up with it all, so tired, and each day dragged on with the same shit, over and over. On top of all that, my hair was starting to fall out. I could see it on my pillow, and on my clothes, and that brought on a whole new heaviness to my growing depression.

Later that afternoon, a care coordinator came in to tell me I had been scheduled to visit the Cancer Center every day for ten days after my discharge in order to continue receiving the Rocephin, which was the antibiotic that had to be administered through my port, and it took about 30 minutes for each dose. I'd been receiving it since I was admitted Wednesday night. I also needed four more days of neupogen. I was thinking to myself, how much worse is this going to get before it gets better?

Then about ten minutes after she left, Dr. Fleming came in to tell me the best news I had heard in almost a month. The tumor markers in my blood were now way down from 200,000 to 26,318! What a feeling of joy and relief that was for me. I smiled at Mom, and we gripped each other's hand in personal celebration as Dr. Fleming continued. I would not be receiving the day's scheduled bleomycin dose, because my blood cell counts were still too low and I needed the continued antibiotic for the infection. That had to be cleared up before any chemotherapy could start. There was still a lot of progress to be made, but to feel that all the suffering I was going through was actually paying off was a great boost to my spirits. After he left my room, I gave my mom a huge hug. I asked her to call Mark and give him the good news. I listened to her as she repeated the details to him, enjoying the sound of it again and feeling some new hope. I held my hand out for her to lend me the phone, and I felt a little bit of a smile on my tired face as I greeted him.

"Hey...."

"Hey, how about it, Stretch!" he started.

I listened, smiling and drawing strength from the sound of his voice congratulating me on my progress.

He said he'd call Kristen and Tracey to tell them the news himself. It had been a long time since we had any happy news to share, and it felt good to be able to do that. After I hung up the phone, though, I felt pretty worn out, and decided to rest for as long as I could. I would tell others later, when I felt more energy to talk.

It soon came time for my dose of Rocephin in my port, and I got some other meds to take orally. My nurse, Trishna, said she would be giving me the shots of epoetin and neupogen later that evening. I wasn't feeling well at all, sick to my stomach, and now nervous about the upcoming pain of the shots. I asked her if I could have something for anxiety and nausea before I got those shots, so around 5:30, she brought me an Ativan tablet.

My dinner came an hour later, and I was actually enjoying the look and smell of my food, eating pretty well in comparison to past weeks. I had ordered a baked potato with cheese, pears, and some chocolate milk. Unfortunately I was still eating when Trishna came to give me the dreaded shots. She couldn't leave the prepared doses in my room while I finished eating, so I had to take them right away.

It didn't seem to hurt quite as bad as the times before. I mentioned that to her, and she gave me information that became very valuable for future injections. She said I should ask the nurse who would be giving me the injection to use a diabetic needle, because they're a little narrower, and especially to let the neupogen or epoetin warm to room temperature before injection, and most important, inject it slowly into my arm... as slowly as possible. I was very grateful to her for telling me this. It was still very painful with a lasting ache, only a little less intense. Even worse, there was still enough pain to ruin what had been a good and rare appetite.

By midnight, my back pain was throbbing really bad. I had rated it at an eight, but all I could receive without a doctor's okay was another oxycodone. My night nurse gave me one, and told me if the pain was still bad after half an hour, she would contact the doctor on call. I dozed off for a little while, and four hours later, she came in to draw some blood for labs. I told her my back still hurt, and she gave me another oxycodone tablet. An hour later I told my mom that the pain was still bad, so she went to find the nurse, who called the doctor. He prescribed a couple milligrams of morphine, and had come in to have a look at me. I had never seen this doctor before, but he said there didn't seem to be anything serious going on that would cause the back pain, that he thought it was muscular pain. Mom tried to ease the pain my massaging my back, but it only helped a little, and temporarily.

My back continued to hurt, and hours passed, and another doctor came in to see me around ten a.m. He said my back pain was probably caused by the neupogen, and suggested Tylenol for the pain. I received another injection of neupogen, and another dose of Rocephin, and was told I would be released to go home later that day. I was to return to the Cancer Center tomorrow for a neupogen shot and a dose of Rocephin, and on Monday for the same, and to see Dr. Van Veldhuisen. We would be making the hour and a half round trip every day in the coming week, for daily doses of Rocephin, and an injection of epoetin on Friday. Heavy sigh... I was getting very tired of the cancer routine.

My friends in the band I played with had planned a benefit show for me that Saturday, to help raise money for my rapidly rising medical expenses. Our band manager and lead guitarist, Pat, had arranged the whole thing, and booked five or more bands to play for free, including Axium with David Cook; Unorthodox, which was Chris, a friend from high school, and his successful band; our band Crimson; and a few more local bands. They had billed it as the "Rock Out Against Cancer" benefit concert in my honor, and Pat had made up these great poster ads and posted them all over the downtown area of our hometown of Lee's Summit and at local businesses. I was incredibly honored that all these guys would get together and do this for me, and I wanted to be there to personally thank them.

Mom wanted to ask Dr. Van Veldhuisen's nurse if I would be okay to attend the benefit concert that evening. She called and left a message, and told me that we would have to follow the doctor's orders on this one. Being around lots of people would put me at risk for getting sick again and ending up right back in the hospital. Nurse Kathy's advice was to stay home, but if I insisted on being present, I was to keep the visit short, wear gloves, something to cover my face if I had to walk through a crowd, and most of all, have no physical contact with others. No hand shaking, no hugging, no kissing, no drinking from any public glasses, bottles, or cans, and avoid use of public bathrooms if possible. She made it very clear that I would be putting myself at risk for another infection. These were strict instructions I could live with. And Mom, weeks ago, bought small bottles of hand sanitizer for both of us to always have on hand. I kept mine in my coat pocket.

I stood before the microphone on the stage, and I was in awe of all the people who showed up for me. After expressing my extreme gratitude, I explained it all, why the gloves, the scarf to cover my mouth, and how important it was for people to resist gathering around me, if they wanted me to get better. I wasn't feeling well that night anyway, very tired and nauseous from the activity and excitement, so I didn't want to stay long. But I was glad to be present and see all those people and feel their support for me, and especially to see the guys in the band. They all cheered for me as I made my way to the door to go home.

That night I found it easier to fall asleep than I had in a week. I hadn't slept well in the hospital the last few days, and the stress of being in the crowd of my friends and trying to look alive and friendly really took a toll on my energy level. I had installed a sliding dimmer switch on the light in my room a couple of years ago and so could keep it at a very low light level. That came to be more of a blessing than I'd ever expected.

I was jolted out of my light sleep in the middle of the night from a nightmare, followed by the intense feeling of falling through empty space at a tremendous speed. I couldn't feel the bed underneath me, I couldn't see the walls in my room, and I couldn't feel my hands as I reached to grip on to anything to hold on to. "MOM!...MOM!"

She sat straight up from the floor next to me.

"Mom...it's happening!... it's happening, Mom!"

She saw the frightened wide eyes of mine that searched the room looking for her face, her voice. She took hold of both my hands in hers.

"Ian, it's Mom... I'm right here, honey, I'm right here with you... we're at home, we're in your room... everything is okay... look at me, just look at me... here I am, Ian... Ian... I'm right here... I'm right here...

just look at me, just look at me, Ian...."

I was looking more at her voice than her face at first. My eyes couldn't focus, but I could follow the sound of her, and I held my gaze to her with wide, scared eyes... "Okay, Mom... okay Mom... okay... okay... okay...." I replied to her words in my weak, fearful voice. I gripped her hands and pulled, as if pulling myself up toward her to keep me from falling farther down into—I didn't know where.

When that episode was over, I was sweating, and trembling a little. I wanted the lights to be brighter, but I wasn't ready to let go of Mom's hands. She knelt beside me and waited for me to calm, and decide how one of us was going to reach the light switch on the wall without letting go of the other. Mom reached for the TV remote with one hand, and turned it on mute so we could have the added light of the TV screen. When I was ready, she started to stand to head for the wall switch.

"Wait..." I said, still holding her hand. "Let me see that remote." I reached out to take it with my left hand. It was just enough extension for my long arm to reach the wall switch without getting up or letting go of my anchor. Mom smiled at my ingenuity, and I told her how I'd done that many times out of laziness late at night. I sat up in bed, and Mom went to my bathroom to get a cool washcloth for me. I rubbed it all over my face and hands, then she freshened it with cool water and I lay down with it folded over my forehead. She dimmed the lights again, but not as dark, and we lay there talking about the way I felt, and how my world was changing against my will. Mom sat leaning on my bed, resting her head near my arm and her hand across my stomach. I held her hand as we both drifted off to sleep.

The next morning we woke late, and I felt rested, but still I had the nausea, which stayed with me through the following days. I threw up regularly, but I actually pooped a couple times in four days, which I know sounds weird, but it was something to be glad about, because I was still usually suffering with daily, very painful constipation. I was also having muscle aches all over my body, but especially in my calves. I had to get up in the night two or three times to pee, and the pain caused me to walk with a stiffness that made me feel like an old man.

Mom woke up every time I did, checking on me to see if I was okay.

My falling hair was all over everything, my bed, my bathroom, my face. Every time I moved my head on my pillow, I had to brush the hair away, and every time I got up out of bed, it sprinkled off of me like hair confetti. And each time, my heart felt heavier and more sad at the loss of this part of myself. All this, and the daily trip to the Cancer Center, plus knowing I'd be going back to be admitted there on Wednesday to start my second round of chemotherapy was causing me to feel pretty depressed. My port site and my right shoulder had been hurting when I moved my arm, so I made a note to ask about it as soon as I saw one of my doctors. X-rays had shown that the catheter was still in place, and Dr. Van and a nurse examined the site, but couldn't find anything wrong. There was one good thing, though. Dr. Van had told me on Monday in the Cancer Center, that my tumor markers were even lower than they had been on Friday. My Beta hCG was now at 26,000, and the alpha feta protein was down from 400 to 28! Just another chemo treatment or two, and hopefully the tumor markers would continue to go down at that rate. I was trying to hold onto that bright spot of hope.

On Wednesday, I was feeling hungry for breakfast, and asked Mom if we could go to Burger King for some bacon, egg, and cheese croissant sandwiches. I took my morning meds while Mom finished packing my duffle bag with last-minute toiletries, games and movies, and we headed off to breakfast. I ate all of it, and it felt good to be able to do that.

We arrived at KU about ten in the morning, and as soon as I walked into the place, I had to head to the bathroom and throw up. So much for a good breakfast. The admitting rep said there were not any hospital rooms available yet in Unit 42, so we went to the Cancer Center, where they were expecting me for a Rocephin injection anyway. After the 30-minute dose, we learned that there still was no room available for me, and no way for the admitting rep to know when I could be admitted. She told us it would probably be a few hours. Mom and I talked it over, and I decided I would rather wait at home, so we arranged to leave my duffle bag and Mom's luggage on a cart in the admissions office, and off to the car we went.

As we walked to the garage, I could feel some of my hair falling onto my face, and I looked down at my shirt and saw my hair all over it. I was feeling so frustrated about it. When we got to the car, I took the opportunity, as I did whenever I was outside to fluff the loose hair off of my head and brush it off my clothes and my hat. I can't express how sad I was about it. It made me feel like I was changing into someone else I didn't want to be. I felt like I was losing... losing a part of me I'd never get back... losing my strength, my fight... losing ME. Mom wished she could make it stop. She looked so sad for me. She had been changing my pillow cases and sheets often. She had vacuumed my hats and my blankets for me, and wiped off the sink in my bathroom every day, so I wouldn't have to look at it.

So our morning spent at KU and driving to and from had me feeling very mad, sad, sick, tired, and fed up with all of it. I got home to my room and threw myself down on my bed in disappointment and total frustration with my circumstances. Mom sat near me, quietly listening to me lament about things, and then suggested maybe we could watch a movie while we waited. I felt better about that, and asked her where we had put the movie that Mark rented for us the other day, which we hadn't had a chance to watch. After looking for it, we both remembered that I had put it inside the pocket of my duffle bag, which was sitting on a cart in the admissions office, waiting for us at the hospital.

I felt completely dark and defeated inside. I just turned the light off in my room, fell back down into my bed, grabbed the remote and turned on the TV. My face reflected how awful I felt inside, as I blankly stared at the commercials.

Mom sat down on the floor next to me and laid her head on my bed. I flipped through the channels on TV a few more times, then I turned it off and closed my eyes. I felt completely dismal, hopeless, and helpless.

I looked over at her and she raised her head to look at me. "Momma,

I'm so depressed... I'm so sad... I feel horrible." I knew she could see in my eyes how awful I felt. I just wanted to be done with it. I was tired of being in my room. I wanted to move forward, and I felt like having to come back home was moving me backward. I rolled onto my back and stared at the ceiling in despair.

"Well, do you feel like going shopping?" she asked.

I looked at her and smiled. I thought about how good it would feel to do that, to get out and do something else.

"Let's do that..." she nodded, "We'll buy you a new hat and a new pair of comfy sweat pants..." She looked hopeful to cheer me, and I actually felt a bit of excitement.

The thought of it made me feel better instantly. But as I got up to put my shoes on, I talked to her about my concern of feeling suddenly nauseous or too tired once we arrived at the mall. Mom said it would do me some good to get out and walk, see some new things, and if I did get too tired or sick, we would leave, no problem. It wasn't risky for me to be around crowds as much any more, because my white blood cell count was high again, so we headed out. As we were driving, I asked Mom if we could stop to see my boss, Gina. It was fun to see her, and she and I talked about when I could try to come back to work again. She was really cool, and wanted me to take the time to get well again, first. Her mom was also fighting cancer, so Gina had a good idea of what I was going through. She was a great boss, and I liked working for her, and with her.

When Mom and I got back into the car, the admitting rep at KU called her cell and said they had a room ready for me. Shit. I had just gotten my spirits up. Now I had to switch gears again. We sat in the parking lot for a minute, and talked about it. I decided that it would be best to skip the shopping trip and make our way back to the hospital. But first, Mom had another idea to make me smile. Steak 'n Shake was across the street, and she remembered that I had been craving what we jokingly called a bacon-freakin'-cheeseburger. So we stopped for a quick lunch, and then headed for KU. Mom called Mark on her cell, and he said he'd meet us there once he was off work.

This was where I had left my attitude of surrender... in the hospital. It's the way I had to work up the will to go through it. I knew I had to be admitted to live there for five or more days while receiving the chemo. And that's what had my emotions so messed up earlier. I had prepared my battle plan, and surrendered to it. Then someone behind a desk told me they didn't have a place for me and my emotions spun out of balance, because my plan was altered without my consent. But finally, I was in my battle station, my bed, my room, with my mom in her chair next to me, Mark sitting beside her, and both of them watching me play a video game on the TV while we waited for my doctors to come and see me.

Dr. Fleming came around 5:00 p.m. He said I looked remarkably better than when I first had come in. I could see in his face and hear in his voice that he meant it and was happy to see the difference. Mark, Mom, and I all felt very happy about that report as well. It made me feel a lot better about being there again, ready for another round to kick cancer's ass. Mom had already hung my inspirational football photo on the wall at the foot of my bed, just below the TV, so I would see it often.

Dr. Fleming commented about the picture, and we talked a little about the game and my high school career in football. We were fans of rival college teams, and we had a few laughs razzing each other about it. It was nice to have that friendly sort of conversation, joking with one another.

He asked how I had been feeling, and I told him of all the things that had become normal for me, like the fatigue, nausea, constipation, hair loss, and growing depression. He said he'd prescribe for me something for depression. He also said I would have another MRI on my head during my stay, and according to all reports from the Cancer Center, everything was good to go with me to start my second round of chemotherapy that evening.

Mark's brother stopped by after he got off work, and we had some laughs with the video games, and he and Mark left for home around 9:30. It was getting on time for me to take all my pre-meds and pre-hydration before the chemotherapy got started, and I could feel the anxiety building up in my gut. Mom prepared her chair-bed next to me, and we both settled into the evening routine, flipping through the channels on TV, and talking about this and that.

The evening-into-morning dosing of chemo went pretty smoothly, and we were both awake early. Mom tried to time her cafeteria visit with my breakfast delivery time, but the food cart had still not arrived when she got back with her box of breakfast. It smelled good to me, and she had picked up a couple of extra pieces of bacon in case I wanted any. I was munching on one when my breakfast came in, and I ate about half of that. I had a pancake, some eggs, and juice. It tasted pretty good, and didn't bother my stomach much, and I was really happy about that.

About ten that morning, a transport person came to take me for the MRI. Mom went to visit the hospital chapel while I was having that done. Dr. Fleming had been to see me in that time I was gone, but we met in the hallway on my way back to my room, and we visited a little right there. I was feeling okay, nothing new to complain about, just still very tired and nauseous. I did okay throughout the day and into the night chemo treatment, except for a constant nauseous feeling. I slept most of the time, although there were times I was jolted awake by a dream or hallucination.

"What was that?!" I would look at Mom with a startled expression.

"What was what?" she'd ask, looking back at me.

I'd look around me and slowly realize where we were, and that what I thought I saw and heard wasn't really there. I'd shake my head, frowning with the idea that I was fucked up. "Nothing..." I'd mumble.

Mom would squeeze my hand reassuringly, feeling very sad about my suffering state.

I would lay there looking at the ceiling, puzzled and pissed off at the nightmarish hallucinations, but eventually would drift off to sleep again.

Other times, I'd think I was awake and lying quietly with my eyes closed, only my eyes would suddenly open wide and look over at Mom with a concerned expression on my face. When she'd look back at me and squeeze my hand gently, I'd just keep looking at her, trying to figure out what the hell was going on. I could never describe to her exactly what had startled me, but it always seemed so real when I first opened my eyes.

On Friday morning, I didn't really have any appetite, but I managed to eat a little breakfast without throwing it back up. Dr. Fleming came around noon and told me that the MRI showed that the small lesion seen in my brain appeared to have grown slightly smaller, while the larger lesion looked a little larger. He said he would consult with Dr. Alvarez and Dr. Van Veldhuisen about these findings, and that I might have to start radiation on my brain. He wanted to make sure we understood that the oncology group was constantly reassessing the plan, its progress and decisions in order to stay ahead of the cancer growth.

I was feeling very bummed out by the news, and restless and tired at the same time. Mom offered to take me on a tour of the older parts of the hospital, to get me out of my room and moving around, seeing and thinking about other things. There was a small library with a few museum-quality medical devices on display at the other end of the hospital, and Mom had found a map of the hospital in the information book hanging on the wall in my room. It wasn't anything to get excited about, but I knew it would be good to look at something else besides the white walls, ceiling, and floors of my room. I decided I wanted to try walking there, and I asked Mom if she minded pushing an empty wheelchair in case I suddenly got too tired or too sick to walk farther. I pulled my blue jeans on, and slipped my feet into my sneakers while she went out into the hallway to ask for a wheelchair.

I unplugged my IV machine from the wall and wrapped the cord around the top to keep it out of the way. It had a two hour battery, and I knew we wouldn't be gone that long. I draped the IV lines over the machine to keep them loose and out from under the wheels. I used my IV pole as my staff on wheels, and we set off down the white corridors to the elevators. Once downstairs on the main level, we strolled past the cafeteria to the older buildings of the hospital. It was after the busy lunch hour, so the foot traffic around us wasn't too bad. It was easy to see where the new building ended and the old building started. The corridors were narrower in the older buildings, and the linoleum floor tiles were a beige color with muted white tones. Around almost every corner, the floor tiles changed, noting another addition to the hospital at one time or another. The main corridor walls were painted white with rust-colored indoor/outdoor carpeting from about mid-wall to the floor. The appearance of the walls also changed from corridor to corridor, some being built of white tile or beige ceramic brick, with doorways to offices and clinics for one specialty or another that stretched down both sides of the halls. We had to take an older elevator to the first level, and that older main corridor was lined with pictures of graduating nursing and med students dating all the way back to 1905.

The library was at the end of the very quiet and rarely traveled hallway, and its double glass and white painted wooden doors opened up to a spacious room that housed a few interesting pieces of old medical gadgets. We strolled around looking at the medical equipment and medicine cabinets, and books that were as old as the school itself. It was kind of interesting and fun, looking at all of the stuff and making jokes about some of the equipment. There was a white metal EKG machine that looked like something out of an old Sci-Fi movie, and a wooden Franklin Roosevelt-style wheelchair, both from the 1930s. And of all things, a wooden birthing chair from Germany, circa 1750. It resembled an old wood rocker, except with a U-shaped seat, like a toilet seat with no bowl underneath, and it looked pretty well used. Someone had tied a rope across it from one arm of the chair to the other to keep people from sitting in it, apparently.

"Why do they think they need to do that?" I looked at Mom. "Who would want to sit down in that thing!? That's gross!"

She laughed, scrunching her nose, and nodded her head agreeing with me.

The room was only about 20-by-40 feet, but after walking around in there for about 15 minutes I got very tired and pretty nauseous. I told Mom I suddenly didn't feel very well and I needed to lie down right away. I walked slowly over to a bench in the middle of the room, and lay myself down very carefully. I didn't want to move so fast that I'd make myself more nauseous and throw up in the library. Mom sat down next to me while I lay still, waiting for the nauseous feeling to pass so that I could move again. When I felt ready, she rolled the wheelchair over to me, and I moved slowly from the bench. She took the folded white cotton blanket from the back of the wheelchair to cover me after I sat down. She helped me adjust my IV machine beside me, then wheeled me slowly through the exit, down the main corridor of the old building into the newer, busier corridors and elevator that led us back upstairs to my room. Once I got settled in my bed, I slept for over an hour. I felt good to have gotten away from my room for a while, but that trip had wiped me out.

That afternoon around four o'clock, I was sitting up in bed talking to Mom when we heard a knock on my door. The door slowly opened and in walked Brent, a guy I worked construction with during one summer at Total Interiors, where Mark worked. He had come over from the office Christmas party just a couple miles down the road. He was carrying a brown paper grocery sack with a gift he'd brought for me. He smiled as he propped it on my bed, and sat down in the chair next to me to watch me look inside. He had bought three of those toy guns that shoot foam rings. I grinned back at him and thanked him for thinking of me, and he said he was hoping to help me still have some fun in the face of my circumstances. He said Mark was still at the office, but he'd be coming over soon, and I could tell when we looked at each other, we both had the same idea. Brent, Mom, and I loaded our guns with as many foam rings as they'd hold, then we aimed them at the door, as we visited and watched for Mark to enter the room. When he walked in, we pelted him with at least 30 foam rings. He started laughing and picking them up and throwing them back at us. We were laughing, and it was fun to forget where we were for a minute. But the "attack" wore me out pretty quickly. Mark and Brent picked up all the rings, and shot them around the room a little more, and I just sat and chuckled at them. It was a good visit. They talked about the party, and about the guys I knew from working there. They had some pretty funny stories. I was glad Brent stopped by. He definitely cheered me up.

After he left, I lay my bed back down to rest a little. Mom updated Mark with the news of my head. I listened, feeling heavy over the reality of my situation. Suddenly Mom's voice seemed to get muffled, and I had that feeling again that I was falling instantly into nothing, with only darkness below me. The room faded, my sight went blurry. All of what I thought was real was spinning around me as I kept falling and falling, and falling, and I called out to Mom and reached for her again. "Mom!... Mom!!"

She knew what to do the second she heard my voice and saw that frightened look on my face. She took my hands and asked Mark to gently press his palms on the bottom of my feet, to try to give me the sensation of standing on ground. She talked to me until I could focus on her face again...

"Okay... okay, Mom... okay... okay...." I said over and over, talking myself back into reality and concentrating on looking at her face and pulling myself toward her. I could feel the warmth of Mark's hands on my feet, and it seemed the episode ended a little faster than before. When I was sure it was over, I asked Mom to adjust my bed so I could sit up more. All that falling made me feel tired, hot, and irritable. After sitting still for a few minutes, I decided to take a shower while it was still kind of early, hoping to make myself feel better. I called the nurse to let her know, so she could come in and cover my port and IV in my arm to seal them watertight.

Washing my hair was one of the most depressing things I'd ever done. I could feel some of my hair just sliding off into my hands as I tried to shampoo it as gently as I could. I finished washing the rest of me, and when I reached for my towel, I looked down at the shower drain. It was covered with a solid circle of my hair. I didn't even want to rub the hand towel on my head to dry off. I just draped it over my splotchy haired head and put my t-shirt and shorts on. My self image was shrunken as I rolled my IV machine ahead of me and shuffled my way back to bed without looking up at Mark or Mom. I didn't even plug my IV machine in. Mom noticed the forlorn heaviness in my face, and she asked about it. I just looked up at her in disgust with the thought that she didn't know and I had to tell her. I turned away to hide myself in my pillow.

She came up to me and put her hand on my shoulder. "Ian... honey... what's wrong?" She was so concerned, but my sadness hurt so bad that I couldn't say what it was.

"Look in the drain," I said to her in monotone, as I stared at the space in front of me, turning my back to the world. I could feel the angry stiffness in my face, a disgusted, horrible pain of shame. I just lay there feeling miserable.

Mark was still and quiet in his chair while he watched her take the handful of hair from the bathroom to the trash by the sink.

Mom came and sat gently and slowly on my bed behind me.

She laid her head on my shoulder, and put her arm around me. She didn't say a word, but I could feel her loving me, and I could feel her sadness for me. I appreciated that she didn't try to talk me out of my feelings, she just let me feel sad, and she shared it with me.

"I want to shave it off..." I whispered after a few minutes of grieving.

"Okay..." Mom said quietly. "Whenever you're ready."

"I'll shave mine off, too." Mark smiled at me. "And I'd bet you Uncle Dale and Uncle Curt would do it."

I felt a little better with that suggestion and, as my dinner tray was being brought in, we started hatching plans for a head shaving party in the next week. Meanwhile, I still had my hats. And when Mom straightened my bed and fluffed my pillows each time I got out of bed, she also brushed off all the hair for me.

I was getting a little nauseous from the food in my stomach, and the knowledge of the upcoming chemotherapy treatment that night. Mark was getting hungry, so he headed to the cafeteria. Since it was Friday, he had planned to stay at the hospital with us. He had brought a clean change of clothes and would sleep in another chair-bed at my feet. Mom started pulling her blankets out for her evening bed-making ritual, and got some extra ones for Mark. She was getting tired, too, and halfway unfolded her chair-bed so she could stretch out. I had packed my favorite green striped Mexican woven blanket and feather pillow from home, so I slept on top of the turquoise cotton hospital blanket, and covered up with my own. I didn't like the cold feel of sheets. And having my own blanket and pillow was one of those little things that helped to make living in the hospital a little more bearable, like having a small piece of home with me. Mom went to the nurses' kitchen to get herself some cereal for dinner, and I turned on the TV, looking for some kind of comedy show. Eventually, the pre-meds came, and the chemotherapy was started, and the night was like all the rest, nightmares and all.

When morning came, I was still very sleepy. I had been getting text messages through the night, and so had eventually put my cell phone on silence mode. I just didn't have the energy for it. Dozens of people wanted to know how I was feeling, what it felt like to have cancer, what morphine and chemo felt like, whether chemo hurts—all kinds of questions. I was beginning to feel like a spectacle, a curiosity, even a stranger, to everyone. I eventually tried to avoid answering any list of questions that wasn't coming from a doctor or nurse.

Through the morning, I let the nurses and aides do their job, but I wasn't much up to any kind of conversation. I was resting with my eyes closed, and the room was quiet, just the way I liked it. I opened my eyes with a start, and looked over toward the door, then at Mom, "Who was that?" I asked, feeling very concerned about them.

Mom looked up at me, "Who?" she asked, surprised.

"Those people who were just here."

"What people?" she asked softly.

"Those people who were standing right there just now." I looked over to where I'd seen them, and pointed toward the door about five feet from my bed so she could see where I was talking about.

"Honey, no one was in here with us just now. You must have been dreaming."

"No, I thought I saw people standing there, they were looking at me and talking about me... they were all wearing those white coats."

She shook her head, "No...no one has been looking at you, honey, and no one has been standing here talking about you, I promise. There's been no one here since Dr. Fleming left. Not even a nurse."

I rolled my eyes and slammed my head back into my pillow. "Fuck!" I whispered. I was so sick of that hallucination bullshit. I hated feeling like I didn't know what was going on, or that I might be missing something because I'd been sleeping. I hated waking up feeling scared all the freaking time.

I looked over at her. "Mom? Will you promise to wake me up if anyone comes in my room? I don't care who it is, if I don't wake up, will you wake me? Please promise you'll wake me?"

"I promise, Ian. I promise I will wake you up if anyone comes in here to talk about you or look at you. I promise."

I knew I could trust Mom's promises. She never once made a promise to me she couldn't keep, and there were a couple I held her to, that I know were hard for her. But I trusted her more than anyone else in my life because of it. "Thank you, Mom." I squeezed her hand and closed my eyes again.

Those kinds of hallucinations happened several times a day, and eventually I just looked nervously around the room and over at Mom without saying anything. Each time I saw her face looking quietly back at me, I knew it had been a dream or hallucination. I would roll my eyes and shake my head at my seeming loss of sanity.

Each day was the same as all the rest, and I was so damned tired of it. I was too run down to do anything, too exhausted to even think or have conversation. The hair all over my hat and my pillow pissed me off. I was in a really foul mood, and I didn't want anyone to see me this way. Each day I asked the nurse for something to help me sleep, and I told Mom that I didn't want any visitors. I was embarrassed about my appearance, my mood, my pale and weak cancer body... I wanted to sleep the time away and hide from the world until it was time to go home again, and I didn't want anyone standing in my room, looking at me while I slept.

Several groups of my friends had come to visit me during that weekend, and Mom said that she hated having to tell each of them that I couldn't have any visitors at that time. She had visited with all of them a little in the hall outside my room to update them on my status, but was honoring my wishes to not let anyone see me in the state I was in. I thanked her each time she told me she'd had to do that. I could see that having to turn my friends away had made her feel bad.

I had one of those falling episodes again, during the day as I was lying quiet, trying to sleep. Mom had tried to get me to sit up in my bed that time, so I could feel more upright. She thought if we could hold each other, the feeling of falling might go away faster, but I had been too petrified to move my body, even though I tried. It was all I could do just to hold on to her hands, listen to her voice and keep looking at her eyes. I knew the episode would end eventually if I did those things. I couldn't risk making it worse by moving a part of me that felt like it was falling off the earth into nowhere. That episode seemed as if it hadn't lasted as long, though. When it was over, Mom suggested that maybe it would help if I kept the head of my bed elevated a little bit more. The doctors said these episodes might be caused by the cisplatin, one of my chemotherapy drugs. Cisplatin can cause hearing loss, and could cause vertigo. Mom thought maybe the hallucinations were caused by my own fear of losing control of things, the morphine, and all the scary things that were happening to me. I thought it was probably caused by all of those things. What was strange was that the more the hallucinations happened, the easier I could recognize when they were happening, and I knew that it was only a hallucination, but I couldn't pull or talk myself out of it. I could not just lie there and experience them, because they were too frightening, even though in my mind I was pretty sure it wasn't really happening. I knew logically I wasn't really falling, but I also knew I needed someone to hold on to until it was over. There was a part of me during the experience that was afraid it was real, and that if I didn't have someone there to hold on to, I might never stop falling.

My last dose of the second round of chemotherapy was on Sunday evening, and Monday morning I told my doctor that I was ready to go home. I couldn't take another day in the hospital. I didn't care about being without the nursing staff, or the IV drugs for pain. I just wanted to be home, where I could hopefully feel more like myself again.

We learned that I had to visit the Cancer Center on the following Friday for an epoetin injection. I also had to have a daily injection of neupogen for the next ten days, but Mom would give it to me at home. She was concerned about giving me the shots correctly, so that afternoon Margo brought in a fresh orange and a few syringes to help teach Mom how to do it. Margo was a very good teacher, thorough and patient. She first demonstrated the procedure for Mom, showing her where and how to hold the skin on the back side of my upper arm. Margo said that injecting a needle into a whole orange feels similar to injecting one into human flesh. I watched from my bed as she coached Mom's practice injections on the orange, until Mom felt comfortable with the feeling of it all. I felt better knowing that Mom was getting some education on the matter, too.

Dr. Alvarez and Dr. Van Veldhuisen each paid a visit to me before my discharge, and talked to me about the possibility of starting whole brain radiation soon. Dr. Van was disappointed that the regression of the lesions in my lungs was not at all what he had hoped to see at that point in my treatment, but the mass in my abdomen was not as easy to perceive with touch, which was a little bit of good news. But that mass was still causing pain sometimes, so I knew it was definitely still there.

Dr. Alvarez talked with us for a long time about my latest MRI results, and his consultations with Dr. Van Veldhuisen and Dr. Fleming concerning my cancer's response to the chemotherapy. Because my tumor markers decreased so much, Dr. Alvarez felt that this indicated a good response in the brain tumors, with the one showing a decrease in size. He said that because there was no shift in my normal brain tissues, the fact that the other lesion appeared to grow larger could have been an error in measurement and placement of measurement points, because there was a little more swelling on the latest exam. But he believed that even if the lesion had increased about two millimeters, there had still been a good response to treatment. He thought I should wait a couple of more weeks and complete the current second cycle of chemotherapy, then get another MRI at that time. Dr. Van agreed, but Dr. Fleming still thought I should start radiation right away. Mom and Mark let me say what I thought, then offered their own opinions. I decided to follow the plan that Dr. Alvarez had suggested. Truth is, the idea of radiating my brain scared me, and I hoped that the tumors would continue to shrink in the next two weeks. I was released to go home, but had to return to the Cancer Center on Wednesday for another bleomycin dose, and again one week later.

When we arrived home on Monday afternoon, my Siamese kitty started meowing at me the minute we walked into the house. He sometimes got on my nerves, but I missed him when I was living in the hospital. I was happy to see the cute, furry little guy, and I could tell he was glad to see me, too. I could see where he slept in my bed while I was away, and he liked to stay close to me for my first couple of days at home. This time upon returning home, I didn't have to go straight to my bed. I actually sat in the living room and felt like a member of the world. It was great to be able to do that, and so weird that I could appreciate stuff like that now... things that I used to take for granted, like sitting on a couch in my living room, petting my cat, and having a conversation.

Mark had a stack of bills on the kitchen counter, awaiting our attention. He brought mine in to me, with my checkbook. His thoughts were, get to it now, pay the bills while I was feeling okay, because nadir might get to me in a day or two, and I wouldn't feel like getting out of bed. I wanted to pay my bills myself, and it actually felt good to hold a pen and write checks, enter all the information in the register, seal the envelopes and write my return address. I was doing something real, something that could make me feel I was still living the life I had before cancer.

The people who cared about us had done amazing things to help us in my cancer fight. Mark's family had taken up a collection among themselves, and given him $200 mixed in with a big box of Hershey's hugs and kisses candy, as an early Christmas gift. Mark had brought it to the hospital and enjoyed watching Mom and me having fun digging through the candy to find the buried cash. Everyone at Total Interiors had collectively donated over $1,200 to help us with our finances. On top of that, each employee in the company was working one hour overtime every day, and that extra money was being deposited into an account that paid Mark's wages when he took time off to be with me. They started that system the day I first went into the hospital in November, and Mark's bosses had told him never to worry about money when he needed time off, because they had taken care of it. I knew there would never be a way for me to express how grateful I felt for their generosity and compassion. Because of those 40 or 50 people, Mark was able to be with me when I needed him most. And that meant the world to me.

The minister at our church had told Mom that people wanted to help, and suggested that she set up an account for me at a local bank, so people could donate money if they wanted to. Mom put the account in my name only, so that people would be able to go to the bank and just mention my name and the money would go to the correct account. People from all over the country were sending me encouraging cards and letters, praying for me, and having Catholic Masses said for me. I was so amazed and honored that people I didn't even know cared about me and wanted to help. Mom had a whole notebook page filled with lists of churches and people across the U.S., even Hawaii, who were praying for me.

The expenses added up all around us. Our prescription insurance was still denying most of my medicines after leaving the hospital, so the household emergency credit card was racking up quite a balance. Mom no longer had an income, and neither did I. But I still had my personal car payment, car insurance, cell phone bill, and credit card payments that needed to be made every month. I had been responsible for my personal bills since I was a senior in high school, and I'd always had enough money to keep everything paid on time, with help from Mark on the car insurance. Mark and Mom told me to just concentrate on getting through the cancer, and not to stress about money, but I worried about it anyway. My family stepped in and helped any way they could. Mark had been depositing some of his money into my personal bank account for me since November, so I could continue writing checks to keep up the payments on my debts. As a Christmas gift to me, my Aunt Denise offered to make my car payments for me until I was able to go back to work, and my grandma said she would pay off my credit card balance. A few of Mom's other family members sent money, too, which she put into my medical fund. Those were burdens lifted from Mark's shoulders, and mine. I called them, and we sent cards, but I don't know if they ever realized how thankful I was for what they did for me.

Lying in the hospital for the last week, I thought a lot about

Christmas, and how it was going to be very different from our traditional Christmases. Mom and I had talked about it, and she wanted to make our Christmas as joyful and normal as always, with lots of pretty wrapped presents, Christmas carols, cookies, and going to church Christmas eve, if I felt up to it. Still, it was depressing, knowing Christmas was coming, and I felt like hell. I had no spending money, and no energy or will to go shopping at all. I knew money was an issue for all of us, so there would be limited gift exchanging. And Mom hadn't even had the time to get out all the decorations that she usually put up to make our home so cheerful and festive at this time of year. Our house looked as if we weren't going to have a Christmas at all. Before, when I felt so sick in the hospital, I didn't care about Christmas, but now that it was getting closer and I was home feeling better, I found I still did have a little Christmas spirit in me.

I set my checkbook down next to me on the couch. "Hey Mom?" I looked at her. "Can we get a Christmas tree?"

She smiled. "Sure we can. Do you want a real one?"

We'd had some good times, shopping for a real tree together in past years. There was a Christmas tree farm not too far from our house where we could chop one down ourselves. I loved wandering through the hills and fields full of different fir trees, trying to find the perfect one waiting just for me. Mom let me choose the tree I thought was best, and then watched, and once even took pictures while I sawed on the trunk. I loved bringing it home and setting it up, a tall, bushy evergreen with lots of colored lights in front of our living room window.

I thought about all the work involved. I knew we had a fake tree in a box in the garage. I used to love putting that together when I was a little kid. But neither option gave me feelings of excitement. "Can we buy a new fake tree... something different?"

"We can do whatever you want, Ian." She looked at Mark to see if he agreed, and I looked at him, too.

He shrugged and shook his head slightly, "Makes no difference to me, whatever you guys want to do...you know that."

I smiled and looked back at Mom. "Can we buy some new

decorations, too? Some new stuff for the tree? Let's get all new stuff."

"Okay," she nodded. "Do you want to go shopping with me to pick out the tree yourself? We can go to K-mart, it's closest."

"Yeah..." I wondered if I had the energy to walk through a store. "Yeah... I'll go with you. Can we go now?"

Mom looked a little surprised. She shrugged slightly, "Sure."

The weather was about 45 degrees, and it was just about four o'clock in the afternoon. I was feeling pretty drained of energy, but I wanted to do something fun, something that would make me feel like there was more to my life than cancer.

The drive there took only about ten minutes, but even that wore me out a little. Mom and I walked through the automatic doors, grabbed a cart, and headed directly toward the seasonal section of the department store. There was a foot-high display island full of assembled Christmas trees of all styles, sizes, and colors. Mom and I walked a slow lap around the island, looking at each tree and sharing our comments. I had my eyes on an eight-foot-tall, solid white tree. I envisioned how it would look covered in white lights, with shiny red and bright green ball ornaments on it.

"I like that white one..." I pointed at it.

"Yeah, that's really pretty. I like it, too." she shared. "I never thought about having a white tree."

We looked at each other and nodded, "Yeah."

We strolled around, looking at the shelves of ornaments, then turned back to the trees. My energy level had been slowly depleting, as we stood looking at the overwhelming assortment of decorations. We circled the tree island again, and I told Mom I didn't think I could shop much longer. I shared with her my vision of the white tree with green and red balls on it, so she left me with our shopping cart near the tree while she walked over to the shelves to choose the balls, holding them up for my approval before carrying them over to our cart. I also picked out a new silver lighted treetop star, and she chose a new bright red tree skirt. She pulled the cart toward the boxes of unassembled trees, lifted the white model into our cart, and very slowly, we shuffled our way to the checkout, me holding on to the cart for stability. I was filled with the joy of getting a new Christmas tree and the celebration of Christmas swirled with disappointment and dread of what cancer and its treatments were doing to my body, and how it was going to have a serious effect on my holiday experience.

Once the tree was up and decorated, it looked exactly as I had envisioned it. It was bright white and sparkled with white lights, accented with the richly colored large ball ornaments, and the shining silver lighted star on top. It was a cool-looking tree, and very different from years past. This Christmas would be one like I had never had before. But having a new tree made me feel some kind of hope that it was all going to get better. Mom had pulled out a lot of our traditional decorations too, including the special ones she put in my room each year. I had a really cool tabletop fiber-optic lighted tree that glowed in the night with changing colors of red, green, blue, white, and purple. On my wall she hung a traditional deep green wreath with lots of gold ball ornaments and a deep red ribbon, and she even had some Christmas towels for my bathroom. Christmas might not be as much fun as before, but I would make the best of it.

During the week I was in the hospital, Mom had been arranging the head-shaving party for me. She had called a lot of my friends and asked them to pass the word that I was going to shave my head, and anyone who wanted to join me could get it done for free at this party. Mom had her hair done at Salon Par, a place she learned about back when Carrie and I were dating. Mom asked the owner if she would be willing to open the salon after hours for us. Veronica, the owner, not only offered to open her salon for the party, but she and two other hairstylists donated their time to shave anyone's head who was willing to do it. So the party was set for Wednesday at 7:00 p.m.

As it turned out, nadir set in on me and I felt like shit that night. I had just received the dose of bleomycin that afternoon, so I had some mild nausea and an overall horrible feeling. I was so exhausted, and definitely did not feel like socializing. But I for sure wanted what remained of my sparse hair completely removed from my head. I was looking forward to not having my hair falling out all over me and everything in my room. And I did want to be with my friends.

Mark bought ten large pizzas, and brought a cooler full of assorted sodas and bottled water. They set the pizzas and coolers in the back room, and someone brought the six chairs from the waiting area into the salon so we could gather for before and after group photos. I wanted to be the first one to be shaved, and I wanted Mom's hairstylist, Sheryl, to do the shaving. Everyone watched as she started at the base of my neck, and shaved upwards on the back of my scull, then took the patchy hair off of my forehead back and around my ears. I watched intently in the mirror as she worked, saying a silent and sad goodbye to my hair, my looks. Both Mark's brothers and his uncle turned up for the occasion, and shaved their heads bald to support me. My Uncle Dale's hair was at that time longer than Mom's, and I wanted to shave that off myself! Sheryl let me do the honors of getting him started, then she completed the process, while Veronica and Kim shaved the heads of several of my friends, including all the guys in the band. Several girls came to support us, and even some parents came to watch the shaving of hair. Mom's brother and his family drove almost an hour from their house, just to be there for us. Several people were taking pictures, and the whole salon was filled with voices, and the sound of electric razors, as the smell of pizza and hair products scented the air. When the floor was covered with hair and the razors stopped buzzing, there were 13 of us with shaven heads. Under better circumstances, something like that would have been kind of fun, but I felt like hell. And even though I appreciated the support probably more than anyone realized, I felt I wasn't very good at expressing my gratitude because I was so sick.

A friend of mine, Tina, didn't make it to the salon, but came by my house afterwards to visit. We had dated during the past summer and had some good times just hanging out. We shared some laughs and took some pictures of ourselves. It felt weird to see a photo of myself for the first time with a bald head.

A friend of ours called me later that night. He had been keeping in touch over the phone since I'd been diagnosed, and had stopped in to see me in the hospital during my second round of chemo. Matt was the husband of one of Mom's friends. He was one of those people who you just automatically get along with. He was an attorney, friendly, energetic, full of ideas, and it seemed as if he knew everyone in town. He was doing a radio show on a local station back in the summer, and I got to do several guest spots on his show so I could highlight my music and get some publicity. Matt was so great to me. He even found a way for me to have some studio time at the station to record some of my music for a demo CD. I often wondered if I would ever be able to repay him for all that he did for me.

Matt had told me that if I needed anything at all, to just call him. I had told him how bummed I was about Christmas, because I didn't feel I'd be able to give any gifts this year to the people I cared about, since I had little money and no energy to do the shopping anyway. He offered to do my Christmas shopping for me, if I wanted. At first, I didn't want to ask such a large favor of anyone, but in my rejuvenated Christmas spirit, I decided I very much wanted to be able to give gifts at least to my family and closest friends. I had hoped I could afford to buy for each of them. Matt was the only person I trusted to do this shopping for me. I asked him if he was still willing, even though Christmas was just days away. In the devoted way that he did things, I felt as if he rearranged his whole schedule to accommodate my request the following night. He devised a plan to call me from the shopping mall nearest my house, and I would read to him my list of people. I had no real notion of what to get anyone, but I gave him some general ideas. Matt was so great. He'd shop around a little, then call me with ideas of things he'd found that might be a good gift for one of the people on my list. He was actually very good at it, and in just a few hours and a few phone calls to check with me, he had bought a gift for everyone on my list. He even had them all wrapped when he brought them to my house. And when I tried to pay him, he refused my money. I don't know if he ever knew how grateful I was, not only for the money part of it, but for what he gave of himself and his time. I was in awe at his generosity and compassion for me. I hoped someday I could prove to be as good a friend.

I was still suffering in the state of nadir when Christmas eve and Christmas day arrived. I got dressed and tried my best to feel okay and be a part of things, but I didn't even feel like sitting up. My Grammy, Mark's mom, had sent over lots of presents to put under our tree, and it all looked very inviting and cheerful, but I really was too miserable to feel much joy. I lay on the couch near the tree and tried to help Mark hand out the gifts. Mom took some pictures, but I could barely smile, I felt so sick. But overall, I was glad that I could be a part of it, however weak I felt. And Mom and I prayed together for the only gift we truly wanted, for me to win this fight over cancer and live a healthy, happy life again.

It seemed as if nadir didn't last quite as long as the first time though, and by a day or two after Christmas I was starting to feel a little better. I didn't know if I was used to feeling lousy, or whether my body was adjusting better to the chemotherapy drugs. One thing that did mess with me, though, was a horrible, torturous pain in my gut that was as bad as when the cancer first started hurting me back in November. I groaned in loud yells, it hurt so bad. Mom called Dr. Van's nurse, who, after asking a few questions, determined that it was a serious case of constipation. She called in a prescription that Mom immediately filled and gave to me, but it still took a couple of days to get through it. After that, my time at home was a lot better than before. I could eat. I could sleep a little better. And I had no pain, anywhere, outside of an occasional headache. I was still taking my daily doses of morphine, and those were working great. Even the nausea wasn't as bad. I had written in my Cancer Mountain journal: "Treatment 2: A little smoother, still throwing up a lot, and can't poop! Tumor markers are down from 200,000 to 20,000....sweetness."

I felt good enough to get out of the house, so I went to the grocery store with Mom and Mark one day. Mom was so enthused about me feeling so good that she brought a camera to the store and asked Mark to take pictures of us doing funny things, like posing with our favorite foods as if we were in a commercial. She's weird like that. She had carried a camera in her purse ever since I could remember, so she could keep a record of the good times.

I started feeling so much better that I felt I could drive my car again. I went outside one day and sat inside it, and realized how much I missed it. I loved my car, a 2000 midnight blue ZX2, with silver graphics down the sides, tinted windows, a ground kit, and silver wheels. It had a great sound system, too, and I had painted parts of the dash and doors bright blue. Yeah, I had missed my car. I hadn't driven in over two months. I convinced Mom that I was okay to drive by taking her out one day to run errands. We drove all around the city, just so I could do it. We turned up the tunes and rolled the windows down just for the fun of feeling the breeze, even though it was chilly outside. We stopped in to see my boss at work, we went to lunch, and when we returned home, Mom agreed that time-released morphine tablets didn't seem to be reducing my response time, like alcohol would. So later on, I went out alone to get together with some friends. It wasn't as it used to be, although I tried to make it all feel normal. I found out I couldn't tolerate alcohol. It made me throw up and feel nasty afterwards. I later learned that was a side effect of one of the drugs I was taking. Most drugs say not to drink alcohol when you're taking them, but that one didn't need a warning. I just could not do it. My body wouldn't let me. I told Mom about that, thinking it might reassure her that I wouldn't be drinking when I went out, but she still worried about me like crazy. But she knew I needed to get out and be with my friends. She had to trust that everything would be all right. I had told her how much I missed being normal... living life, and she tried to be okay with me being on my own with so many drugs in my system.

I didn't go out a lot, but I tried to get together with my friends whenever I could. It never felt the same, though. I felt kind of alienated by my cancer experience. I felt different from everyone else now. I felt as if no one could relate to me anymore. It was weird. When people asked me what cancer felt like, I knew they wanted to understand, but the question made me feel so different, because there was no way I could make them understand how I felt. They'd never know unless they went through it themselves. I felt like there was this room full of people, normal people drinking, laughing, and having a good time... and then there's the guy with cancer... in his own world looking out at them.

I had started seeing a girl named Afton. I was amazed that any girl would take interest in a cancer case like me, but it was great that she did. She was hot, very pretty and very sweet. She didn't mind just sitting or lying in my room with me watching movies. She came to visit me three or four times a week when I didn't feel well enough to get out, and it was nice having her around. She didn't expect the time to be filled with conversation or anything at all. She was okay just hanging out with me, and I appreciated that more than she'll probably ever know.

They say relationships are the biggest part of a young person's life, but that is no comparison to the importance of a relationship between someone and a cancer patient. I was learning what true loneliness felt like, being in a cancer-filled body, full of 20 different drugs. And I deeply valued the few people who were willing to just sit beside me and be present with me hour after hour.

6

Cancer Shame

On Wednesday, I had an appointment to see Dr. Van Veldhuisen in the Cancer Center, have blood drawn for labs, and get a bleomycin dose if my blood count was okay. I dreaded the long days at the Cancer Center. I hated the way that just being there always made me feel worse than I did at home.

The University of Kansas Hospital was an ever-growing medical center. Entire wings, floors, and updates had been added since the building first opened at its present location as a medical school in the early 1920s. Every department in the hospital had its own personality, its own decor, with one exception. What smelled like a kind of sweet cinnamon cotton candy scented every corridor.

The Cancer Center was located near the main entrance to the hospital, though it also had its own outside entrance about ten yards south. The main waiting room was very large, with over 50 chairs and a couple of couches in it. For me, it was like the first holding chamber for those of us awaiting our torture. Yes, it was a center for curing cancer, not torturing people, but for me, there was no good feeling in being there. Cancer and cancer treatment felt like torture to me. Usually though, I had only to give my name at the desk, and they'd tell me to go right in.

My first stop was the lab. I knew the drill. Sit quietly in the chair while the nurse finds a vein to draw three or four vials of blood. I could never get used to having a needle jabbed in my arms, and knowing my blood was being sucked out of me. It made me feel weak and nauseous. Mom tried to keep a conversation going with me and that helped sometimes, but after the dozens of times I'd had to have it done, I decided to just lay my head back, close my eyes, and try to pretend I didn't know it was happening. It usually took less than ten minutes, and afterwards I felt a little dizzy, and depressed that I needed to have that done so often.

After my blood was sent to the lab, I had to go sit in the waiting room where Dr. Van Veldhuisen's office was, also inside the Cancer Center, but down the hall from the main waiting room. The Cancer Center as a whole was a pretty nice place, considering what it was. The nurses were always pleasant and friendly. But sitting in that waiting room for two hours waiting for the lab work on my blood to be finished and sent to the doctor, while surrounded with a dozen or more people suffering just like me was as bad as sitting in a hospital bed. I felt drained of all energy, nauseous with the smell of others around me, and once I sat down, I didn't even want to keep my eyes open to see my surroundings. No matter how well decorated it was, it was still a place especially for cancer patients, and being there painfully validated the fact that I was one of them. It was all too depressing. Most every time I went there, I threw up in the bathroom before taking my seat with Mom and Mark in the waiting room. My head pounded from heaving, my body ached, though limp with exhaustion. I did my best to get comfortable in a casual chair with stiff wooden arms. I used my coat for a blanket and Mark's shoulder for a pillow, and slept the time away until I heard the nurse call my name.

Slowly I rose out of my chair, gave my coat to Mom, and shuffled my way nauseously toward the door where the nurse stood waiting for me. The nausea was too strong, and the nearest trash can in the closest exam room was the best I could do. It was so damned tiring. But also embarrassing, throwing my guts up in a small wastebasket while the nurse and Mom and Mark waited. I sat down in the chair in the room, knowing there was more coming up. I felt so weak, crumpled, and disgusting. When I felt like the vomiting was over, I grabbed a few tissues from a box on a nearby table to wipe my mouth, and walked back to the nurse with my head low and eyes to the ground. The nurse tried to console me by telling me that people getting sick was a common sight around there, and assured me there was no need to feel embarrassed, but her words didn't sink in deep enough to get past my shame of having cancer in the first place. She asked me to step onto the scale to get my weight, then I sat in a nearby chair while she checked my vitals. I was down to 172 pounds. My jeans drooped off my hips, clumping in folds around my leather sneakers.

She ushered us down the hall and around the corner to room number 260, across from Dr. Van Veldhuisen's office. I took my place on the examination table, laying my head on the pillow while Mom covered me with my coat. My legs were so long that they hung off the table, so Mom pulled out a short extension at the base of it. It wasn't very comfortable, but it was better for me to be horizontal. She unfolded a blanket that had been set out, and draped it across my legs. There was a dispenser with foam hand sanitizer hanging next to every door in every room we visited in the hospital and in the Cancer Center. Mom always took a puff of foam onto her hand, and shared it with me to clean my hands from any germs we may have contacted on door knobs or surfaces. She and Mark sat in chairs next to me in the small room and waited with me, while I rested with my eyes closed. When Dr. Van entered the room, he smiled at me, and shook my hand as he quietly said hello. He always greeted me first, then greeted Mom and Mark with a handshake and a nod as well. He then turned his attention back to me, asked me how I was feeling, and listened intently to my answer. After I finished talking, he waited, and watched me for a good long moment, just looking at me in silence as if he was studying to see beyond my answers. I sometimes wondered what our spirits were busy doing during that silence. It wasn't that kind of uncomfortable, distant silence that people often have with those they don't know very well. It was a working silence, a connecting silence. Mom and Mark sat watching and waiting, hoping for good news. Dr. Van and I just looked at each other, and I pondered what he might be thinking. Maybe he had memorized all my numbers from my new labs and was organizing them with the rest of my data in his head. Maybe he was mentally sifting through my file for the most important facts to tell me. Or maybe he was really looking deeper, waiting to feel or see something else in me beside what I told him. Heck, maybe he was just thinking about his golf game, but only after that momentary silence would he start telling me what was on his mind. "All right..." he started. He examined me, listening to my lungs and my heart, and feeling around on my abdomen. He asked about the intensity of any side effects I was experiencing, and reminded us what symptoms to consider serious enough to call his nurse. He said my blood counts were still low, but high enough that I could receive the dose of bleomycin. He said the tumor markers were showing a positive response to the chemotherapy, and that was always good news. I'd be getting a chest x-ray during my next appointment with him in five days, to see the visual effects, if any. He waited a few moments, looking at each of us, silently waiting for questions or concerns, then he took a visible breath, "All right...." He gave me another look that seemed to say the same, confirmed my next appointment, nodded goodbye to us, and left the door open for us to leave after him.

I sat up and slid stiffly down off the table, and slowly shuffled my way out the door, down the hall of exam rooms, through the waiting room, and down the art-filled corridor to the other waiting room in the treatment area. Mark claimed three chairs for us, while Mom went to the desk to let them know I was there. I was feeling more nauseous with the thought of receiving the bleomycin dose. It was as if my body was trying to tell me, "No, I don't want that, it makes me feel sick." I headed to the bathroom near the treatment rooms, and as soon as I opened the door, my throat opened up and I started gagging. I had thought that I'd already thrown up everything in my stomach earlier, but more fluid came out of me. It tasted nasty as hell, and burned my sinuses. I flushed it away and grabbed some paper towels to wipe my mouth. I turned on the sink and splashed some water on my face, and took a little into my mouth to rinse out that foul taste. The taste of the water brought a grimace to my face, but it wet my throat, and that felt a little better. I pulled the collar of my t-shirt up to cover my nose and mouth, to guard me from smelling anything as I walked back to the waiting room. I wanted to lie down, but there was nowhere to stretch out. I sat down heavily, and leaned over and rested my head on Mom's shoulder. Mark reached his arm around Mom and laid his hand on my back and gave me a gentle rub.

"I can't take this, Mom. I'm so tired of throwing up." I could barely take a breath to speak, I was so exhausted.

"I'm so sorry, Ian..." she sounded very sad. She kissed my head, and spoke softly. "I have some peppermint candy, do you want one? It might help you feel a little bit better."

"Yeah, thanks Mom..."

She took the candy from the front pocket of her purse and aimed the open-ended package at me to take one.

"Will you take it out for me?... I'm too tired..."

She thumbed the piece of candy out of the wrapper and dropped it in my hand. It tasted a hell of a lot better than my breath, and helped to stave off my thirst.

"Hey," she spoke in a very quiet, soft tone, "Remember one time we went to California to visit Aunt Denise?"

She was trying to take my mind off of my misery. "You were 12." She nodded, "You were already taller than me, about five foot eight, I think. You and I went to Newport Beach one afternoon, and we were playing and body surfing in the waves, and you were chasing flocks of seagulls, just to see them fly away together..." she smiled, "You loved doing that..."

I just slouched there in my chair with my head on her shoulder, trying to let the memory float in.

"Do you want me to go on?" she paused to ask, knowing that I generally didn't want any conversation.

I gave her a weak nod of my head.

Mom continued to paint the memories for me, "... we walked over to the boardwalk, and we were playing all those games on the midway." She paused to remember... "We took the ferry over to Balboa Island, and walked around looking at all the cool bungalows there. There was a walking path, all the way around the island, trimmed with perfect green grass that spread only a few feet to the sand... and that sand was so soft, we took our sandals off and walked around in it for a while, and dug our feet into it. And on the ride back to the boardwalk, we were sitting on a bench... there was a pelican riding on the end of the ferry, and those two seagulls were flying around, pestering him... then he spread his long wings to scare them off, but they always came back...we were laughing at those birds, and you were so funny, Ian." I could hear in her voice, she was smiling.

"Yeah..." In my own head, I remembered making her laugh by saying funny things as if the birds were talking to one another.

"And when we got back to the boardwalk, we got into one of those photo booths and took pictures making funny faces together..." she paused, and smiled... "I still laugh when I look at those pictures."

I just kept listening, drifting deeper into the memory, as she spoke softly about our fun, "We got some blue and pink swirled cotton candy to share, and walked around while we ate it...talking, watching people... and we played more games in the arcade...didn't we? And you were on that one new video game where you stood up on that platform and had to balance on it while you were playing...and you had such a high score, so you kept playing, and a crowd of guys gathered around you to watch and cheer you on, because you had the highest score ever on that machine.... oh, that was so much fun... and the sun went down and all the carnival lights were on, and the place was getting so crowded with people, laughing and walking together."

I felt a weak smile as I recalled the night atmosphere and the excitement I had felt in the admiration and celebration of the other gamers watching me, and giving me high fives. "Yeah..." I was thinking how fun that memory was, but my body was too tired to speak the words out.

"Ian..." The nurse called my name from the doorway, snapping us out of the past.

Mom and Mark stood, and he offered his hand to help me up. Fear suddenly gripped my stomach, and my muscles all felt tense. I knew what was coming, and it was as if I could already feel the effects of poison running through my veins. I felt kind of shaky, a little from feeling cold, but also kind of a tremor as if my body on its own was feeling afraid. I'd been through it enough times that I knew the protocol. The worst part was having the nurse access my port, and then I could sleep through the rest. But my body knew the stuff was toxic, and physically remembered the side effects that would soon follow.

We trailed behind the nurse to the treatment room, and I set myself down slowly into the beige leather recliner. I pushed backward to pull up the footrest and lay still for a moment, watching the aide as she came with her cart to check my vitals. When she was finished, Mom noted all the information, then went to the nurses' station to ask for an extra pillow and two warmed blankets. I was still trembling a little. She unfolded the blankets and laid them over me, and the warmth felt soothing.

"Mom, could I please have a little water?... no... ice, just ice and a little bit of water..." My throat was so dry it felt like it was closing up on me. But I remembered the taste of the water in the bathroom. I didn't want to chance making myself throw up again. She retrieved the ice in a small Styrofoam cup, and set it on the small table attached to my recliner. Mark had adjusted a couple of chairs for them to sit with me, and hung our coats over the backs of the chairs. He sat watching all the goings on in our space.

The nurse soon came in and began to prepare the tray of items needed to access my port and start the IV. She covered her hands with plastic gloves, hung two bags on the IV pole, adjusted the lines on the IV unit, and opened the needle package. As she started to tear open the alcohol swab to clean the skin, I pulled my right arm out of my sleeve to lift up my t-shirt, so she could get to the port without stretching the collar. I asked her if she would please numb the port site before sticking me with that needle. The needle they use for chemotherapy is a lot bigger than those they use for a shot. The skin just under my collarbone was tender in that spot from my port being accessed so much in the last couple of months. She said she would, as she prepared the IV unit to first deliver my pre-chemo fluids. She left and brought back my pre-meds, which was acetaminophen and something for nausea, and rubbed an ointment called Emla cream on and around my port site. It felt very cold. She had to wait about a minute for the numbing sensation to take full effect, then sterilized the site. I could still feel the stick, but the initial puncture of my top skin wasn't quite as painful. She attached the bag of fluids I had to receive first, programmed the IV unit to calibrate the time and dosage, and reminded us, "It will be about a half an hour, then we'll get you started with the bleomycin, okay? Call me if you need anything at all," and she whisked out of the room.

Once I was able to lie back and close my eyes, Mark went for a walk to call other members of our family to tell them the news we learned from Dr. Van. Mark couldn't sit for hours the way Mom could. He had to get up and move from time to time. Mom settled into her chair next to me and just waited. That last hour and a half went by pretty fast for me, because the meds they gave me for nausea also helped me to sleep through it. The nurse flushed my port with saline solution and heparin, pulled the needle out, cleaned the punctured port site, covered it with a sterile bandage, and I was free to go home. Mark went to get the car from the garage and meet us outside the entrance. Mom and I walked slowly to the door and waited inside, watching through the glass doors until we saw him drive up.

There was something different about lying in the back seat, and lying with the front seat lowered back. Being horizontal in the back seat and moving sideways made me feel more sick than reclining backwards in the front seat and moving straight ahead. My equilibrium was very sensitive. Mom offered to sit in the back seat so I could recline in the front seat next to Mark. I couldn't tolerate the radio, and they both knew I preferred minimal conversation when I was feeling so bad, so it was a long quiet drive home for all of us. Once home, I just wanted to sleep as long as I could, and hoped I would feel better whenever I woke up. The coming weekend was all I had to try to catch up with friends and have some kind of a life besides cancer. I had already seen that I'd missed a few calls, but I was way too tired to try and call people back that night.

Friday was New Year's Eve, the last day of the year. Mom and I had an annual ritual of attending a special New Year's service at our church. It was my favorite service of the year. I was feeling mildly nauseous and generally tired, but I especially did not want to miss it this year. Mom was thrilled that I felt well enough to go. My doctors had said that church is a place where I could easily come in contact with various germs and viruses, so I asked Mom if we could sit in the balcony away from the rest of the congregation. It was just her, me, and the sound man up there. I liked having the space around me.

During the service, we affirmed as a congregation that we are made new in Christ, that the old had passed away and the new had come. We wrote down all the things we wanted to be forgiven for, and people we wanted to forgive. Mom and I shared our lists with each other, and as it turned out, they had many similarities. Then as a congregation, we prayed about it, and filed outside to put the list into a large fire and watched it pass away, as if the smoke was taking our prayers to God. Mom and I waited to be the last ones, so I would be less likely to come in contact with any germs or viruses. When we and the rest of the congregation had returned to our seats, we each wrote a list of our own goals for the coming year, ways to become better people, positive things to accomplish in our life. At the top of my list: "Being 100% back to normal and cancer free." My list was a long one, and my intentions were solid. Mom and I shared our lists of goals before folding them up, and I wrote a note on the outside of mine, asking myself, "How good have you been?" As a congregation, we each put our list of intentions for the coming year into a self-addressed envelope, and placed them all in a prayer box where they would remain in a special space to be prayed over every day for the next 11 months. The envelopes would be mailed to us at the end of the year, so we could check our year's accomplishments against the list we'd made. At the end of the church service, we prayed for each other, and for ourselves, and affirmed again that we are made new in Christ. Our minister was surprised to see me after the service, and amazed that a young man of 19 years, sick with cancer, would spend his New Year's Eve in church. I figured what good was my faith if I didn't put it into action? Mom and I drove home talking about how wonderful it was going to feel in achieving my main goal, and how important it was to keep praying, and visualizing myself in perfect health. We were feeling certain, strong, and full of faith that God was supporting our intentions.

A friend was having a New Year's Eve party that night. It was a great chance to see a lot of my friends, and be a part of the world that I lived in before cancer. I went with a girl I dated for a little while the summer before, named Jess. It was good to get out, and I tried not to let it show when I started feeling like shit after a while. I was feeling a lot of pain in my stomach and my back, and the extra oxycodone I took with me wasn't enough. Jess had an old prescription of liquid oxycodone, about half a bottle, and she gave it to me. I took about half of it and saved the rest for later, but it didn't get rid of all the pain. It was embarrassing that I couldn't keep up with my friends anymore. The party was fun, but I couldn't laugh and tell stories like I used to. I was so very different from who I used to be. I wasn't the same guy at all, at least from my point of view. I felt like cancer had segregated me, singled me out, and no one could see it but me. But it was still good to be able to ring in the New Year with my friends, everyone raising a toast to share hopes and best wishes for my full recovery.

Mom hated letting me go out, but I had made a promise to her that I would send her a text message every few hours to let her know I was doing okay. At first it bothered me that she worried so much, but I was grateful to her for all she was doing for me, so I eventually came to realize it was the least I could do for her. Of course, I didn't tell her about the extra pain reliever I had at the party, but she found out about it months later. If she had known about that at the time, she certainly would have had more to say about my going out. She had already told me her fears of my getting a possible overdose if I was out with friends and not paying attention or forgetting how much I had already taken. She was also more worried than I was at the possibility that I might come in contact with a cold or flu virus. I knew my white blood cell count was okay, and I didn't want to be concerned about germs. I just wanted to be with my friends. But I assured Mom that I would stay away from anyone who was sick.

As the weekend progressed, I steadily felt worse, more nauseous, more fatigued. I slept through football games during the day, waking up once in a while to ask Mark what I'd missed, and I flipped through the channels on TV through the night. Mom tried to stay awake with me, but usually fell asleep in my room around midnight.

I had a followup appointment with Dr. Van on Monday. I was glad I wouldn't be receiving a dose of bleomycin, and I was looking forward to getting the chest x-ray and having a look at the lesion situation in my lungs. As usual, though, the drive to KU wore me down, and arriving at the hospital still caused a sickening feeling in my stomach. I did feel well enough to walk from the parking garage to the Cancer Center with Mom, though, and that was a pretty good measure of accomplishment. She parked as close as she could get to the stairway, and when I got out of the car and smelled the cement-enclosed damp scent of car exhaust in the air, it didn't even make me gag. We walked at what felt to me like a pretty reasonable pace, and I didn't feel completely drained as we descended the stairwell and walked across the catwalk into the hospital. As we approached the door to the Cancer Center, I turned to Mom with a prayer in my head. "God, please let the x-rays show that the cancer in my lungs is going away," I said to her.

"Yes! Let's hope!" she said as she rubbed her hand along my arm. She opened the door for me so I would be less likely to contact any germs from the doorknob. The main waiting room was pretty full of people. We walked up to the desk and the woman there recognized us.

"Hi, Ian," she said, smiling and handing me the forms to take with me to the lab. "You can go on back."

We walked to the lab and Mom sat in the small open waiting room in the lab. She was about eight feet from me, and I saw her rubbing sanitizer on her hands. The nurse greeted me and made some small talk. I joked with her that I didn't think I would ever get to a point where I was comfortable with getting blood drawn. She chuckled that some people do, and some people never do, as she prepared her items and gloved her hands. I concentrated my attention on looking only at Mom as the nurse strapped my upper arm, sterilized the site, stabbed my vein, and drew four vials of blood. Mom kept her gaze on me, too. She knew what I was doing. I was putting myself eight feet away from where I was actually seated, escaping the uncomfortable reality that I was so tired of experiencing.

We walked side by side down the corridor toward Dr. Van's office, sharing comments on the artwork as we continued past the pictures hanging on the wall. We both had the same favorite, a 20-by-24 framed print of an evergreen forest. It offered a feeling of comfort, a promise of a better place, peaceful and fun. The cinnamon cotton candy scent grew stronger as we passed the treatment area waiting room. We both glanced into the waiting room as we passed the large black framed panel of windows that lined the room from door to door. There were a few sorry-looking people, sitting and waiting. I knew their pain. I was glad I wouldn't be joining them on this day. The next double doorway was the entrance to the exam office waiting room. We checked in at the desk, and Mom followed me as I chose our seats. The place was mostly empty, to my satisfaction. Mom asked me if there was anything I wanted to make sure to ask or tell Dr. Van, and I couldn't think of anything. She always wrote our questions down in her notebook that she carried with her everywhere. We affirmed our hopes for good news, then I told her I wanted to just rest for a while. I suddenly felt a rush of tiredness. I rolled my coat up and made a pillow to place behind my head, laid back a bit, and closed my eyes to wait. We knew it would be a long while before the results from my blood work were finished and sent to Dr. Van.

After about half an hour, a nurse walked up to us and told us they were ready for us to go over to the x-ray lab. Neither Mom nor I could remember how to get there, so the nurse offered to escort us. I got up kind of slow and stiff, and Mom followed behind me, trailing the nurse out the double doors to the left, then down the corridor to a door on the right, around a corner to another tiny waiting room with sliding glass doors. She told Mom and me to wait there and the x-ray therapist would be with us soon. She reminded me to take my jewelry off, so as usual, I removed my earring and gold necklace and gave them to Mom for safe keeping. Mom was still nervous about my upcoming x-ray, and asked if I minded if she went with me as far as she was allowed. The idea of radiation going through my cancer-scarred lungs scared her. When the x-ray therapist came to take me in, Mom asked her where the x-ray room was. It was a couple hundred feet down the hall. The therapist said there was another waiting room nearby, so Mom could wait in that one if she wanted. Mom carried my coat, walking behind me in the narrow hallway as I followed the therapist to the x-ray room. I looked back and reached for Mom's hand before going in.

"I love you," she said quietly.

"Love you, too," I whispered quickly. I entered the room and the therapist closed the heavy door. I was in there for about 20 minutes, while the therapist x-rayed me on all four sides. When I came out of the room, Mom was standing in the doorway of the waiting room across the hall, watching for the door of the x-ray room to open. Her face relaxed with a smile of relief when she saw me. She was kind of cute, being scared for me and of something like a simple x-ray, and I told her that. She wasn't afraid to show her fear when she knew I wasn't afraid, and x-rays didn't bother me at all. It was actually the entirety of my cancer situation that caused her fear, though she tried not to let me see it most of the time. When she knew I was scared, she stood strong for me, and pushed her fear to the ground.

We wandered our way back to the exam waiting room, and checked back in at the desk. We would be waiting, and waiting some more, for the x-ray report, images and lab report to be sent to Dr. Van. I was starting to feel hungry. A sign posted near the desk clearly stated, no food allowed. I didn't want to risk missing my chance to see Dr. Van if they called my name, so I asked the nurse at the desk if it would be safe for me to take a short trip to the cafeteria. She said it would be about an hour before I would be seen.

It was past the lunch hour, so there wasn't much fresh food available in the cafeteria. We settled on two orders of french fries from under the heat lamp, and a couple of half pints of skim milk. Mom paid at the cashier, and we went to find a table. The entire outer wall of the cafeteria seating area was built of floor-to-ceiling windows. It came with a view of a couple of small, bare trees in the middle of a small snowy hill, lined with flowerbeds of now dormant canna plants. Several picnic tables sat in the cold shade of the building on an outdoor patio off to one side, and just across from the small space of nature was a four story brick wing of the hospital. Inside the cafeteria, the windows were lined with large booths, and the center of the room was crowded with tables and chairs on a multicolored carpet. White painted support beams crisscrossed from end to end below the high ceiling. There were only about ten people in the place. We sat in a booth near the snow-covered hill, eating our salt and peppered fries, talking about life and how we were both feeling as if KU was becoming like another home to us.

Mom kept watch on the time, and after about 30 minutes, we headed back to the Cancer Center. There was an entrance from inside the hospital also, so we didn't have to walk all the way through the main hospital lobby and main waiting room of the Cancer Center. The back door, as we called it, was at the end of the main corridor in the Cancer Center, just about a hundred feet from Dr. Van's waiting room. We settled in and waited about an hour, then the nurse called me in for the routine weighing and vitals check before leading us down the hall to room 260. I was pleased to learn that I had gained weight. I was now at a full 176 pounds. Still fifteen pounds too skinny, but at least my pants fit a little better.

Dr. Van asked me the usual questions, and I didn't have anything bad to report, other than mild nausea and fatigue. I told him that I'd been feeling better than before, I was getting around pretty good, and had just had some food. He said my lungs sounded clear, my heart was strong, my abdomen sounded fine, and overall, it looked like my health was improving. He talked about the report from my x-ray, and explained that even though the lesions seen in my lungs were still too numerous to count, the findings were that they did appear to have decreased in size and number from my previous examination. It was the news I'd prayed for. The cancer appeared to be going away, although not as much as I had pictured in my mind. We talked about my next course of chemotherapy starting on Wednesday, when I would again be admitted into the hospital. Mom and I left feeling happy about the x-ray results, but also sharing the looming fear that it was not over. On the way to the car, we talked about staying on it, about my efforts to keep eating healthful foods, and doing my best to get some exercise every day. Mom said she would do her best to help me stay on the right track. We took the stairs instead of the elevator, to get to the third floor of the parking garage. It was a slow climb, but exercise that I needed.

During the drive home, I turned the radio on and switched through the stations. I came upon a favorite song of mine, by a band named Dashboard Confessional, and Mom and I sang in harmony to the chorus. It was good to feel like singing again. When the song was over, I turned the radio off and told Mom about some guitar chords that had been going around in my head while we had been waiting at the Cancer Center. I hummed them out for her, in the rhythm that was sounding in my mind, as I strummed my air guitar. It was a new song forming, and I wanted to get home and work it out on my twelve string. It had been a long time since I'd had the energy to do that.

I was excited to tell Mook about the news of my x-ray. He was home when we arrived, and I went straight upstairs to find him in the kitchen. He smiled and gave me a huge hug and a heavy pat on the back. We all sat down in the living room and Mom and I filled him in on the events of the day. Then I retreated to my room to put those chords together on my guitar.

Playing my guitar and writing songs was one of my favorite things to do. I could sit and play for hours, all by myself. Mom loved sitting and just watching me play or create new songs. She told me she could see by the concentrated expression on my face and the distant look in my eyes, that I was hearing a chord and a rhythm in my head. And she loved watching me try to find it on the guitar. Sometimes I couldn't find it, right off, exactly what I was hearing, so I'd sit and listen in my mind, then search for it on the guitar... sit and listen again, then search on my guitar again. Once I found what I was looking for, I listened for the next chord in my mind, and repeated my process until I found the second chord, then I played them both together, then listened for the third chord in my head to find it on my guitar, and so on. Sometimes, within 15 minutes, Mom had watched me create a whole song. She was both tickled and amazed at my ability to do that, and she said that watching me compose like that gave her great joy. I liked having the admiration, and of course she was my most devoted fan, but when I wanted to practice singing, I wanted to do that alone. When I was pleased with my final cut of a song, vocals and all, Mom was the first person I wanted to hear it. I'd call to her from my room, and she'd come thumping down the stairs. She got such a happy smile on her face once she'd entered my room and saw me sitting on my bed holding my guitar.

I couldn't help but smile back at her, feeling pride at what I was about to share with her. "Hey Mom, I got something to show you..." I'd always tried to keep my smile humble, but I knew Mom would be proud, and I was always excited to present a new song. She would sit down just about three feet in front of me, usually off to one side on the floor.

"I just finished it..." I'd start. "I'm not sure yet if I'm gonna keep the middle eight the way it is, but tell me what you think..." I'd take a moment, looking at my fret board, to put myself in the mood of the song. I'd start playing, and Mom sat watching...then I'd stop. "And tell me what you think of the chorus, if it sounds too familiar..."

"Okay," Mom would say, smiling and nodding with anticipation. She would sit attentively while I started. Her face always looked so proud as she watched me. Usually, after about the fifth bar, she'd close her eyes, so her ears could hear better, she had once said. I played, and she sat very still, absorbing my voice and the chords, and I could feel her loving my song.

At the end of the song, her eyes were usually tearful, and she had a very proud smile on her face. And when I asked her what she thought, I meant it. If she loved it, she truly loved it just the way it was. She was always honest if she thought a chord or note would sound a little better another way. She wasn't a musician herself, but she did have a good ear for it. I always valued her opinion, and usually took her advice, on music anyway.

She asked me once, how do I go about writing a new song. "Do the words come to you first? Or do you get a melody in your head, and then try to find words to fit it... or do you just come up with it all together?"

I told her it was all of those, but only one at a time. Sometimes, a mood I was in would cause me to think about stuff, and the feelings I was experiencing in that point in my life. Then while I was thinking, I'd notice that the words in my head had a rhyme or rhythm. When that happened, I wrote the words down, and tried to work it out to make a song out of them, then come up with a melody to fit it.

Then other times, I heard chords in my head, and the more I thought about them, they started forming themselves into a melody. Then I either wrote down the chord progression or picked up my guitar and played with it until I liked the way it sounded.

Then there were other times when it all seemed to come together at once. The words in my head already had a rhythm and a sound at the same time. "Something To Remember" was one of those songs. I felt so happy in love with Carrie, that song just came right out of me.

Well, the chords that had been going around in my head that day didn't form into a song as easily as songs did before cancer. I grew a little depressed that my mind didn't function as well, and my creativity had been stifled due to the chemotherapy and all the other drugs in my system in the past two months. I did write the chords down though, and it would still be a song, eventually. Mom came down to listen to me play after I'd had a while to play alone, but I could only play a few minutes longer. I didn't feel like playing old songs. I had been in the mood to write one, but it wasn't happening, so I just shared the chords and thoughts with her about the forming song, then had to put my guitar away for a while. Playing it made me so sad that my creativity was fading, and that I didn't have the energy to keep playing like I used to.

On Tuesday night, Mom had all my favorite comfortable clothes washed and packed into my duffle bag, ready for the hospital. She made sure all my toiletries were in a Ziploc bag on the vanity in my bathroom, so I could add them to the duffle after using them before we left for the hospital. I couldn't sleep that night, dreading the next day. There was that feeling that if I didn't fall asleep, morning wouldn't come. But, when it did, I was exhausted from staying awake until three that morning. Mom made a sandwich for me of peanut butter and honey on toast with a tall glass of cold milk. It felt good to have been able to eat for the last few days. I was going to miss that feeling in the next couple weeks. While I was eating, she loaded the car with our luggage, my feather pillow and green striped Mexican blanket, and the green throw pillow in case I wanted to rest my head against the window in the car.

In those times when I wasn't feeling so well, I preferred to take the smooth ride of the highway all the way to the hospital. All the stopping and going, bumping and turning of city driving made me feel so nervous and nauseous. But the highway seemed to take longer, so I asked her if we could take the city route to the hospital. That meant taking the highway half way, then jumping off to a straight shot down 39th street to KU. I thought it was a shorter drive, even though we had to travel a good five miles through the inner city, and some not so savory parts of town. As we drove through what was known as the Hyde Park area, we passed near the three story house of one of my friends from Longan elementary school, Eric. Mom and I both thought about him and his family every time we drove past their street. Eric's father had been fighting another kind of cancer a few years ago, called non-Hodgkins lymphoma. Mom and I hadn't known until a year later that he had passed away. Now with all my travels back and forth to KU, we thought of him at least once a week.

Arriving at KU was a little like arriving at a busy airport sometimes. Mom dropped me off at the main entrance with our luggage, then drove away to park the car in the garage and walk back to meet me. The place was bustling with people coming and going, and some waiting in wheelchairs along the inside of the hospital entrance. There was always a porter standing outside to assist the many arriving and departing travelers. He hauled our bags into the entrance of the main lobby for me, and went back to his work while I waited there for Mom.

When she came in, she piled my duffle on top of her rolling luggage, and we walked together toward the admitting office.

After about 30 minutes' wait, the admitting rep said she didn't think they would have a room available for me until later that afternoon. I just rolled my eyes and looked at Mom.

"Oh, my God," I muttered. I slumped into my chair and laid my head back against the wall. We just sat there. Mom was patient and tolerant, and I felt totally impatient, uncomfortable, restless, and irritable.

"What time is it?" I asked, without even opening my eyes.

"Almost noon," she said quietly.

I heaved a heavy sigh, "Can we go somewhere?"

"Sure we can," she nodded, looking over at me.

I opened my eyes and stared upward with glazed eyes. "Where can we go that's not too far away... I don't feel like driving all the way home. Is there somewhere we can go and just sit, just so we can be somewhere else but here?"

We talked over the possibilities. We had to go somewhere indoors, because the weather was too cold and damp to sit outside. There were no shopping malls in that part of the city, and restaurants tend to frown on you if you just go in and sit down without paying for something.

"Are you hungry at all? We could go get some lunch, and kind of hang out there for a while." She offered. "How about Winstead's? It's not too far away."

I pictured it in my head. My friends and I had been there a few times. A nice, old fashioned burger and fries, soda fountain kind of place. "Yeah, let's go there." I sat up.

Mom arranged with the admitting rep to store our belongings inside her office while we went for lunch, and the rep offered to call Mom's cell phone when a room was ready for me. I shuffled alongside Mom as she walked to keep a slow pace with me, through the bustling lobby, up one floor to the catwalk, across the street to the parking garage, then up two more levels and around the corner to our car. I felt exhausted as I fell into the car and closed the door, and laid the green pillow against the window to rest my head while Mom drove.

By the time we arrived at Winstead's, I actually did have an appetite. We had a good lunch, and sat talking, sharing memories and thoughts about one thing and another. We were there for about an hour and a half, but the admitting rep hadn't called. We opted to go out to the car and try to think of somewhere else to go. The sun had come out, and when we got inside the car, it was nice and warm. We sat there for a minute, but neither one of us could think of anywhere else we could go.

"Actually, Mom, you know, I'm getting kind of sleepy." My eyes felt droopy.

"Yeah, me too," she said. "The warm car is making me feel like a nap," she smiled.

"Well, do you think we could just stay here in the parking lot and take a little snooze?" I thought it was a great idea.

She looked around. We were behind the restaurant, in a more remote parking spot, and there was a small tree right in front of our car, blocking us from view a little bit.

"Come on, Mom, I'm so tired... I just want to sleep for a minute."

She laughed as she thought about it, "Well, I guess we could lock the doors and take a little nap."

"Yeah, and you can set the alarm on your phone to wake us up in like 15 minutes, okay?" I laid my seat back, adjusted my travel pillow, and closed my eyes. "Okay, Mom." I had already made the decision. I was going to nap, no matter what she decided to do.

I heard the power door locks set, and she laid her seat back. She shifted to lie on her right side facing me, and with her arm curled up under her head, she closed her eyes.

It was about 20 minutes later when we both seemed to wake up at the same time. We looked at each other, then at the clock. Mom checked her phone for any missed calls.

"We should probably get back to the hospital," she said. "They didn't call, but it's past 2:30."

"Yep, okay," I stretched and set my seat up a little. I felt a little rejuvenated for the events ahead, and set my mind to just doing it.

When we arrived, there still was no room available yet for me, so again, we planted ourselves in the admissions waiting room chairs. Waiting there for nearly an hour became too much for me, having given me time to sink into the hospital experience again. I was feeling nauseous and sleepy, and I told Mom I needed to lie down. I left her sitting amidst the crowd of others, while I lay down on a cushioned bench near the windows of the office. I had plenty of time to take a nap, and Mom woke me when a room was finally ready for me up in Unit 42. Mom made a comment about how sad it was that a hospital cancer unit was completely full.

A transport assistant came for me with a wheelchair, and upstairs we went, riding on the main elevators as they squeaked softly toward our destination. The silver metal doors opened, and I could hear the thumping of Mom's luggage rolling along the textured black rubber elevator floor behind me, as the transport wheeled me out onto the familiar white tiled fourth floor. The cancer floor smelled of sweet cinnamon like the rest of the hospital, only with an added scent of what Mom and I thought smelled a little like Play-doh. We rounded the corner and saw the familiar bold overhead sign for the Bone Marrow Unit straight ahead. My room would be just around the next corner and down toward the back of the unit.

The transport first lowered the hospital bed for me, then held the wheelchair steady while I stood up. I thanked him as I sat down on the bed, he gave me a salute, then off he went, checking his radio for his next stop. I adjusted my bed so I could be sitting up when the nurse and aide came in. Mom called Mark to let him know what room I was in, and then began putting our belongings in place. She left the room and brought back an extra blanket and pillow for me, and some for her as well. When she was finished building our nest, she turned off the lights, shut the blinds, and drew all the curtains closed, just the way I liked it. That was it, we were officially moved in, and sat talking and waiting for the nurse and Dr. Fleming.

Mom had written down a few questions she wanted to ask Dr. Fleming concerning how much morphine I was taking, what he thought of the latest x-ray results, and when I would have another MRI on my head. And I was looking forward to learning what my current tumor markers were showing.

Mark had been able to leave work a few minutes early, and was in the room with us when Dr. Fleming came with his entourage at 4:30 that afternoon. Dr. Fleming first greeted me, then Mark and Mom, and introduced us to the two new resident doctors, and the group of five student doctors standing behind them. He asked how I had been feeling the last couple of weeks, and I was glad to be able to tell him I'd been getting around better lately, and the nausea wasn't quite as bad. After our brief personal visit, he turned to the resident doctors and motioned for them to come stand near him. The crowd of students scuffed slightly closer and stared at me, the cancer specimen that I was, a 19-year-old in the critical care unit normally filled with elderly patients. They each leaned in to watch intently as he examined me. I sat obediently while he listened to my heart, lungs, and abdomen with his stethoscope. I laid quietly while he pressed gently, lightly tapping his fingers on different points in my abdomen, feeling around my lymph nodes, pushing inward to feel around on my internal organs, and I told him when a particular spot was painful. Once or twice during the exam he would turn from me and look at the students, telling them exactly what to write in their notes about cancer patients, or treatment observations as they scribbled frantically to keep pace with his thoughts. Once he was finished, he turned his complete attention to me, as the rest stood waiting. He told me I would be getting an MRI done soon, to check the lesions in my brain. He said my complete blood count was slightly low, and my white blood cell count was even lower, but I would still be able to start chemotherapy. The tumor markers were not as low as he'd like them to be, but still showing a response to treatment, as the beta hCG was holding at around 26,000. He shook my hand, gave me a couple pats on my now bony right shin, and led his trail of white coats out of the room.

Mark headed to the cafeteria in hopes of getting ahead of the dinner crowd. Mom had placed her order with him, and he would bring their food back to my room. I felt pretty hungry, and liked the idea of all of us eating dinner together without any nausea to ruin things for me. My dinner arrived just as Mark got back with a tray of food. I had a bowl of chili, cheesy potatoes, and a bag of sliced apples. It smelled delicious, it looked yummy, and the taste wasn't too bad either. The potatoes were so good I ate all of them first. We were having some decent conversation over a decent dinner, but as I was half finished with my bowl of chili, my stomach started to have ideas. I put the bag of apples on my bed table and covered my tray of food. "Mom, can you please take this? I don't think I should eat anymore."

She looked sad for me as she picked up my tray of food and set it on the vanity across the room. I felt at the head of my bed for the TV remote, and flipped through the channels, looking for something funny to watch. My stomach churned. I was bummed that nausea had intruded on my perfect meal.

But apparently that discomfort wasn't enough to satisfy the cancer's torture on me, because a few minutes later, one of the resident doctors whom we'd just met came into the room and said she needed to check my scrotum. She said she wanted to check the incision site, and make sure everything had healed up well. That's all I needed. Another stranger poking and pulling around on my lonely one. Mom and Mark left the room, and took all our trays to the meal cart at the end of the unit near the service elevators. The doctor pulled the curtain closed and I had to pull off my shorts while she waited on the other side. I covered up with my shorts, and then told her I was ready. Humiliation and embarrassment sank heavy in my stomach as she pulled the plastic gloves on her hands, lifted my shorts and leaned over me. All I could do was lay there and watch her inspecting the site, lifting my poor separated twin and the empty loose skin that was shriveled up to it as if it was still grieving the loss of its package. Fortunately, she was very quick and business like. She said it all looked good, and off she went, leaving me to dress and lay alone to think about how awful it felt to have only one ball.

When they returned, Mark closed the door quietly behind them, and Mom immediately noticed the mood written on my face. I was quiet for a minute while they sat, waiting.

"Well, what did she say?" Mom finally broke the silence.

I looked over at her, "I want to get a fake one as soon as possible." I said without room for argument.

"Okay," Mom said, agreeably.

"Will you remind me to ask Dr. Fleming how soon I can get it done, and who do I need to talk to?" I asked.

"Of course." She looked at me with compassion, but I wasn't sure she really understood my reason.

"They'll probably want you to wait until you're done with treatment, when they know the cancer is gone," Mark offered.

"What ever, I don't care, just so long as I can get it done as soon as possible, that's all." I looked at them sternly. I was going to get it done, no matter what. "I hate the way it looks now, that loose skin just hanging off my good one.

"You'll get it done, Ian, okay? I promise, we'll make sure. But don't worry about it right now. We'll find out more about that when it's time." She waited a moment before asking again. "But what did the doctor say? Is everything okay?

"Yeah, it's all good."

She saw that I didn't want to talk about it. I laid my head back with a sigh, thinking to myself the same questions that I'd asked myself over and over... 'Why the hell hadn't any of my doctors told me about checking myself for testicular cancer through the years? Why didn't I know something was wrong? I could have avoided all of what I was dealing with now.'

The nausea was working on me. My stomach started to hurt, and I was feeling the urge to take a nice big dump. I asked them if they'd mind leaving the room for a while again, so I could poop in private. I got out of bed and unplugged my IV unit, sprinting with it to the bathroom. I was in there with the door closed before Mom and Mark could make it out of the room.

When they came walking back into the room, I was already lying in my bed. They both tried not to show any notice of the smell, but I had to smile at them. I was expecting a reaction due to the serious stench. They both broke into a big smile when they saw me smiling.

"Damn, brother! That's ripe!" Mark joked.

Mom covered her smile and her nose with the collar of her sweater. "Feel better?" she asked, squinting.

"Yeah. A lot better. Thanks for the privacy."

As they sat down, I was still smiling at them. "You wanna hear something funny? When I was in there, I heard the door open, and I thought it was you guys, but nobody said anything... so I said hello, and that one guy, that resident doctor, said he just stopped in to see me and he'd be back later... then I couldn't help it, I just had to rip a loud one, and it echoed in the toilet and in that little bathroom..."

I paused to laugh at the thought of the situation... "and all of a sudden I heard the door close really fast..." I chuckled again.

They both chuckled with me, and Mom asked if I was going to be embarrassed when that doctor came back in.

"Naww! Are you kidding?" Mark looked at her.

I shook my head, "No, no..."

"That's like a badge of honor!" Mark teased. "A guy's proud of a good stink... even with strangers!" He laughed.

Mom just smiled at us. It was good to feel like laughing, a stress relief valve for all of us.

There was nothing on TV, so Mom went to the nurses' desk to ask if the movie cart and VCR were available. They had several donated movies to choose from. She wheeled it back to my room, Mark hooked it up, and we watched Beverly Hills Cop until it was time for Mark to go home. Mom and I started another movie, but I had taken my premeds about 8:30 and was starting to get sleepy, so I missed most of it.

Carol was my night nurse, so she was the one controlling my chemo regimen... running the IV lines, using a little blue clip to pinch them in the precise spot to slow or speed up the drip, programming the IV machine, changing out my different IV bags, watching the timing and checking on the dosage process through the five-hour treatment. I knew the night would be all right, with her taking care of me. Not that other nurses didn't take care of me, but I have to admit that I did have my five or six favorites, and I always asked the aide which nurses were working each day, and if they knew who all my nurses were for the second and third shifts. My favorites all knew who they were, as I had told each of them at one point or another. And over the hours and days I'd spent with nearly two dozen nurses in Unit 42 in the last month and a half, I'd asked each one of my favorites if they would please be my nurse whenever I was in the hospital on their shift. It meant that much to me. One of the nurses once told me that sometimes a few would try and rush to take my room on their shift when they learned I would be there, before another nurse could have me. I guess in relation to a lot of the elderly patients in that unit, I was pretty easy going. That, and no one had to change a diaper on me.

I was always grateful when I learned that one of my favorite nurses had made sure to be the one to care for me. It made my days and nights in the hospital so much more bearable, having a nurse with a cool personality, compassionate, and nice to talk to, like a friend. Some nurses just barged into the room, startling me out of my restful state, moving around the room hurriedly and noisily taking care of their tasks. As I'd mentioned before, I knew I was irritable and particular, but also all the more appreciative of the people who were calm, mellow, friendly, and nice to me, who took the extra time out of their busy nursing schedule to stand and quietly visit with me about my questions, my concerns, and to talk with me about general stuff, and joke around with me once in a while. I don't know if I ever thanked them enough, Margo, Mark, Tracy, Angela, Stacey, Janet, and Carol. I had too much opportunity to see how different nurses can affect the way I felt, about my illness, my situation, and about myself. Some nurses made it harder to cope with those things, but the others made all the difference in showing me that they genuinely cared about me, the person inside the cancer-filled body.

All this was not to take away from the incredible responsibility that every oncology nurse bears in a daily routine. I had great reverence for every nurse that accepted that obligation, educated to follow my prescribed treatment regimen, accessing my port and plugging me into the chemotherapy drugs in an effort to save my life. To those who dedicate themselves to the work, know that you do make a difference, even if some of your patients don't live long enough to thank you.

I had been sleeping after my chemo hook-up late that night, and Carol took care of things with hardly a peep. Just like Nurse Mark, she used a tiny little flashlight so she wouldn't need to turn on an overhead light, and when I woke while she was working, she whispered to me what she was doing, and I was able to drift back off to sleep with not much trouble at all.

The night was barely over when my morning nurse, Angela, came in at 5:30 to let me know I was scheduled for the MRI at 7:45. I mentioned to her about the last MRI that I had, when I had just started with the procedure and had to be pulled out to throw up. Angela said she would see if the doctor would approve something for nausea and anxiety. After she left my room, Mom looked at me with concern.

"Ian, you never told me that happened," she said, trying to be calm.

"It's no big deal," I said. "It wasn't worth talking about, it's just something that happened and I don't want it to happen again, that's all. I don't really want to think about it. It's too depressing."

"Okay," Mom said. She nodded that she understood and breathed a quiet sigh.

I closed my eyes, and she dropped the subject.

After a short while, Angela came with a pill for me to calm my anxiety and nausea. A transport came at 7:30 to give me a wheelchair ride to the radiation oncology department downstairs for the MRI. Mom waited for me in my room. I wouldn't be gone but 30 minutes, and I felt okay going on my own.

When I got back to my room, I was sleepy and kind of testy. The MRI procedure and the whole trip through the hospital and back, being wheeled onto elevators and down so many stretched corridors full of hustling doctors and other patients in wheelchairs had beat my spirits down. I just wanted to be left alone to sleep, but I didn't get that wish. The two resident doctors came in and wanted to check the lump in my left breast. I sighed as they both leaned over me, and I lifted my shirt. With gloved hands, they both felt around on me along my upper chest and all around the nipple. They looked and conferred with one another, and touched around on me some more. It made me feel disgusted...with the lump, with them, and with my own state of being. It hadn't decreased in size since I was diagnosed, but it wasn't that large, really. Mom said it wasn't even noticeable by looking at me, and I scolded her for looking. "No, don't look at it..." I covered my chest with my hand. I didn't want anyone looking at my cancerous parts. It was bad enough my doctors had to look. It was just too embarrassing. She apologized, and said she was just trying to help me feel better about it, and I shook my head, scoffing at the idea. She really couldn't understand how horrible I felt about my cancer body, and myself.

Dr. Fleming came in shortly after the residents left. One of them had expressed concern about the size of one of my lymph nodes in the previous exam. Dr. Fleming wanted to check for himself, and he found everything to be normal. He said I would have another pulmonary test that afternoon, and he would be in to see me again, once he had received the results of the MRI.

I asked Mom to get my jeans out of the closet. I didn't want to sit through that pulmonary test wearing shorts, it was too cold. I put on my shoes, and waited for my transportation. Mom asked if she could come with me, but I wanted to feel more independent, the way a guy my age should feel. I didn't want to need her, and if I could handle things on my own, I wanted to do that. She understood, but it didn't change her feelings of wanting to be with me anyway. But she stayed in my room and waited for me, making phone calls, straightening my bed, and tidying up while I was gone.

After I was finished with the pulmonary test, the therapist wheeled me to the waiting room next door, and I sat waiting for the transport to come and return me back to my room. I was feeling a bit impatient as I watched the clock for five minutes. The pulmonary therapist was with another patient, so I thought, to hell with this, I'm not waiting any longer...what the heck, I can roll myself back. After all, it's just a few hallways and a couple of elevators... I could remember my way once I got going, and the exercise would be good for me. I was just mad enough to do it. I positioned my IV unit between my legs and rested my feet on top of the wheel base. The heavy asterisk-shaped metal base had five wheels, so it was good and stable. I tested it to see if I could roll along that way, and it worked fine.

I rolled out into the hallway and looked both ways. I turned left and rolled toward the nearest corner, where I turned left again and saw the elevators about ten yards away. I rolled along, no problem. I read the sign at the elevator and figured I had to go down four floors to the main level. When the elevator doors opened, I wheeled myself in backwards, the way the transports did, so I'd be facing the door, and hit the main level button. I watched the numbered lights above me, as the elevator moved downward floor by floor. The motion took my nausea up a notch, and I swallowed hard to push the feeling down. The smell of the enclosed space was just starting to get to me, when the doors opened to fresh air and access to the main corridor. I wheeled myself out with three big shoves on the wheels, while others waited to board the elevator. I rolled myself to the corner, looking right and left for familiar sights. I remembered the long stretch of hallway connecting the two buildings, with windows that extended all the way to the ceiling the full length of it, and the wheat-colored floor, unlike any other floor I'd seen in the hospital. The corridor led to the cafeteria and the main lobby. It was at a slight decline, and made it easy to roll along, and I thought, 'I'm glad I did this... this is good... on my own, finding my way....'

The ground leveled off as I approached the cafeteria, and my nose caught a strong whiff of lunch food wafting through the doors from inside. It made me feel both nauseous and hungry. I kept my focus on keeping my IV unit locked in front of me, my hands gripping the wheels on my chair, trying to get quickly beyond the scent of food. I found that moving myself along level ground took way more energy at that point. There were about 15 yards of hallway to get past the cafeteria. I rolled myself along near the wall so I wouldn't attract too much attention to myself or slow the traffic of people walking behind me. I just rolled along, one shove of the wheels at a time, and eventually I made it to the main lobby elevators. The space between the six silver doors was swirling with a sea of all kinds of people, some wearing green or blue scrubs, others in groups wearing white coats, or visitors in street clothes, some carrying gifts, rolling flower carts, or baby strollers. Some patients coming in wheelchairs, and some going out toward the main entrance. Elevator doors opened and more people spilled out, as the crowds funneled into available elevators. I paused at the corner of my corridor crossroads, and wondered how I would ever squeeze myself into an elevator with all those people without throwing up once the doors had closed. I looked down the seemingly endless corridor to my right. I remembered that was the way toward the back entrance to the Cancer Center, and there were two service elevators there that Mom liked to use instead of the busy main ones. The corridor was about 25 yards long, but it looked quiet and peaceful. I decided it didn't matter how long it took me to get to the elevators. I could take my time in the near vacant hallway, ride the elevator by myself, and pretty soon would be back to my room.

I gave the left wheel a strong push to aim me in the right direction, and then both wheels several good pushes to get past the main thoroughfare. Once I reached the quiet of the less-traveled corridor, I stopped to rest a moment. After I felt I had gathered my strength, I slowly rolled myself down that hallway. I had to stop a couple of times to let myself breathe and rest, and by the time I reached the elevators, I was getting pretty short of breath. "Just a little bit further," I kept telling myself. I rested a minute, then I rolled to back myself up to the elevator. I pushed the up arrow button to open the doors, and they opened right away. I pulled back on the wheels to roll myself backwards onto the elevator. I pulled as hard as I could, but I couldn't get my wheelchair all the way into the elevator. The doors tried to shut, but my feet were still in the way. It pissed me off enough to get a little adrenaline going, and I breathed as hard as I could to help my body pull myself the rest of the way in, my feet holding tight to my IV unit. The doors closed, and I was so exhausted I didn't think I could reach to push the button to the fourth floor. I just wanted to sit there, but I suddenly felt claustrophobic and more nauseous. I forced myself to stretch for the button. I sat praying as the elevator rose, floor by floor, "God, just get me back to my room." I built up my mental strength, telling myself that all I had to do was roll my chair off of the elevator. Then I could take my time to get around the corner and finish making my way down the last two corridors to my room. The elevator doors eased open, and I forced all my strength down onto the wheels, pushing and pushing, until I inched my way off of the elevator. I had to stop right there. I couldn't breathe well enough to go on. I sat crumpled in my wheelchair, my body exhausted, and my lungs gasping for more air. It was pretty scary, and I had a thought in my head asking for God to help me. I took as deep a breath as I could get, and started rolling myself forward, toward Unit 42. I wasn't making much headway, when an aide saw me from down the hall, and rushed toward me. She asked me where I was trying to go, but I couldn't remember my room number. I tried to point toward my room. She looked at my hospital bracelet, then she checked my pulse right there. She stepped behind me to push me along, and stopped by the nurses' station to find out where I'd been and where I was supposed to be. They asked about the transport person who was supposed to have brought me back, and I explained to them briefly that I had tried to wheel myself back.

Mom was sitting in her chair when the aide opened the door and wheeled me into my room. She stood right away, startled at my white face and weak appearance. "Oh my gosh! What happened? Where have you been?" she asked in a panicked voice.

The aide helped me into my bed.

"It's a long story... I'll tell you later." I was way too exhausted to talk.

"He's okay," the aide assured her. "I think he just tried to wheel himself back from the Pulmonary lab, which is a long way...I found him down the hall... his aide is on her way now, to check all his vitals."

"Thank you for your help..." Mom offered.

"Yeah, thanks..." I gave a weak wave to her as she backed the wheelchair away from my bed.

"You're welcome. I hope you feel better soon," she said as she left the room.

"Honey!..." Mom was concerned. "You came all that way, rolling yourself and your IV unit?"

"Yeah. I thought I could do it." I said with my eyes closed, and my head tilted toward her. I was so tired my eyes wouldn't open.

"I wish I would have known you needed help..." she said quietly, as if to be punishing herself for not knowing. "I would have brought you back myself."

I opened my eyes slightly and looked at her, hoping she'd understand it was no fault of hers, "Mom, I wanted to do it. I didn't want somebody to help me. Besides, the freakin' transport didn't show up, so what the hell was I supposed to do? I was tired of waiting, so I decided to see if I could make it...I thought I could... it just sucks that I couldn't."

"I'm sorry, Ian," she said sadly. She hated that she couldn't fix it.

"Yeah..." I closed my eyes again. "I'm gonna rest now, Mom. I'll tell you about it later. Tell me when Mook gets here."

She took my hand and kissed the back of it, and pressed it to her cheek. "I love you, Ian."

"Love you too, Mom..."

7

WBR = Whole Brain Radiation

Mark called and asked if we wanted him to bring some food. He was at the office, and would travel past my favorite Mexican food restaurant on his way to the hospital. I told Mom I wanted three beef enchiladas and she relayed my order to him. When he walked in, my whole room instantly smelled like good food. Mom pulled the table up to me with my dish on it. I took the lid off, and it smelled amazing. The steam came rising up, filled with the scent of garlic and enchilada sauce. It made my mouth water. "Mmmm! Thanks, Mook!" I smiled at him and licked my lips as I grabbed my plastic fork. I couldn't wait to dig in, I was so hungry. It was the first enchilada I'd eaten in months, fresh, soft and cheesy, with salty ground beef, and spicy sauce with fresh cilantro. I hadn't quite finished the first one, when my stomach started to hurt. I took a couple more bites, but then feelings of nausea crept up in my throat. Almost suddenly, the food in my mouth felt heavy, and sour tasting. I swallowed the bite I had taken, then put my fork down and took a quick drink of ice water. I didn't want to taste it coming back up. I pushed the table away from my bed in case I had to make a quick exit, and announced that I was sorry in the event that I suddenly had to ruin dinner by throwing up. Mom put the lid on my remaining food and saved it, hoping I could eat some more later, then she went to the unit kitchen and got some fresh ice water for me. I reclined the head of my bed slightly, adjusted my pillows, and sat disappointed and weary of always being sick and tired. Mom and Mark quickly finished their dinner and we watched some random stuff on television, and Mark shared some funny stories about his work day.

Dr. Fleming came in at about seven o'clock that evening. He stood near my bed and prepared us by saying that he was not pleased by what he had seen in the MRI results. Mom stood up, solid beside me, gripping my bed rail and silently praying for strength to receive the report. Mark sat forward in his chair, and clasped his hands in front of him. I felt a lump in my throat, and fear in my chest. I didn't move. I felt my breathing get faster, as I tried to mentally brace myself to hear the bad news.

As usual, Dr. Fleming's explanation of my situation was detailed and thorough, but it was way more than I could mentally absorb. The MRI showed there were more tumor lesions...several more...very small. He said we would most likely be looking at whole brain radiation. He said my team of doctors would consult on it, but I would without a doubt need to start radiation very soon. I sat looking at him from my bed, listening to him with all my attention, but all the words sounded the same... more cancer growing in my brain... radiation on my brain... more cancer... radiation... cancer... radiation... radiation... damn it... shit.

Mom didn't budge. She stood strong for me, determined not to shrivel. And Mark didn't show his emotions either. His eyes were steady, and his mouth stiff with concern. And all I could think, was 'Fuck.'

Dr. Fleming answered all of our questions, but the information was too shocking for us to process. After he left the room, Mom sat back down, and the three of us looked at one another, our heads swimming in the horrible news. We had tears in our eyes.

"This sucks..." I voiced my thoughts, "My whole brain...radiated. What if it fucks with me, I mean mentally?"

Mom looked at me, empathetically. She was wiping her tears with the sleeve of her sweater. "I know, Ian. I'm scared too. I'm sorry, honey..." she took my hand. "We'll learn more about the side effects tomorrow... everything's going to be okay."

"Lots of people have radiation, Ian," Mark offered. "It's not all bad. It's a common treatment for cancer, and people live through it just fine."

"But it's going to make me feel like shit, I know it." I said. "It's going to suck."

"Well, yeah, probably," he said. "But if you need it to save your life... I mean, it looks like there aren't any other options. It's a matter of saving your life, that's it right there. So you'll get through it because you have to. You can do it because you want to live. And me and your mom will do whatever we can to help you get through it, you know that."

"Yeah..." I laid my head back and closed my eyes. I couldn't believe my fate. All this because I didn't tell anyone I had a lump in my nut a year or so ago.

After about an hour, the nurse came in and brought my pre-meds, and I asked her if I could have something extra to help me sleep. I just wanted to forget about everything that was happening to me and sleep through the night. Carol would be my chemo nurse, so I wasn't going to worry about it. Mark gave me a long hug, then he had to go home to rest up for work the next day. Mom pulled all her blankets and sheets out of the cabinet and transformed her chair into a bed, while I replied to a few text messages on my cell. My pre-hydration and chemo stretched on through the night, and Mom and I woke up groggily each time Carol came in to check on me.

Mom was awake and sitting in her chair drinking a cup of hot tea when Dr. Van Veldhuisen came in at 7:30 the next morning. Mom woke me by gently touching my shoulder. "Ian," she whispered. "Dr. Van is here to see you."

He waited for me to acknowledge him, as I shifted from my side to my back so I could face him. "Hey..." I said weakly. I was too tired to extend my hand.

He stepped closer, smiled kindly, and in a gentle voice asked how I was feeling.

"Well.... I've been better..." I said, trying to stay positive.

"Yes..." he said, with his genuine smile. He looked at me the way he did, as if looking for me to say something else, or listening to his thoughts about me. He moved closer and, facing me, sat slowly on the edge of my bed near my legs, his hands folded in his lap. He looked at me compassionately, "So you've talked to Dr. Fleming about starting radiation..."

"Yeah," I said in a disappointed tone.

Mom sat quietly listening and watching. She nodded as he looked over at her, still seated in her chair.

Dr. Van gave a very slight head nod to acknowledge he'd understood. He sat quietly looking at me for a few seconds... "Dr. Alvarez will come and talk to you about it this morning... he will be the one overseeing your radiation. He will be able to answer any questions you might have about your radiation treatments."

There was a pause, a quiet in the room while the three of us sat looking at one another.

"All right..." he said quietly, as he stood up. "Just lie flat for a moment." He leaned over me to gently feel around on my abdomen. He took his stethoscope out of his coat pocket, and listened to my gut. "Can you sit up a little?

I pushed myself to a sitting position and adjusted the head of my bed. Mom and I sat silently while he listened to my heart, and my lungs, front and back, asking me to breathe deeply, and then normally. He said it all sounded good. He stood still and looked at us for a moment.

I felt I looked beaten with fear in the news of radiation.

"All right," he said with a sigh. "I will check on you later."

"Thanks," I said as I lay back on my pillow.

He bowed his head slightly and smiled politely, then left the room as quietly as he had come in.

I rolled onto my side with my left arm under my pillow supporting my head and looked at Mom. She sat sideways in her chair and leaned her head on the back of it, looking at me. For a brief moment, I remembered how we used to lay still and look at each other when I was a little guy in grade school. I'd crawl in her bed to snuggle after Mark left for work, and when it got light outside, I'd roll over to face her and stare at her until she woke up. Once her eyes opened to see my face looking back at her, she always smiled and gave me a great big hug, and it made me feel so good. Then we'd lay there for a minute, just looking at each other, neither one of us saying a word. I had loved doing that. That happy memory slipped away in a blink of my eyes, and there we were, in my hospital room looking at each other. I felt her love now, and her sorrow. And I knew she felt my heavy fear, and I hoped she felt my appreciation.

"Thank you, Mom... for being here with me."

She smiled a little and gently squeezed my hand. "I would never want to be anywhere else on earth, Ian. I love you more than everything."

I lifted her hand to my face, kissed her fingers, and held her hand close to me. I closed my eyes, and we stayed resting like that for a few minutes.

As I lay there, it suddenly occurred to me that I had an empty feeling in my stomach. I opened my eyes again and looked at her. "Mom?"

"Yes, Ian?" she asked, with her kind, tender smile. I called that her mommy smile.

"I'm hungry...will you see if the breakfast cart is in the hall?"

She went to the door, opened it, and peeked out, looking both ways. "I'll go down the hall a ways, I don't see it around here," she said, as she stepped out the barely open door.

She returned a minute later with two cartons of milk, one white and one chocolate. "The food cart is at the end of the unit, it should be here in a few minutes, but here's some milk from the nurses' kitchen to tide you over, if you want it," she said as she held them out to me. "Whichever one you don't want, I'll drink, or you can have them both."

I chose the chocolate milk, and Mom walked over to the window to peer out through the blinds.

"Ian! It's snowing!" She looked over at me. "Do you want to see?"

I looked toward her, and she pulled on the cord to raise the blinds, revealing the outside world. I rarely looked out the window while I was in the hospital, because doing so was a cruel reminder of where I was, and why. Today, though, the scene was pretty. The snowflakes were big ones that floated down peacefully onto the tops of buildings and the parking garage full of cars across from us. Everything was covered in sheets of white. But the light of it was too bright for me, and I asked Mom to close the blinds again. It looked cold, anyway, and seeing it was enough to make me wish even more that I was home.

Dr. Alvarez came to see us a couple of hours after we'd eaten breakfast. We greeted each other with a handshake, and I joked that it wasn't anything personal, but I'd hoped not to have to see him again. He smiled, and said he understood exactly what I meant, and that he knew it was hard to hear the news I had been given. He pulled a chair close up to my bed, and sat down, holding my file that he had brought with him. He was a tall man, with coal black hair, and a friendly smile. He had an intense, busy energy about him, and being from the Dominican Republic, spoke with a strong Spanish accent. He was easy to understand, though. He said I would be starting radiation within a couple of hours, and as soon as I heard his words, I felt like there was a heavy brick sitting in my stomach. He went on to explain that I would be receiving whole brain radiation, on a low dose for five consecutive days, and continuing for five consecutive weeks. Then I would have another MRI on my head after the fourth course of chemotherapy.

That sounded like a ton of radiation to me. I asked him if it would hurt, if I'd be able to feel it going into my head. He said I would feel nothing at all, that it was just like getting an x-ray and it would take only a few minutes. I asked him how that much radiation would make me feel, what were the side effects. He said the most common side effects would be fatigue and nausea, just like with chemotherapy. However, I would be having both radiation and chemotherapy at the same time, so I figured my side effects would be double the fun. I just couldn't imagine feeling worse than I already had.

Mom asked if he would explain a little about how radiation works. I wasn't sure I wanted to know, but I listened anyway. We learned that a radiation treatment is given using small amounts of gamma rays that can break the DNA strand of a cell. That causes the abnormal cell to recognize that it's damaged, so it stops trying to multiply and it dies. Dr. Alvarez explained that gamma rays are high energy light waves that can penetrate almost any substance, and that the earth's atmosphere constantly absorbs gamma rays that come from all over the universe. I would soon be finding out how it would feel to have small amounts of those waves going directly into my head, and the thought of it had a paralyzing effect on me.

Once Dr. Alvarez was sure he had answered all of our questions, he stood and shook my hand. He said I could call him anytime with questions or concerns, and gave me his business card with his direct number on it. I had hoped his answers to my questions would help me feel better about radiation, but with every minute, my thoughts of radiation treatment and its side effects made me more and more afraid of how horrible I was going to feel.

After he left, Mom listened to me while I voiced my fears. I had never heard anything good about radiation, and I was dreading the thought of beams being zapped into my brain, leaving me feeling more sick than ever before. Mom just held my hand and listened.

She sighed and looked at me for a moment, then asked, "Can I go with you?"

"Yeah. I want you to. I'm afraid of how I'll feel when they get done with me. I'm afraid of all that's going to happen."

"Do you want to wear your jeans? I'll get them out for you."

"No, thanks. I want to stay in my sweats. It's cold down there. But can you get my blue hoodie?"

She went to the nurses' station to freshen my ice water while I dressed and washed my face. It wasn't long before a transport person showed up with a wheelchair for me. I asked Mom to grab a thin blanket for me. Sometimes I would get a chill as I got out into the hallways. Mom draped the blanket over the back of the wheelchair, and off we went with the transport.

There was a maze of corridors the length of a football field leading to the radiation oncology department. As we arrived at the radiation therapists' desk, both therapists, Leslie and Michelle, greeted us. Mom introduced herself, and asked if they would be able to show us around and explain the radiation process for us. I got up from my wheelchair and followed them into the room with the heavy lead door, Mom behind me. Leslie showed us the treatment table and the machine, called the Varian Linear Accelerator 2300. It actually looked like a giant room-sized cake mixer, without the beaters, of course. She explained that I would be fitted with a radiation mask that would hold my head in perfect alignment on the table, and showed me by placing another patient's mask where my head would be. Michelle operated the movement of the machine for us, to demonstrate how the front end of the cake mixer could be moved above and around my head from side to side, in order to dose the radiation according to my personal prescription.

First I had to go into what is called the Simulation Room to be fitted for the mask. The therapist asked me to lie on the slab table, and she guided me to place my head in the precise position and close my eyes during the fitting. She had a thick plastic net with a U-shaped bracket around the edges, and placed it in hot water to soften the plastic net. She and Dr. Klish, the resident in Radiation Oncology, stood on opposite sides of my head, and together they placed the warm soft plastic netting over my face and pulled the thick plastic bracket of it downward toward the table. One of them pressed gently at the bridge of my nose to pull the net in for a close fit. It was a weird sensation, because the entire plastic netting instantly molded itself to my face, sinking into my eye sockets. I could feel it pulling to fit around my chin, my jaw line, cheekbones, and scalp. I had to lay there with it on my face for about five minutes while it cooled, and when she lifted it off, it was an eerie-looking shape of my face, in powder blue-colored plastic netting. Because the heavy U-shaped bracket had been pressed all the way to the table, the netting stretched straight back about two-and-a-half inches past the shape of my head. It looked like something out of a science fiction movie, a human face stretching out beyond the grid of another dimension. The bracket would be secured to the treatment table to hold my head perfectly still. I had a feeling it was going to feel pretty strange.

They had to take a Polaroid picture of me and my mask in position on the treatment table for my medical records, and I asked Leslie if she could take one for me to keep. She lifted her camera and asked if I was ready. I opened my eyes to see, hoping they would show for the picture, and gave two thumbs up. I made a few joking remarks and we had some laughs, but after that, it was time for radiation, and the seriousness of the procedure settled in.

Lead blocks, two inches thick, were precisely placed on the radiation machine, to block the radiation from my whole face, especially my eyes. The rest of my head would be radiated. That thought made me feel nervous and scared. On the mask there were short pieces of masking tape with markings on them, to help with perfect alignment of the blocks and radiation. There were two cameras in the room, both aimed at the treatment table, and an intercom system in case we needed to communicate during the treatment. Leslie and Michelle would operate the linear accelerator from computers and monitor my treatment from behind the desk outside of the treatment room.

I laid there anxious to get it over with, but afraid of what was about to happen, though I hoped to exude a cool exterior. I tried to trust what Mom had often said, that God was in all of it, and I prayed it would be okay. The commotion exhausted me, the activity, the communication, the emotions, the nausea. I even grew tired of thinking, and actually drifted off into a light sleep during the treatment. When Michelle came in to tell me it was over, I thought maybe it wasn't going to be too bad after all. But when I sat up from the table to stand, I realized how tired I really was. I was glad to see the transport waiting for me with the wheelchair.

When we got back to my room I got out of that wheelchair and fell into my bed, I was so wiped out. It had been a busy, stressful day. I lay in my bed and slept from the moment I got back to my room, while Mom sat next to me listening to the ticking of the clock on the wall and the constant mechanical clicking of my IV machine. At 3:30, Tracy, my nurse, came in to give me some acetaminophen and hook me up with a dose of bleomycin in my port. I was feeling sick to my stomach from the thought of it dripping into me, but I felt so tired I just slept the afternoon away.

I didn't wake when Mark came in the room after his day's work. I woke up and he and Mom were both sitting there in the quiet. Mom had one hand holding mine, and her other hand holding Mark's, on the arm of her chair. I had awakened with a jolt, and reactively squeezed Mom's hand as I woke. I looked over at her with my sleepy eyes. She and Mark both looked at me.

"What are you guys doing?" I asked. "Are you just sitting here watching me sleep?"

"No..." she smiled, "we're just sitting here being with you." Mom said, "Mark got here maybe 15 minutes ago. He actually was resting his eyes, and I was sitting here between my two boys, loving you."

"..kay ..." I said, tiredly. I closed my eyes again for a minute, then I looked back at her. "What day is it?"

"It's Friday. You just had your first radiation treatment this afternoon, and a bleomycin dose a little while ago. It's almost five o'clock in the evening. How do you feel?"

"Tired."

I lay limp in bed, staring at the air space, listening to the sound of the IV pump, and the quiet around us. Minutes ticked away to a quarter past, then half past, then ten minutes to the hour.

"I'm getting kind of hungry," Mark said, quietly breaking the silence.

"Yeah," I agreed.

But still, we sat in the quiet, me staring off into space thinking random thoughts, Mark resting his eyes, and Mom, with her head resting on my bed beside me. Fifteen minutes later, our quiet world was opened up when a friendly black woman knocked on the door and stepped in to deliver my food tray.

"Hello!" She sang her greeting softly as she entered. "How're ya'll doin' today?" She smiled at each of us.

We greeted her and thanked her. "Got a nice dinner for you today, sir," she said in a soft cheerful voice, and set the tray on my table. She pulled the table over to me, and I raised my bed to sit up. She stood still beside me, her lips pursed together with a compassionate smile. She rested one hand behind me, on the top of the head of my bed, and tilted her head a bit to look at me. "You been coming here a long time, haven't you?"

"Yeah," I smiled, looking under the lid on my plate, then back up to her.

She patted my shoulder, "Well, you just keep on fightin', honey. The Lord gonna take care of you. Just you don't give up."

I nodded, grateful for her encouragement. She had a kind smile, and her dark eyes looked as if they held a promise. "Thanks," I smiled. "And thanks for the food."

"Oh, you're more than welcome, sugar. You all have a good night, okay?" She softly sang a gospel song as she walked toward the door.

"Thank you," Mom said before she closed the door. "She sure is nice, isn't she? What a pretty voice."

"Yeah, she's cool," I had the cover off my plate, tearing open the packet of salt for my food.

Mark stood to stretch, then announced he was taking the opportunity to make a trip to the cafeteria. He and Mom were more used to the hospital food than I was, and Mark made his trek downstairs to fill a tray with home style food for both of them. I had always been a picky eater, so it was a little harder for me to find food that I liked, not to mention, food that I could keep in my stomach.

We whiled away the evening in stages of visiting, and sitting silently, until around 8:30, when it was time for my pre-meds. It was a little early for my liking, and I asked my nurse if it was necessary for me to take them so early. Some of the meds I took were for nausea, and they made me sleepy. It was hard to stay asleep, so I also received a sleep aid, but I at least wanted to wait and stay awake until 10:00 p.m. or so. That made it a little easier to stay asleep later.

At ten o'clock I got my bag of fluids for my pre-hydration drip, and my chemotherapy was started when that was finished, around 10:30. Mark stayed the night with us, on his chair-bed at my feet, and I managed to sleep through most of the night, waking only when the nurse came in to adjust my chemo meds and check the IV machine, and when the aide came in to check my vitals.

I was awakened abruptly by one of the resident doctors at 6:30 in the morning. She practically exploded into the room, talking loudly, asking me half a dozen questions, and pushing too hard on my abdomen, feeling for the cancer. She pissed me off so bad I pulled away from her and told her to stop it, and she got a little bit snooty with me in defense of her method of examining me. I looked at Mom, and saw in her eyes the signs of a mother bear about to defend her young.

"Please get Dr. Fleming or the other resident doctor," Mom said firmly.

She looked at Mom. Mom sat with her hands in her lap, looking straight back at her. She offered a polite smile to show she was serious. "I'm asking for a different doctor," Mom repeated.

The resident doctor paused and glanced at Mark, sitting quietly looking back at her, then she looked at me.

"Can you just get Dr. Fleming?" I suggested flatly.

She nodded, then she turned and left the room.

"Gawd I hate that bitch," I said. "She always barges in here like she owns me, and she's always so freakin' loud."

"I know, honey," Mom said.

Mark just frowned and shook his head.

"I'm telling Dr. Fleming not to let her come in here anymore. I can't stand her. I don't want her touching me."

Mom sighed. "I'm sorry, Ian," she said in her sad voice.

About half an hour later, the other resident doctor, Pete, came in to see me. He was a nice guy, and seemed to be very empathetic toward me and my health situation. I respected him because he showed respect to me, not just as a cancer patient specimen, but as a human person who was suffering... a human person fighting cancer in his body. That demeanor made all the difference to me. He had regard for me... for my feelings. I could see the compassion in his face and humility in his presence. Mark, Mom, and I agreed he was a good doctor.

I had a special appointment for a radiation treatment on Saturday, while I was still an in-patient. My second treatment was set for ten o'clock that morning. Mom and I thought we could remember the way, so we told the nurse we would not need a transport, and the three of us set out in that direction without my usual tour guide. I wasn't sure I could walk the entire distance, so Mark pushed my empty wheelchair just in case I needed it. I rolled my constant companion IV machine along between Mom and me, the five wheels rattling their way across the tile floors, announcing my presence everywhere I went. The corridors were well marked with signs to each department, so we had no trouble finding our way. The radiation department was quiet and empty, since I was the only one due for a treatment on a Saturday. Leslie greeted us, and I followed her into the radiation room. Mom came in behind me, as she wanted to see me in the whole setup. Mark waited for her near the desk.

Leslie lowered the table so I could lie down, then she adjusted the height for my treatment. She slid a foam pillow under my knees. She took my radiation mask from the shelf of others, and placed it over my face, securing my head to the table for the ten-minute treatment. She covered me with a light blanket to keep me from getting chilly and turned on the radio to a station I told her was one of my favorites. She made sure the blocks were perfectly in place, that everything else was aligned just right, and she checked with me to see that I was comfortable. Mom gave my hand a quick squeeze, whispered that she loved me, then she and Leslie disappeared from my sight. I heard her close the one-foot-thick lead door that separated me from everything else, leaving me alone inside my radiation world. The room was well lit, but not too bright. I closed my eyes, my hands folded across my stomach, the prescribed position for my treatment. Nausea grew stronger each time I swallowed, and I felt more and more nervous with the knowledge that there would soon be radiation directed right at me, into every one of my brain cells. That thought was so sharp in my mind, I kept feeling more sick, so I tried to focus on listening to the music on the radio.

I heard the accelerator hum as it started up, and the air filled with a very faint smell and taste of something I could only describe as bleach. It was the scent of the radiation, and it became a taste at the back of my tongue and throat. It made me feel very nauseous, even though I couldn't actually feel the radiation itself in my head. I was glad for the music. It made being there a little bit easier to handle.

When it was all finished, Leslie came in to free my head from the table, and that was it. I felt just slightly nauseous, but overall, not too bad. As I walked out the door, Mom and Mark were standing a few feet away waiting for me. I opted to try walking back to my room, so Mark pushed the empty wheelchair and I gripped my IV unit, and down the empty halls we strolled, the three of us and my wheeled companions. When we got to the cafeteria, we stopped in to find a snack. I actually had an appetite, and it felt good. Mom and I each got a strawberry shortcake ice cream bar, and ate them on the way back to the room. Mark and I joked about this and that, and I enjoyed the long walk. I was a little tired by the time we got back to my room, so I rested quietly for a while before taking my shower.

The day was pretty uneventful, except for the pain in my stomach. I tried to sleep most of the afternoon, while Mom and Mark sat by, watching football on TV, with the sound turned down. But I had my usual day-long restless cycle of waking and dozing, waking and dozing. I could never get any real solid sleep. The nurse came in around 9:00 p.m. to give me my pre-meds, honoring my request for a later start time. I knew the meds they gave me prior to chemo should help ease my stomach pain, and help me to sleep a little. I was growing so weary of my cancer and treatment experience, I asked her if I could have an extra dose of Benedryl and something extra for pain. I wanted to be taken away from it all for a while, and to be able to sleep a deep sleep through the night. When she came back in with a dose of Benedryl to put in my IV, and an extra dose of oxycodone, I knew I'd be feeling okay pretty soon. In about an hour, I was flying high and feeling really good. Mom and Mark were cracking up at the funny things I was saying, I was making jokes about everything. I felt good for the first time in weeks, and I enjoyed that short time. I could sit and laugh, and smile with no pain and no worries, and it was a freedom I didn't get to enjoy very often. I felt so good I wanted to take pictures of myself smiling, but my phone's photo file was full, so Mom gave me her phone. I took a couple of pictures of myself, then I wanted her in the photos with me, so she crawled on top of my bed and we squeezed our heads together for a few good pictures. We were laughing, joking around, and making funny faces. I just kept clicking the pictures and laughing at what they looked like. It was so much fun just to feel carefree and pain free for a while.

Eventually, though, the sleepiness kicked in, and I was feeling too groggy to carry on much of a conversation. My pre-hydration was started about 10:30, and by 11:00 that night, I was getting my routine chemo of cisplatin and etoposide. I did manage to get some fairly good sleep through it all, even though I woke each time the nurse came in.

Sunday morning I was still very sleepy, and continued to sleep through the morning without very many interruptions, except for the aides checking vitals. As I started to wake up more, I was too aware of the pain in my stomach, and I told that to the doctor when he came to check on me. I had been feeling pretty nauseous and eventually threw up around noon, but after that I felt okay. I actually was in the mood for a double bacon cheeseburger and fries, so Mark left for Wendy's and came back with my feast. It tasted awesome, and I ate all of it, no problems at all. That felt wonderful to be able to eat so much. I hoped it wouldn't cost me later. Uncle Dale and Tracey came for a visit that afternoon, and we all had some good laughs, although my stomach pain was still hanging tough and the nausea was getting worse. I asked my nurse, Stacey, if I could get an extra med for the nausea. She came back a while later with some Compazine to inject into my port. She also listened for bowel sounds, and said everything sounded okay.

Late that afternoon, my stomach still hurt, but the nausea had subsided a little, so Mom and Mark offered to take me for a wheelchair ride just to get out of my room. There was a Health Walk Trail inside the hospital that Mark had discovered on one of his walks, and we decided to check it out. A long, long hallway led to a modern brick-and-tile concourse with a big waterfall fountain in the center, and lots of cool-looking tropical plants. Surrounding the concourse were two stories of open offices, for what, we didn't know. But the whole place looked like a plaza that was probably used for receptions and the like. We continued on the Health Walk, where a catwalk took us across the street to the library, something to do to break up the boring hours of living in the hospital. We strolled around, taking in a new atmosphere, then eventually headed back toward my room in Unit 42. We made a stop into the cafeteria to pick up some boxed dinners for Mark and Mom. I rested in bed while they ate. Food had no appeal to me in my tired state. My dinner tray arrived later, but I was feeling too nauseous to eat much of it. I tried to sleep away another night, as the tiring routine of pre-meds, pre-hydration, and chemotherapy rolled on.

The next day, Dr. Fleming told me that he had placed the order to have my blood drawn for labs twice each week, on Tuesdays and Fridays, with neupogen every day in the radiation unit when I went there for treatment, and I was to travel to the Cancer Center to receive it on weekends. My insurance was refusing to pay for it if I needed it outpatient, so Mom couldn't give it to me anymore. That was not a big problem, because she didn't like injecting me anyway. The good news was that my tumor markers had gone down, from 26,000 to 25,000. It wasn't as good a response as we had been hoping for, but it did show the chemotherapy was still working.

When I had seen Dr. Alvarez the day before, I told him I wanted to see the lesions in my brain, and asked if there was any way he could show the MRI images to me. He said he would be happy to do that, and asked only that I remind him about it when I went for my next radiation treatment on Monday, and I could see them at that time. I told Mark about it, so he took the afternoon off from work to meet us there. Mom and I left my room early, and walked the stretch of corridors to the radiation unit.

As it turned out, Dr. Alvarez had been called away, so Dr. Klish showed us the images. Mark met us at the nurses' desk in the radiation unit, and the three of us followed Dr. Klish down the hall to the conference room in the unit. Dr. Klish was really cool. He offered each of us a chair in front of a 20-inch computer monitor. He pulled up my images on the screen, and pointed to the lesions seen in my brain from several different angles. He showed us the original lesions deep in the occipital lobe, which had not grown in size since the last report, then he showed me the six smaller lesions, scattered in other various lobes of my brain. Each lesion measured about one centimeter.

I felt angry when I saw what cancer was doing in me. I wanted to go into the radiation room and just blast the radiation at my head. My mind, my thoughts were spinning in disarray at my worsening fate, but I kept my composure. I sat looking at my brain on the monitor, and in a way, couldn't believe it was my head I was looking at, with all that cancer in it. Dr. Klish said that he was optimistic that my radiation treatments would completely kill all those lesions in my brain, including any that may be there that were too small to be seen by MRI. I took another long look at the lesions, and asked Dr. Klish again, "So you really think they'll all be gone by next month?"

"Absolutely, Ian," he said assuredly, looking me straight in the eye, "It's completely possible, and I feel very confident about it."

Dr. Klish had a cool way about him, a friendly manner, and I knew he cared about me, as did Dr. Alvarez. I appreciated them as much as I did Dr. Van Veldhuisen and Dr. Fleming.

Mom's Uncle Jim had survived cancer, and he told me that I had to form a strong ally with my doctors, but I also had to be educated about the cancer and my treatment. I was glad I had all those guys on my side. They each helped me, in their own way, to feel trust in all of it.

As I stood from my chair, I thanked Dr. Klish for taking the time to show the images to me. After a few thank you's and hand shakes, it was time for my radiation treatment. The four of us walked down the hall toward the radiation therapists' desk, and Dr. Klish wished us a good evening as he left us there. Leslie greeted us and took me back to the radiation treatment room, while Mom and Mark waited in the hallway just outside the unit.

Just walking into the radiation treatment room brought up the nauseous feelings in my stomach and my mouth. We chatted a little, and I tried to ignore the nausea, following the routine of lying on the table with my hands across my stomach, while Leslie covered me with a blanket and secured my head in place under my mask. She checked to make sure everything was in order, then let me know she was leaving the room to start the treatment. I heard the huge door shut. The radio was playing one of my favorite songs, so I tried to keep thinking about it, singing the lyrics in my head. The hum started up, and the bleach-y scent of radiation was instantly in my mouth, my throat, and the nauseous feeling grew worse. The smell lasted only about a minute, but its effects seemed to linger. I knew I would only be in there for ten minutes, so I had to keep listening to the music and hold on a little longer.

I was not feeling well at all when the treatment was over. I went to the nearest bathroom to throw up. Mark asked one of the nurses if there was a wheelchair we could use to take me back upstairs, and he rolled me back to my room. It was an awful ride. I told Mark to take it really slow, and we strolled down the corridors like sightseers in a museum. It was the best I could do. Motion wasn't agreeable with my stomach. We even had to stop a couple of times because I thought I was going to throw up right there in the hallway. The elevator ride was miserable, and it was all I could do just to hang my head and hope the nausea could wait at least until I made it back to my room.

Once we entered my room, I got out of the wheelchair and went straight to the bathroom. I threw up a whole day's worth of liquid, heaving for more than ten minutes, and it drained all the energy out of me. Mom prepared a lukewarm damp washcloth for me and placed it on the vanity. I rubbed it all over my face, then rinsed my mouth in the sink. I was so weak after that, Mark had to hold my hand to help me back to my bed only ten feet away. Mom stood by, and held my IV lines while I fell into bed, then covered me with my own blanket. It was only two o'clock in the afternoon.

I still felt like shit when Kim, our insurance liaison with the hospital, came by about an hour later, but it was a relief to hear her good news. She had been working with us tirelessly through the last few months, making sure the insurance company continued to cover my treatment. They kept trying to back out on me due to the requirement that I remain a full time college student in order to keep my coverage, but cancer had made it impossible for me to do that. It had been a constant struggle for me to get insurance to pay for my prescriptions as an outpatient, too, so she hooked us up with a couple of people Mom had to call for help every single time I needed another prescription filled. Kim helped to ease my stress about the incredible medical expenses that I knew were racking up each day.

After she left, the three of us had hours to pass, me lying limp in my bed, and Mom and Mark sitting quietly next to me. It was all I could do to just look at them. I was too exhausted to think. I knew I looked miserable, but my appearance was nothing compared to the way I actually felt. My body felt old and worn out, but with a burning feeling all through my muscles, my veins, my chemical-filled blood. My bones and joints ached all the way through to my bone marrow. It hurt when I moved, but if I didn't move, I got stiff, and that hurt even worse. My entire body felt so weak, I couldn't even lift one leg. Mark stood and offered to stretch my legs and arms. I told him I was too tired to move, but he lifted one of my feet anyway, saying that he would move my limbs for me, because it would be good for my circulation and my joints. He knew to move slowly, and after ten stretches on each limb, I did feel better.

I had one more night of chemotherapy to get through, and I was hoping to be able to go home on Tuesday. Mark stayed as late as he could, then left for home to rest up for the work day ahead. Mom and I settled into our evening routine once again... my pre-meds were given to me... my pre-chemo hydration... then my chemotherapy through the night... waking every four hours for my vitals check, or when the IV machine beeped for one reason and another, or when the nurse came in to adjust chemo doses on the machine, or when I had to go to the bathroom to pee or throw up.

I had my first of ten daily neupogen injections in the radiation oncology department before I went in for my fifth radiation treatment as an inpatient. I still hadn't gotten used to the pain of those damned shots. I sat in a small chair in the nurses' area where they checked my vitals each time I came in. The nurses were very nice, and the process went along quickly. I felt the usual nausea in my gut and throat just before going in for the radiation. And the ever-present smell and taste of the radiation itself as the Accelerator started up was becoming something I started to dread each day.

Fortunately, I got released to go home that afternoon, so once we arrived back at my hospital room, Mom started packing up all of our stuff so we would be ready to leave when the time came. She called Mark to let him know so he could arrange to pick us up. I lay in bed, feeling nauseous and tired the whole afternoon, but looking forward to being home in fresh surroundings.

I had two appointments at the Cancer Center to receive bleomycin during the next two weeks in addition to the daily trips to KU for radiation treatment. Mom and I talked about how we would cope with the daily drive. Just like Mark had said, we'll do it because we have to... we will just do it. I had to get my mind set on that.

My home routine was not much different from the one at the hospital. I was more comfortable at home, but I stayed in bed most of the time, and got up frequently to throw up. Mom gave me all my medications at the same time every day, and took care of everything I needed. She made sure my room and bathroom were clean, changed the sheets on my bed, made sure I always had fresh ice water to drink, and brought nutritious food to me whenever I felt I could eat. I was glad I had her to care for me. I wouldn't have taken such good care of myself if I had to do it alone. I hated to cook, and even when I was healthy, I was usually too lazy to prepare food that didn't come in a box marked "pizza." I was the kind of guy who would rather drive to McDonald's than get the peanut butter and jelly out and make a sandwich. I once told Mom about my theory on the make-to-eat time ratio when I had asked her to make a sandwich for me. She had wondered why a healthy young man like myself couldn't make his own sandwich.

"If it takes longer to prepare than it does to eat it, it isn't worth my time to make it." I stated reasonably.

She had smiled at me in disbelief.

"What? How long does it take to make a sandwich?" she had asked.

"Okay, you gotta get the peanut butter out of the cabinet. Then you have to dig through the fridge and find the jelly. Then you have to open that twist tie on the bag, which you always lose because you set it down somewhere on the counter and can't find it again. Then you have to stick your big hand in there and pull out two pieces of bread and close the bread bag up again. Then you have to get a plate from the cupboard. Then you need a knife from the drawer. You gotta open the jars... and just try to spread the peanut butter without tearing the bread!" I could get pretty animated in my explanations... "...so you've got torn bread, then you have to spread the jelly, and you know, I can't spread jelly... it just moves around the bread in a big clump. So now I have a dirty knife, a dirty plate, torn bread, lumpy jelly, and then I have to put the peanut butter and jelly away again and clean up my mess. And it took me a whole five minutes or more..." I looked at her, waiting for her to agree.

She stood there, smiling at me.

"And how long does it take me to eat the whole thing?" I continued, my hands in the air for extra emphasis. "One minute... one lousy minute, and after all that work my sandwich is gone, and I'm still hungry."

Mom just laughed, looking at me and shaking her head. "What about frozen pizza?" she asked. "It takes ten minutes to cook. How long does it take you to eat that?"

"Yeah," I argued humorously, "but there's very little effort, you just take it out of the box and put it in the oven, set the timer and wait. You can do other stuff while the pizza is cooking. Then you just take it out and slide it on top of the box it came in and roll the slicer over it a couple times. So it takes me only one minute to fix it, I don't dirty a dish, and it takes me more than five minutes to eat it! See?" I raised my hands in the air again, emphasizing the weight distribution of work effort in the make-to-eat ratio.

Mom just smiled and shook her head, but her eyes told me she really was amused. "That's a lot of thought you've put into just getting a bite to eat... and you don't mind having someone else do the work for you, do you..." she laughed.

I gave her my most charming smile, and a look on my face that I knew she couldn't resist. "So... will you make me a sandwich?"

I couldn't even joke around like that anymore, I was way too tired, much too sick to even think funny thoughts. I missed who I was before cancer, and the way I felt about myself back then. Friends called, but I was too tired to get together with anyone. It seemed like all I did was sleep and throw up, sleep and throw up some more. I was sleeping off and on through the days and nights, and many times in a day had to ask Mom or check my wall clock to see what day it was, or whether it was a.m. or p.m. I hated losing track of time like that. I felt like I was living in my own cancer time zone. It felt like I was actually losing time itself. I didn't have enough appetite to eat meals at the same times each day, so there was no way of keeping track of time by the food I ate. Mom gave my meds to me at the same times each day, but with sleeping all the time, taking the doses all felt the same. There was no hospital regimen. The only thing that kept me oriented in world time was my daily trip to KU for radiation treatments. My appointments were set at 1:15 p.m.

Exhausted doesn't even come close to describing the way I was feeling by Wednesday, after only 11 radiation treatments. I felt too tired to swallow water. The continuous heaving and throwing my guts up had beaten my will to try to swallow anything except for the medications I took to prevent nausea. Mom laid my jeans on the floor in front of me so I could slip my feet into them. She went outside to warm the car, then she found my shoes and coat and brought them to me. I could smell the wintery outside air as it followed her from the front door to my room, and the scent brought a heavy feeling of dread with it. I didn't want to go where I was going. She picked up her purse and notebook to leave, and I grabbed a package of Strawberry Pop Tarts from the box on my shelf in case I got hungry along the way.

I tried to make myself comfortable to sleep through the drive, but the nausea got worse after being on the road for about half an hour. I sat up for the rest of the trip, but as we grew closer to the hospital, I grew even more nauseous. I told Mom how it felt so weird, that the closer we got to the hospital, the more sick and dreadful I felt. It really did feel like my body was thinking for itself, and knew instinctively that something bad was about to happen to it.

There was limited parking in front of the radiation oncology department entrance. We had to have a patient pass hanging on our rear-view mirror to avoid being ticketed for parking there. As I crawled out of the car, I felt a heaviness in my stomach, a feeling of anxious resistance in my body, as if my insides were pleading, no...no...no. I stepped up on the curb and waited for Mom to join me, and we walked toward the entrance together. The air was cold and misty, the ground was kind of damp, and the sky was a solid cloud of gray. It all looked as pallid as I felt.

The sliding glass doors opened for us, and we proceeded down the 20 steps to the main waiting room. I headed directly to the couch to lie down, while Mom walked to the receptionist to let her know I was there. I felt like I was going to throw up, so I got up and shot into the men's room a few feet away. When I came out, Mom was waiting on the couch. I lay down with my head on her leg and covered up with my coat. I hoped I wouldn't have to throw up during my treatment while my head was bolted down. The thought of that was frightening, and I told Mom I was a little worried about it. She gave me a peppermint candy and suggested I tell Leslie or Michelle before they took me in. I remembered they had cameras and an intercom in the treatment room in case I needed help. Once I was in there, Michelle let me sit on the treatment table until I was sure I felt I was okay enough to lie down, and said just to speak out if I needed to get up, and she'd be right there to help me.

As it turned out, I got through the treatment okay, once I was able to get past that first smell of radiation. She helped me off the table and walked with me to the nurses' station, where I needed to get the neupogen shot. While Vici, my nurse, was giving me the shot, Mom was telling her about my unbearable nausea. Mom thought it was not normal. She felt it was too much, even considering the chemo and radiation I was going through. Vici said she would make note of it and check with the doctor, and after I stood up, I felt even more nauseous than I had before. I felt I had to lie down right away, and I stumbled over to a row of three chairs in a small waiting area near a bathroom across from the nurses' desk. I just lay there feeling like I must be in hell. Mom knelt beside me, waiting. One of the other nurses brought over a small cup of cold water for me. Mom took it and offered it to me, but I couldn't move, I didn't want to move or swallow anything even though I was thirsty.

"I'm sorry, Ian..." she whispered.

I stayed in that position for about five minutes, afraid to move for fear of throwing up. All of a sudden, lying still was not enough, and I leaped up past Mom and into the bathroom. I heaved and heaved, and the sound of my stomach lurching through my throat echoed like catacombs in the small bathroom. My stomach was empty. There was nothing to throw up, but my gut just kept heaving and lurching, forcing my body into a painful crouch over the toilet. I braced myself with one hand on the back of the toilet, and one on the wall in front of me, and heaved nothing but pain, until my knees started to buckle and I could barely stand up. My eyes were watering, from the bitter burning of stomach acid and bile that was forcing its way up through my sinuses. When the vomiting subsided, I opened the door and stumbled out, crumbling onto the row of chairs where Mom was waiting. She knelt down beside me again, and put her hand on my shoulder.

"I'm so sorry, Ian..." she had tears rolling down her face, "I'm so sorry...."

"Why is this happening to me, Mom?" I slurred, tears streaming out of my eyes, and spit running out the corner of my mouth. I couldn't even hold up my head. "I don't understand why God wants me to suffer so much... I feel like I'm dying, Mom... if I'm dying, why won't He just let me die?"

Mom's tears filled her eyes. She graced her fingers across my cheek,

"No, no, Ian... don't say things like that." She leaned in and kissed me on my shoulder, and I felt her warm hand on my back. She laid her head on my arm. "Ian, I love you so much. I'm so sorry that you're suffering like this... I'm so, so very sorry." She sat up and took her knitted scarf off from around her neck. She folded it, then lifted my head slightly and placed it under my face.

"Thank you, Mom..." I was limp, wondering how much more I had to suffer, and how much more could I take.

Nurse Vici came over to us and said she wanted to check my blood pressure again. It was fine when I arrived, but Dr. Klish told her to check it again, once with me sitting, and once with me standing, and once with me lying down. If my blood pressure was inconsistent in the three positions, a condition called "orthostatic," it signaled I was severely dehydrated, which would cause the excessive nausea. He was right. I was in deep need of fluids.

Vici took us to one of the exam rooms and I settled into the heavy padded leather recliner. Mom hung her coat over the treatment chair next to me, and laid her purse and notebook on the small table attached to the arm of the chair. When Vici returned, she prepared to access my port, and Mom asked where she could get a blanket for me. Vici offered to get one as soon as she had me hooked up. I would be there for two hours, while the fluids and glucose dripped into me. I covered up with the blanket, and Mom closed the door, turned off all the lights, and sat in the dark with me while I dozed.

Suddenly, I woke up not knowing where I was. I called out in the dark, "Mom?"

"I'm here, Ian," came her voice from my left. I felt her pat my arm, and the familiar rhythmic click of the IV machine on my right came into my awareness.

At that point, I remembered the events leading to my sitting in a comfy chair in a dark room. "How long have we been here?" I asked, my eyes open in the darkness.

I saw the light of her cell phone barely illuminate her face as she checked the time. "About 45 minutes."

"Have you been here the whole time?"

"Yes."

"Just sitting here, in the dark?"

"I wrote some things down in my notebook. But other than that, yeah."

"Mom, you don't have to stay here. You must be bored out of your mind."

"If you want me to go, I will, just let me know what you want, honey. Whatever you need, I will do."

"Is there a way we could get a little light in here now? Maybe like just open the door a crack?"

I heard her stand.

"Wait..." I said quickly. I pulled my cell phone from my front pocket, opened it up, and held it up to illuminate the room a little. "There." I smiled. "Now you can see where you're going."

She opened the door very slightly, and the light from the hallway was just right. "How's that?" she asked.

"Yeah."

She sat back down in her chair. "Really, Ian, I don't mind staying here with you at all."

"Well, I like having you here with me, you know... I really don't want to sit here alone... but I'm just sleeping, so you could go if you want."

"No, Ian. I really truly mean it when I say there is nowhere on earth I would rather be than right here with you. There is nothing I'd rather be doing than sitting right here with my son."

I smiled and reached my hand out to her, and she leaned over to me and took my hand. I pulled her hand close and kissed her fingers, and held her hand to my cheek. "Thank you, Mom. I don't know how you do it, just sitting here, but I'm so glad you do. Thank you so much for being my mom."

I could see she was smiling. "Thank you for being such a wonderful son, Ian," she said. "You're the best son a mom could ever ask for."

"Thanks, Mom." I squeezed her hand.

"Are you hungry? Do you want me to see if I can get you some food?" she asked, hopefully.

"Yeah, actually, I am." I was happy to be able to say that.

"I can go see what's in the cafeteria..."

"No, that's too far. Do you think there's a vending machine close by anywhere?"

"I'll ask one of the nurses." She stood up and grabbed her purse.

"Okay, but come back and tell me what they say before you go, okay? I want to tell you what to look for that I might want to eat, ok?"

She smiled and said she'd do that.

The nearest place to buy food was the Sunflower gift shop on the next floor up, about five minutes' walking distance. Mom got directions and came back to get my suggestion list. I wanted some kind of juice, a healthy snack, and something salty.

She left the door open just a sliver to let in a little shaft of light, and I laid there in the dark with my eyes open, listening to the clicking rhythm of my IV machine. Only an hour ago I thought I was dying... I truly felt like I was dying. And now, because of this machine with a plastic bag of water and glucose hanging on it, pumping through the needle in my vein, I was feeling alive again... feeling okay. I closed my eyes and thanked God for getting me through it, and I drifted off into a little nap, with a strong request to please not let it happen again.

Mom came in quietly, but the rustle of her paper sack woke me. I looked up at her smiling at me, and adjusted myself to sit up a little. I was looking forward to seeing what she found for me to eat.

"Well, I found some apple juice for you..." she pulled it out of the sack and handed it to me. "And some cold bottled water." She set it on the table attached to her chair.

"Mmmm, thanks Mom..." Apple juice was one of my favorites, but I sipped it slowly.

"I bought both kinds of trail mix so you could choose..." She handed both bags to me, and I chose the one with raisins in it.

"And for your salty snack," she said with a smile, "how about crunchy Cheetos?"

"Ohhh, thanks Mom!" I reached out for the bag and ripped into them.

She had bought some chips and soda for herself, and we sat in the dim-lighted room having a kind of picnic and talking about how much better I felt already, just from having some fluid added to my body. She made me promise to drink more water, no matter what.

It was arranged that for the next five days or so, I would arrive two hours early for my radiation treatment in order to sit in the exam room while I received much-needed fluids. I gave a quick wave of goodbye and thanks to the nurses and radiation therapists as we walked toward the main waiting area and the exit. I felt way too tired to walk up all those steps to the door, so we took the small elevator to the left of the stairway. It seemed a little silly, because it was only a stairway of about 20 steps, but it was just too much for me. We stepped into the tiny elevator, just big enough for a couple of people and a wheelchair. The elevator doors opened a few feet from the main exit, we strolled out, and I wearily planted myself in the car for the 50-mile drive home.

I still felt nauseous through the night, with no energy to do anything but lay in bed. The next day was the same routine, shuffle out of bed and head to the hospital. We arrived about 11:45, and they took me straight in to check my vitals, draw some blood for labs, and get me started on fluids before my treatment. I weighed 158 pounds. I'd never been so skinny. My blood pressure was low, my pulse was high, and my temperature was 96.5, so low that my nurse, Beth, checked it twice. I received another neupogen injection, and some extra Zofran to try to help with the nausea. I asked for Benadryl so I could sleep while the saline dripped into me for two hours, and Mom sat beside me in the quiet darkness. I ended up sleeping through my appointment time for treatment, but since I never slept well for very long, Mom and Beth thought it was okay to let me sleep and rescheduled my treatment for 2:15 that afternoon. I woke about 2:30, feeling as if I'd been asleep for days.

"What day is it?" I asked Mom.

"It's still Thursday..." she whispered.

"What time is it?" I felt like it must be evening.

"It's 2:30."

"Thanks...so now what?" I didn't hear the clicking of my IV machine. "I still have to get radiation..."

"Yeah, Beth said she could keep pushing your time back until you woke up. I could go and check with them... maybe you can go in now that you're awake."

"Yeah, just ask her to come in, so I can talk to her." I liked all the nurses in Radiation Oncology. They were friendly and easy to talk to, and didn't mind taking the extra time to talk with me if I had questions and concerns.

Mom went to get Beth, while I adjusted myself in the chair and took a drink of ice water from the Styrofoam cup.

It was about three o'clock before I was able to get in, but I was glad to have had the solid two-hour nap. It's not like I had anywhere else to go, anyway. When I came out from the treatment room, Mom was waiting by the nurses' desk. We learned that my white blood cell count was high enough that I wouldn't need any more neupogen shots for the week. That was decent news.

Mom could see I was feeling like crap, so she didn't say anything as she walked a little behind me. I headed straight for the elevator, then ambled to the car without talking. She walked ahead and opened the car door for me. I adjusted the seat to recline and lay my head on the small throw pillow we kept in the car. I shifted to one side, trying to make the nausea go away. "Thanks, Mom," I said.

She looked over at me. "Want some peppermint?"

"Yeah, maybe."

She took a box of Altoids from the console and opened it up. The sweet smell enticed me, and I took one from the box. "Thanks."

"You're welcome." She looked at me, making sure. "Are you feeling okay for me to drive now, or should we wait?"

"I'm okay. Let's go." I dreaded the long drive, but I just wanted to be home.

8

Winning is Everything, but Everything is about Cancer

I slept most of the night, and still felt like shit the next day. Mom woke me for my morning meds. I sat up on one elbow in my bed, swallowed them with a single drink of water, then lay back down, thinking about the day ahead. I had a noon appointment at the Cancer Center to receive a dose of bleomycin before getting my daily radiation, and I was dreading it big time. Mom brought me a piece of lightly toasted bread and a small cup of apple juice, and encouraged me to sit up and try to eat. The feeling of nausea churned from my stomach all the way up through my esophagus to the back of my throat, but I munched on the bread in small nibbles like a rabbit. I took tiny sips of the juice, hoping my stomach wouldn't recognize that any substance was being put into it. I wanted to lie down and sleep again, but Mom kept on me to move, stretch, get my blood circulating.

"Mom. Enough." I snapped at her. "You don't understand. I can't. You don't know how bad I feel."

She looked sorrowful, but concerned, "You asked me to help you, Ian, to keep on you to do what the doctors say. You said you knew you would need me to push you, remember?"

I looked at her, giving her a slow blink and slight roll of the eyes as

I turned away. I sighed, agreeing with my thoughts that she was right. "All right, I will," I said in a not-so-grateful tone, "but I just want to lay here for a minute."

I lay quietly and thought about the fact that I had to keep pushing myself. No matter how bad I felt, I had to keep moving. I eased my legs over the side of the bed and sat up again. I prepared myself mentally to stand and walk to the bathroom without getting sick. I washed my face and brushed my teeth lightly. My gums had been sore and swollen from the chemo, so brushing was painful. Instead of asking Mom to get my clothes for me, I did it myself. I opened my closet and pulled out some clean underwear, socks, jeans and a shirt, and took them with me to sit on my bed. I needed to rest a minute before getting dressed. I was just sitting there thinking, when the nausea suddenly became too strong to hold back. I dashed to the bathroom a few feet away and threw up on the sink, on my way to the toilet. I spewed yellow vomit across the floor, the toilet paper, and the toilet seat. I was pissed as hell, but too sick to express it. I pulled my dirty shirt off and hung it over the shower door, rinsed my face and mouth, then stumbled my way back to bed. I just laid there, head throbbing, stomach aching, back hurting, and thoughts of frustration cluttering my mind.

Mom had been upstairs getting dressed and ready to take me to KU. When she came in my room and saw me lying there, she knelt down beside me and looked at me compassionately. She felt my face with her hand, then the back of her fingers to see if I felt hot or cold. "I'm sorry, Ian. I'm sorry you feel so bad. I was just trying to help you." She pulled my blanket up over my shoulders.

"Sorry..." I said weakly, "I threw up all over the bathroom. It's still there."

"Don't worry about it... I can clean it up." She adjusted herself to sit on the floor. As she looked at me, I saw a sorrow, her love and the pain that she couldn't help me. She took my hand and held it close to touch her face. "Can I get you anything?"

"No, thanks."

She kissed my hand and stood to go clean up my mess. I heard her in there, spraying, wiping things, and flushing it all away. She came back to sit on the floor near me again, and rested her head on the bed next to me for a while.

"Mom, I'm so tired of this," I said, weakly.

"I know, honey. I'm sorry," she whispered. She kissed the back of my hand and held it to her cheek for a second. "I know you don't feel up to it, Ian, but we'll need to leave in about 20 minutes," she reminded. "I'm going upstairs so you can change clothes."

The car was warm, but I still felt cold during the drive to KU. I covered up with the afghan Mom kept in the car for me, and tried to sleep my way there. The closer we got to the hospital, the more sick I felt. I sat up during the last five miles or so, and as we pulled in toward the hospital entrance, my stomach was ready to leap out my mouth. I asked Mom to drop me off at the Cancer Center entrance before she parked. I thought I could make it to the bathroom in the main waiting room, but I didn't even get inside the doors. As soon as I closed the car door, I could feel it coming up. I stopped near the wall at the entrance, and there it all came, pouring out of my mouth, right in front of everyone walking outside. I felt weak and dizzy, and braced myself with one hand against the cold cement wall, to keep from falling over. My stomach hurled everything it had, leaving a puddle splash of yellow green colored matter on the concrete sidewalk just in front of the glass doors.

One of the receptionists saw me, and ran out to help me. She first asked if I thought I could walk on my own, and when I nodded yes, she took me straight back to the treatment rooms so I could recline in a treatment chair. She said I could wait there and my nurse would be in soon. The staff wasted no time in getting my vitals checked, and making sure I was comfortable. Mom had trouble finding a place to park, so by the time she came in and found me, she was a bit unraveled with worry. My nurse came to get me started with Zofran in my port to help with the nausea, along with the fluids I had to receive before chemo. After talking with her for a few minutes, the nausea came over me again, and Mom saw the look on my face. She reached for the trash basket near me and held it up for me. I leaned over the side of my chair and the smell of the plastic in the basket made me feel even worse. I felt so embarrassed with her and the nurse standing there, but I couldn't help it, I just kept vomiting. Finally it was over, and I pushed the trash basket away. The nurse left and Mom walked over to the hand sink nearby and ran some cool water over a couple paper towels and brought them to me. She went back and retrieved a few more to wipe off the arm of my chair, then she washed her hands. I was so embarrassed it pissed me off. I just laid my head back and closed my eyes. I wanted to scream obscenities at the world. I wanted to disappear. Mom knew that mood, and didn't say a word. She knew not to even touch me when I was so upset with myself. She went to get me a warm blanket and extra pillow, as she always did in the Cancer Center. She offered the pillow to me and unfolded the blanket to cover me up. I loved those heated blankets. I felt instantly relaxed as she draped it across me. She pulled the curtain closed, shut the window blinds, turned off the light above me, and sat quietly next to me. We sat silently for a few minutes, and I rested my eyes, trying to get my head to stop thinking about how bad I felt. My embarrassment and frustration subsided, and I looked over at her. "Thanks, Mom." I extended my hand to her.

She squeezed my hand and smiled, "You're welcome, Ian," she said softly.

I just laid there looking at her for a couple of seconds, then I shifted my head and closed my eyes again. I could hear all the noises and voices of the Cancer Center going on outside my little treatment space, and as I drifted off to a light sleep, the sounds faded into nothing more than background clatter. The nurse woke me when she came in to hook my little bag full of bleomycin up to my port line, but after that, I tried to doze until it was over. Mom gave me some earplugs to help muffle the noise of the busy cancer treatment center.

After the bleomycin treatment was finished and my port flushed, Mom and I trekked through the winding corridors to the other side of the hospital for my radiation treatment. I didn't feel too bad, and the walk was good for me. It was the usual drill. I had to first receive the fluids for two hours, then my radiation.

The monotonous routine was draining. The drive to and from KU each day was getting to both me and Mom. There were a few days when the snowstorms wouldn't stop, and travel advisories were to stay off the roads if driving could be avoided. Mom hated driving in bad weather, and navigating the icy, snow-packed blizzard on the highways tied her up in stressful knots. But we never considered missing an appointment. Every day, we just got up and did it. Mom drove in silence while I slept. I still didn't want the noise of radio or conversation. I didn't even want to be aware of the drive, because I hated the routine and the reason. She told me once that she sometimes felt like a transporter of precious cargo, which had to be treated just right, no bumps, no noise, no sharp turns. When we finally reached home, she felt she could relax and be Mom again. I missed driving my car, but I did not feel like driving at all. I felt too sick, too weak to think about it, pushing in the clutch, shifting, steering—that was way more work than I felt I could handle.

One day, I woke feeling pretty hungry, and pleased that I didn't feel very nauseous at all. I asked Mom if we could leave early and stop at Burger King for breakfast. On our way there, we drove past the Hy Vee grocery store where I had worked in my junior year in high school. I gazed over at the parking lot, the row where I used to park my car for work, and at the building, the entrance, and in my mind, I saw the produce department where I put in my time. "That was fun working there," I said to Mom.

"Yeah?" she looked over. "It sure was fun shopping there and seeing you! I loved it when you would find me in the aisles and put things in my cart that you wanted me to buy for you!" She smiled at me.

"Yeah." I chuckled. "That was fun. Good times..."

The parking lot at Burger King at ten o'clock on a Tuesday morning was empty, so Mom parked the car right in front of the entrance. We sat near the middle of the restaurant with our bacon and egg croissant sandwiches, milk, and cinnamon rolls. It felt so good to have an appetite and to be able to sit in a restaurant like a normal person having a nice conversation and enjoying my food. I wasn't able to finish my cinnamon rolls, though, and offered them to Mom. She noticed the subtle look on my face, the look I took on when I felt nausea creeping in. She asked if I was going to be okay, and I said that I thought I'd be all right as long as I didn't eat any more. I pushed my tray aside, while Mom quickly finished her food. We sat for a minute or two, just talking. I looked over toward the play area where we used to take our food when I was a kid, and it seemed like a different lifetime ago when I climbed around in the giant tubes and ball pit, playing hide and seek with Mom as she ran around the structure to catch me coming out of one tube or another.

I looked at Mom. "That was so long ago...when we used to play in there. I can't believe I was ever that little."

"Yeah," she smiled at me, "more than ten years ago... it's hard to believe, isn't it?" She thought for a moment. "Remember all those times we went to play at Tunnel Town?" she chuckled, "My knees hurt for days after an afternoon crawling around in that place, but it sure was fun."

I went there in my memory, the seeming miles of twisting and turning giant hamster tubes, slides, ropes, and a variety of adventure and play areas. "I loved that place."

We sat quietly for a moment, then I decided I was ready to go. I felt okay when we got up, threw away our trash, and walked to the car. Mom unlocked the passenger door for me and walked around to the driver's side. I had just opened the car door to get in, then threw up everything I had just eaten.

As Mom opened her car door, she looked at me from over the top of the car and saw me leaning over a little. She looked through the car to where I was and saw that I was standing there with all my breakfast pouring out at my feet.

I wiped my mouth, sat down in the car, and closed the door. I covered my face with my hands, hiding in disgust, and rubbed my face as if trying to wipe away the stress, then I just sat there, completely depressed and fed up. "This is so fucking embarrassing," I mumbled. "I'm so sick of this shit."

Mom was sitting quietly, waiting for me to tell her what I needed. Her car door was still open. "Do you think you're okay for me to drive?" she asked cautiously.

"No." I said drearily and shaking my head slightly.

"Okay, I'm just going to move back, away from here, okay?" She gently closed her door, put the car in reverse, and slowly pulled straight back to a parking space at the other side of the lot, near a row of trees. "Now at least you have a little privacy." she said.

I opened my door and swung my legs over to lean out. I felt like I was about to throw up again.

We sat for a moment. "What do you think made you sick all of a sudden?" she asked.

"I don't know. Just the smell of the car, I guess. I opened the door and the air came out at me, and it made me throw up."

"Is it a bad smell? I don't smell anything."

"No, it doesn't smell bad. It's not even a smell, really... just like air, only different from the outside air, and it bothered me for some reason. I don't know how else to explain it."

"I'm going to run inside and get you some ice water, and tell them there's a mess to clean up there."

"No, don't tell anyone! They'll look out here at me."

"Don't worry, honey, they can't see you way over here, now. But they need to know, so they can clean it up. I can't just let it set there, right in front of the entrance. I'll explain it to them, that it wasn't the food. You wait here, I'll be right back."

I sat in the car, my feet on the blacktop, my elbows on my knees, looking at the ground. I felt like a moron, spewing up my entire meal right in front of the entrance to a restaurant.

She came back and handed me a napkin and a small cup of ice water, and said the workers inside had been understanding. We stayed there for a minute or two, making sure my nausea had subsided. When

I felt ready to get moving, she drove us out through the back of the parking lot, and we headed to KU.

By the time we got there, my head had started hurting again, and the nauseous feeling was hanging on, unfortunately. But the routine droned on, receiving fluids, Zofran and Benadryl, and having blood drawn for labs before my radiation treatment. Dr. Alvarez and Dr. Klish both visited with me, and I told them about my headache and the ringing in my ears for the past couple days. Neither was concerned greatly about those things, saying that the ringing was most likely caused by the radiation and expected it to stop after treatment was over. As for the headache, I should report one that does not go away. Other than that, they are to be expected. There was an MRI and a CT scan in my near future, though.

I was resting while the fluid dripped into me, when Dr. Klish came in and asked if I was hungry. I was, actually, since I'd left my breakfast in the Burger King parking lot. He said he had some pizza that he'd be happy to share with me if I was interested. That sounded pretty good, and I accepted his offer. He asked what kind I liked best, I told him pepperoni was my favorite, and he soon returned with two big pieces for me on a large napkin. We visited while I started on the first piece. He said a patient had bought pizzas for the entire department as a thank-you gift, and there was plenty if I wanted more. I ate half the first piece, but couldn't finish because I felt very tired and a little nauseous. I put the pizza down on a stool next to me, and stretched my recliner back, and slept the time away.

The next day I was feeling better, and found when I went early to receive the fluids, I didn't need them anymore. I weighed in at 168 pounds, and my temperature and blood pressure was back to normal. So Mom and I sat in the car, passing the hour in various ways, resting, talking, listening to music. Mom asked me what I was going to do first when I was told I was officially cured of cancer.

I looked over at her and thought about it for a second, imagining the joy we'd be feeling at that news, hearing those words from Dr. Van... then I smiled at her and said, "The very first thing I'm going to do is hug my mom."

She smiled back. "Yeah," she said, "that's going to be a great day. That'll be the first thing I want to do, too. What's the second thing you want to do?"

"I want to go to one of those places that has a lot of food, you know?... where you go and eat anything you want?"

"You mean a smorgasbord?"

I looked at her like she had lost her mind. "What the hell is that?"

"It's where they have all kinds of food."

"No, not that, I mean like a place you go to eat, where there's a lot of food and you eat as much as you want."

"That's a smorgasbord."

"No, no.... I mean like a restaurant."

We just looked at each other. I saw her realize what I was thinking.

"OH! A buffet!" She laughed.

"Yeah! That's it. I want to go somewhere like that and just eat and eat and eat."

"Yeah... okay," she nodded, "Well, a buffet then... yeah, we'll find the best and biggest one." She shook her head and smiled, "I don't know why that word wasn't in my head. That's what a smorgasbord is, but nobody calls them that anymore," she mused. "Hey, remember that one time, you were about ten years old, and you found what you thought was nacho cheese on the buffet, and you got yourself a big bowl and some chips..."

A smile came to my face as I remembered the moment. "Yeah..." I laughed. "I'll never forget, I dipped my corn chip in it and took a big bite... freakin' French salad dressing! Mark and the girls were cracking up at me, the look on my face..."

"You were so cute, but I felt sorry for you. You were looking forward to eating nachos, and then you looked so sad!"

"Yeah..."

"So what after that? Think of two more big things you want to do to celebrate being cancer-free."

"I think I'd want to go rock climbing or something, you know, like we always talked about doing in Utah or Arizona? Then I'd probably go on another trip with my friends. That was fun, me and Jared and Keaton, when we went to Daytona Beach our senior year. I'd like to do something like that again, only maybe go to the west coast this time."

Mom smiled and nodded. We talked about what kind of rocks we'd like most to climb, and about our plans to one day hike into the Grand Canyon. Ever since I was a little kid, Mom and I had often gone on trips to find large rock formations to climb and play on. We learned to belay and rappel at a rock climbing gym, and often talked that someday we'd use those tools out in the real world, on real rocks. Eventually all that dreaming made me tired, so I laid my seat back to rest until it was time for me to go in. I knew the routine would take me only about 15 minutes, so I told Mom just to wait in the car while I went in for the treatment. When I was finished being radiated, I scuffed back to the car, and we endured the long quiet journey home again.

On Friday I had another appointment for a bleomycin dose in the Cancer Center, and Dr. Van met me in the treatment center for a checkup. He said my blood counts were low, and I would be getting one of those delightful epoetin shots in my arm to help with red blood cell reproduction. I would still get the dose of bleomycin, though. And the best news of all, my Beta hCG count was all the way down to 641! That was the best news ever! It was still too high to call myself in the clear, but it was actually in the hundreds, not thousands! It was very close to zero, from my point of view. The fact was music to my ears.

Mark, Mom, and I celebrated the reward of my perseverance, hugging and smiling as they cheered me and I soaked up the good feelings of relief and excitement of getting close to my goal.

I actually didn't feel too bad during the weekend following. I was getting more active, no shortness of breath, no nausea, and no bathroom trouble. On Monday, I asked every doctor I saw if it would be okay for me to drive. Dr. Alvarez had told me that I should not drive while being treated with radiation, but I felt fine. I couldn't get it through my head that having a seizure while driving was an actual possibility. It seemed very remote to me, so I tried to find a doctor who would agree with me. Mom was amused at my persistence, because each time I asked another doctor or nurse, they had the same answer. No.

That same Monday in the Cancer Center, I learned that my white blood cell count was too low, and my tumor marker, beta hCG had shot up to 1,244. Dr. Van was not overly concerned at that slight increase, even though it had doubled in only four days. Tumor markers will jump and drop frequently, and an increase by six hundred or so was not that much to worry about. The numbers rising by a few thousand would be a cause for alarm. He said I was looking at potentially two more courses of chemotherapy after the one coming up, but that treatment plan would be re-evaluated after this course and another CT scan. My platelet count was too low to receive the upcoming chemo on Wednesday, but he would re-evaluate that with more labs in a week. I felt fine, so we didn't worry about the numbers. I just tried to keep doing what I had been doing, and hope the numbers would look better in a week.

I wanted to try going back to work. I missed having a normal life. Believe it or not, I missed going to work. On top of that, my boss, Gina, had said she was going to have to hire someone to fill in for me, and that scared me. I was afraid that once my position was filled by someone else, I wouldn't have a job when I was ready to work again. I had already lost all my hair, my muscular strength, and the life I was living before cancer. I didn't want to lose my job, too. I asked Dr. Van if I could return to work on a limited basis, and I called Gina to talk it over with her. She agreed to let me try working while she was there with me, but needed a note from Dr. Van saying it was okay. I was looking forward to feeling real, like the old Ian again. I thought being at work would be a great thing.

Since I couldn't have my chemo treatment on Wednesday, Mom dropped me off at work, and just walking in made me feel better. Working as a shipping clerk there was an easy job for me, over all. I was good with math, computers, money, and small talk. All I had to do was think, pay attention, and get along with all the customers. Gina was like Mom, standing by, watching my every move to make sure I was okay. I was there for about 45 minutes, then I started to feel weak and nauseous. I wanted to fight those feelings, to work through it and stay, but Gina said I was looking pale and sick. Even though I argued with her that I was fine, she called Mom to come pick me up. I had to admit, it was way more draining on my energy than I ever thought it could be, and that was extremely depressing to me. After that, Gina suggested I take care of the cancer first, and she would make sure I had a job when I was ready to go back.

My daily radiation treatments got me out of the house, but I was feeling restless to get out into the world. Just walking around the block for exercise was pretty boring, and by Friday I told Mom I thought I was going to go crazy if I didn't get out and do something normal.

"Hey... want to try going to the mall?" Mom asked. "We can get you a new hat or something... and if you feel like it, we can get a pretzel or have some lunch!"

My white blood cell count was normal, so I didn't have to worry as much about contacting germs in a public place. I knew not to touch surfaces like doors, banisters, and drinking fountains. And I had a good habit of using the hand sanitizer that I always carried in my coat pocket. I figured going to the mall and walking around would help me to feel a little better.

I thought for a moment... could I handle walking around the mall? I loved those giant hot pretzels. I tried to remember who I was with, the last time I had been to the mall. "Yeah, let's go." I looked at her. "Can we go right now?"

Walking into the giant shopping center was like walking into the past for me. "I can't believe it's been like four months since I've been here," I commented to Mom as I looked around. It felt unfamiliar, yet familiar at the same time. "I want to get some sunglasses while we're here, too." I glanced around at the nearby kiosks.

"Is there any particular store you want to hit first?" Mom's intent was all about me.

"Let's go to Hollister's... it's over there." I pointed to the other side of the mall. We didn't keep pace with the shopping crowd, but shuffled a little slower. I did not want to run out of energy. I felt great to be in the midst of what felt like the rest of the world, and I wanted to hold onto it as long as I could.

"I love this store," I told Mom as we walked in. "It's my favorite."

She smiled as she followed me and looked around, letting me lead the way through the racks and tables of clothes. We used to have a lot of fun shopping together when I was younger. She was good at choosing clothes and colors that looked best on me, and I always found ways to make her laugh with my joking comments, character impressions, or silly antics. Of course a guy gets to the age where he feels uncool shopping with his mom, and she missed doing that. She used to ask me if she could go with me once in a while, back before I was diagnosed. The answer was always, "No, Mom. A guy my age can't shop with his mom."

It was different now. I felt older than I was. I felt more like I was shopping with a good friend, than a parent. It was nice, just hanging out, doing something in the real world together.

I came to the shelves of baseball caps and stood looking at them all. One by one, I tried them on, and looked in the mirror, then at Mom for her thoughts. We narrowed the choices down two by two, and the winner was a white hat with Hollister embroidered above the left side of the bill.

We stopped into one of those novelty shops with all kinds of weird gifts, and wandered through, sharing comments about all the funny things on the shelves. I picked up a Jamaican-style hat that had dark brown dread locks attached to it, and I put it on my head and stood behind Mom waiting for her to turn around and see me. I made a silly face and she laughed and took a picture of me with her cell phone. We got a few laughs from the clerk, and had some fun joking around with him.

We stopped at a DSW shoe store, and Mom bought me a new pair of shoes with a gift card she'd been saving for me. We also went into a couple of my other favorite stores, and across from one of them was a kiosk of sunglasses I had been hoping for. I went through the same routine, trying on a couple dozen pairs, checking in the mirror, then looking at Mom for her opinion. She liked most of them, but I settled on a pair of turquoise mirrored ones, and some amber night driving lenses.

We were on our way over to the giant pretzel stand when we passed Lady Footlocker, a store I had applied to for a second job about a month before I learned I had cancer. I had received a call from the manager of the store when I was in the hospital the day after my diagnosis, asking me to call back to set up an interview. I had completely forgotten about it until that moment.

"Hey, Mom... I want to stop in and see if the manager is in there, I want to talk to her and tell her that I didn't just blow off the interview. I want to see if she still wants me to work there, you know, once I get done with all this."

I peered into the store from the mall to look for the manager. "She's there. I'm going to go in. Just give me a minute, okay?"

Mom said she'd wait for me on a bench outside the store. She watched as I walked up to the pretty brunette manager and introduced myself again, thinking that she wouldn't recognize my thinned out face and bald head. She did remember me, and smiled a big smile as we shook hands. I explained to her why I had not been in touch with her, and that I was still interested in the position once I had fully recovered from the cancer in the spring, if she still wanted me there. She assured me she still felt I was right for the job, and asked me to check back in with her when I felt ready to work. I came out of the store feeling promise for my future, and proud of myself for having made such a good first impression.

On the way to the pretzel stand, Mom and I talked about how we both thought I would like working there, and how it would be a good opportunity for me to meet all kinds of new people. I would look forward to it.

The pretzels were warm, fresh, and salty, and especially good with warm cheese dip. We pulled a couple of chairs up to a small table at the stand, talked and ate, and watched the people go by. It was a really good day, but even though we had only been there a couple of hours, I was getting very tired. I decided it was time to go home after we finished our pretzels.

As we walked toward our car in the parking lot, I asked Mom if she'd let me drive home. I was so tired of being chauffeured around. I wanted to feel driving again. Mom wouldn't break down.

"All the doctors say no, Ian. They all say no. Let's respect that, okay?"

Well, I tried. Usually I could persuade Mom to do almost anything, but she wasn't folding on this one. I slid into the passenger seat, put on my new hat and looked out at the world through my new mirrored shades. I flipped through the radio stations as we drove homeward, and as we were sitting at a traffic light, I looked over at her.

"Thanks, Mom... for everything."

She looked at me and smiled. "You're welcome, Ian. Thank you for thanking me."

When we arrived home, I had to take a nap before trying to call any of my friends. I felt very fatigued, but I still wanted to get together with some of them. I didn't want my life to go on without me, my friends getting together without me. I didn't want to be left out, even though I already felt that way. And even while a few of us were hanging out on Saturday, I never really stopped thinking about my situation.

I looked forward with angst and excitement to my Monday

appointment in the Cancer Center. I was due for a chest x-ray, blood work, and to see Dr. Van Veldhuisen. If my blood counts were all right, I'd be admitted to the hospital to start my fourth round of chemotherapy. Dr. Van had discussed with me earlier that I would not necessarily need to be admitted for continued treatment, since I had tolerated previous treatments pretty well, but I didn't feel good about that idea.

Sunday night, Mom and I sat in my room talking about the coming course of chemo and the idea of having radiation each day, the effects of it, and the possibility of having to endure the chemo treatments as outpatient this time. Just the thought of driving home from KU after having both radiation and BEP treatments made me feel very sick. I didn't know if I could do it.

"It scares me so much, Mom." My eyes filled up with tears as I continued to share my fears of the unknown with her. This would be my first experience with having five straight days of four-hour chemo treatments plus radiation every day. We voiced our thoughts, wishes, and still wondered why. Why me? Why now?

"What have I done to deserve this, Mom?" I asked, mournfully. "I mean... I think I've been basically a good guy, happy, fair, honest for the most part... I just wonder why cancer chose me..." I paused, gathering the whirling thoughts in my head as Mom waited and listened. "I feel like an outcast, like I've been segregated from everyone else because of cancer... not because of the way my friends are, but because now I'm so different from all of them. I feel like I don't belong anymore, like I don't fit."

I could see the compassion in her face, and the sorrow in her eyes. "You're not being punished, Ian. I think you've been given a strange gift that is making you stronger and wiser. You're going to come out of this stronger than you ever thought you could be, and you'll love life even more than you did before."

"Well it definitely has changed me and the way I see things and think about life." I nodded thoughtfully. I looked at Mom, and could tell she saw my deep thoughts were about to be spoken. She looked intently at me. "Mom, sometimes I feel like I'm not even in my body like I used to be. I feel like I'm not really a part of anything around me, like none of it is real, except me, like I'm in another dimension. The only place I ever feel like it's real is here at home..."

She smiled slightly with the corners of her mouth, looking sad and sympathetic, but listening closely and compassionately to my every word.

"And I don't even feel like me anymore... I mean when I look at pictures of me from the past, even August and September, it's like I'm not looking at myself, but at some other guy, like an old friend of mine, but not me. That guy... I'm nothing like that guy anymore... and even when I look at myself in the mirror, I look so different than I did before. Not because I don't have hair, but I look like a completely different person... I've changed so much that I can even see it on my face..."

I noticed Mom was biting down on her lower lip to stop her eyes from crying, a trick she told me she learned almost ten years ago when I left for that trip to Belgium with my fifth grade class. She kept listening.

"Then there's those times like when we're driving down the highway and I'm just looking out the window at the trees and all the clouds, taking in the scenery... and I get a tingling kind of rush down my spine... because I'm realizing how beautiful it all is, this world, and how cool it is to be here. I never felt that way before. I was just living my life, so busy and kind of taking it all for granted, you know, the trees and the grass and the sky. I didn't take the time to really look at the world. But now it looks so different."

"Do you like it?" Mom asked.

"Yeah! It's really cool.... I appreciate stuff I never thought about before... I can't explain it, really... I just feel so different now... everything looks different to me now."

Mom kept looking at me, listening. I looked off in thought for a moment as we sat quietly.

"You know it's nice to have someone to reflect things back to me, someone to just listen.... Thanks... sometimes when you're asleep I'm just lying here talking to myself. I do so much thinking now."

She smiled, "You know I have always loved listening to your voice, your words, your thoughts. That will never change because I love you so much. You are my son, Wonderful You."

"Thank you, Mom." I smiled at her. Wonderful You was one of her nicknames for me, ever since I was in about the fourth grade. I liked it when she called me that.

We sat still, looking at each other for a moment.

It was about one in the morning. We had to be at the hospital at 10:00 a.m., and decided we should get some sleep. I was too tired to move from my couch to my bed three feet across the room, so Mom handed me a couple of blankets from my bed, turned off the lights and made herself comfortable on her floor pallet of blankets near me.

"Good night, Ian. I love you." She took hold of my hand and kissed it.

"Good night, Mom. I love you, too." I felt grateful as I looked at her, then closed my eyes and hoped to sleep through the night.

9

Uncertainty, Cancer's Offense

Mom had our bags packed in the car, in case we needed them. I hoped the hospital would allow me to be admitted to start my chemotherapy instead of having to endure it as an outpatient. As long as insurance would pay, and they had a room for me in Unit 42, it could happen.

Mark left work and met us in the Team Center waiting room after I'd had my blood drawn. I semi-slept while he and Mom waited, playing hang-man games on the back pages of her notebook. I was getting crabby and uncomfortable at the long wait, but it was as routine as all the rest. My port site had been sore for a few days, so Mom made a note to remind me to ask Dr. Van about it. There was also another question she wanted me to ask.

Smoking marijuana was a subject that Mom had concerns about since I'd been in college. We'd had plenty of anti-drug talks through my years of growing up, and she knew I drank alcohol, but I had never had a problem with serious drug abuse. I knew how she felt about my smoking though, and she sometimes still warned me about it. I assured her I was just going through a phase, that I wouldn't smoke for the rest of my life, and that I'd get tired of it after a while. "Everyone smokes pot when they're in college," I reasoned. "Don't worry about me, Mom, I'm smarter than that... I won't keep doing it." I had never smoked around her, or in our house, but one very nauseous day, I decided it didn't matter anymore. She had gone to the store, and I hoped she'd understand.

I was lying in bed when she came down into my room. "Ian, why does our house smell like weed?"

"Why do you think?" I muttered. I wasn't really looking forward to the conversation.

She sat on my couch, biting her lip and looking sorrowfully at me. She didn't know what to say.

"It makes me feel better. A lot better. It makes the nausea go away." I looked at her hopefully.

She was quiet.

"Mom, please... it's not so bad, is it?"

"I'm not sure what Mark would say about it. But I don't really like our house smelling like a drug house."

"I'll try to find a way to keep the smell down, okay? Then will you be okay with it? Please, Mom. It really helps."

Because of the cancer in my lungs, she wasn't sure it was the right thing to do. "Let's talk to Dr. Van about it first. If he says it's okay, then, I'll be okay... okay?"

"Thanks, Mom." I reached my hand out to her. She knelt down beside my bed. I took her hand and looked her in the eyes. "Thank you."

Finally, my name was called, and the three of us shuffled through the waiting room to the doorway where the nurse greeted us. I knew to step on the scale first thing. I weighed 169 pounds, and all my vitals checked out okay. She ushered us down the long hallway to the exam room, where we waited for Dr. Van. Mom reminded me of my questions for him. Dr. Van had arranged for me to have a chest x-ray immediately after our office visit, and said he would look at the port site when viewing my lungs to check for healing progress. He asked me other routine questions about how I'd been feeling, and when the subject of nausea came up, I looked at Mom.

"Well, Mom wanted me to ask you about this..." I started nervously, "About... marijuana..." I stopped and looked over at him to catch his first expression.

He just looked at me, thoughtful, waiting and listening. I continued, "I think smoking marijuana has helped me to not feel so nauseous, but she's afraid it will make the cancer worse. I was thinking that it wouldn't hurt me, because other cancer patients do it, but she wants your opinion." He paused to consider his thoughts. He told me that as far as they know, there are no adverse effects with treatment, and it won't deplete the immune system, so if used in moderation, it may even help to boost my appetite, which would be helpful. He did not recommend it though, and that made Mom nervous about allowing me to smoke. Mark felt the same way and was concerned about legal issues, but I heard what I wanted to hear, and they both tried to be okay with it. Mom admitted that it was good not to see me throwing up nearly as often as before.

Dr. Van suggested Marinol tablets, a synthetic version of the THC in marijuana, as an alternative to smoking. Mom and Mark were more comfortable with that option, and I agreed to try it. Dr. Van said he would give me a prescription for it. After a pause to make sure we all agreed, he then said my blood counts were okay, and that I could be admitted to Unit 42 after my x-ray and radiation treatment, if that was what I wanted to do. Again, I handed my jewelry to Mom, and she and Mark waited while I had the x-ray in the Cancer Center, then walked with me to Radiation Oncology.

After my radiation treatment, Dr. Alvarez met with us in one of the exam rooms. He was concerned about the x-ray report he had just read, which indicated a right lung pneumothorax, also known as a partially collapsed lung. He said he was still checking on the information and would be back as soon as he knew more.

"I don't feel so good..." I murmured. The news had made me feel sick to my stomach, weak, cold, hot, and dizzy. Mom commented that I suddenly looked like I felt sick, and moved the trash basket close to my chair. She laid her coat over me, and went to the sink to moisten a paper towel and put it across my forehead. I reached up and touched her hand, and pulled the paper towel over my closed eyes. "Thank you..."

"Can I get you some water... a peppermint or something?"

"No... thanks."

Dr. Klish stopped in, and I shifted the paper towel to see him. He said after the CT and MRI evaluation, they would plan a boost radiation treatment for me, which is extra strong radiation targeted to visible lesions. It's technically known as an IMRT, or Intensity Moderated Radiation Treatment. I had become fairly okay with the idea of radiation by that time, so extra radiation didn't scare me too much. It actually made me feel a little confidence that the overall treatment would be more successful with it.

Dr. Alvarez came back in. He said only five percent of my right lung was collapsed, according to the radiologist from the x-ray department upstairs. It was a small portion, at the top of my lung.

"What exactly does that mean?" Mom asked, hoping it wasn't actually as bad as it sounded.

Dr. Alvarez explained that a pneumothorax is basically accumulation of air in the pleural cavity, the space between the lung and the chest wall. There is supposed to be a little air, but sometimes it accumulates in one spot and causes pressure in that area of the lung, which can cause shortness of breath and chest pain.

I asked what would cause it. He explained that sometimes it is caused by injury, but that was not the case with me. He added it could possibly be an issue with the catheter in my chest, or could also be caused by the cancer itself, and that sometimes, there is no known cause at all. In any case, the CT scan scheduled for the following day would reveal more detail if there was any to be seen. Dr. Alvarez said it was known as a "non-tension" pneumothorax, meaning there was no ongoing accumulation of air, but a pocket just stuck there. It would have been severe if the air continued to accumulate with each breath I took, but he said that was not occurring, so it was not an emergency situation.

Mark, Mom, and I all looked at each other with a little bit of relief, but still very concerned. Dr. Alvarez assured us that as long as it doesn't get worse, it could resolve on its own. He instructed me not to do anything too strenuous if I still feel chest pain or shortness of breath. He excused himself to leave the room, we shook hands, and I assured him I would follow those orders.

I looked up at Dr. Klish, and thought back to the day when I first noticed the pain in that area.

"Do you think doing push-ups would have caused it... I mean a problem with the Port-a-cath that would have caused it?" I asked him.

He looked at me with a little concern as he took a breath. "You were doing push-ups?" he asked.

"Yeah," I admitted, "They told me not to lift anything or strain my pecs, but one day I got so depressed that all the muscles in my arms are gone. I felt like such a weakling, and so mad about it, that I rolled out of bed and started doing push-ups." I looked up at him, feeling guilty.

He smiled sympathetically, "How many did you do?"

"Only about five. It started to hurt really bad right here, so I stopped." I pointed to the area just below my port site where the pain was.

He nodded that he understood my frustration, "Well, that may have been what caused you some pain there, but I don't know if it caused the situation with your lung. I haven't seen evidence that the catheter has been disturbed or moved at all to cause a problem in the lung, and that would have shown up on the x-rays..." He thought for a moment, then continued, "But I would lay off that heavier type of exercise until the catheter is removed. You want to be careful with that. You can try lifting small five or ten-pound hand weights without straining those pectoral muscles."

I gave him a disappointed roll of my eyes and looked back at him. "Five pounds?"

"I know," he sympathized... "What did you used to bench?" He asked with a smile.

"One-ninety."

"Impressive." He gave me a nod. "What was your max?"

"I don't know, like two-thirty."

"You'll get back there," he encouraged. "You will, just give it time."

"Yeah..." I smiled a half smile. "Thanks." I stuck out my right hand.

Dr. Klish shook each of our hands, then he left the room and we headed upstairs to the admitting office.

It was about 6:00 p.m. that evening when I was admitted to room 4220. Mom was still getting us settled when Dr. Fleming came in. He first said he wanted to test my beta hCG levels again, and that Dr. Van wanted to re-stage the cancer before starting this round of chemo. He said they would review everything after my CT and MRI the following day. There were concerns that the lesions in my lungs were not shrinking fast enough.

I was pleased to see that my nurse for the night was Mark. While he was getting my IV set up, an x-ray tech came in with a portable unit to x-ray my chest while I lay in bed. Mom looked at me sympathetically and held her hand out to receive my jewelry. This x-ray would give a different view from the one I'd had earlier. Everyone else had to leave the room for a couple of minutes while that was done, and then Nurse Mark continued to access my port to start me on hydration about ten o'clock that night. Mook left for home, Mom prepared her chair-bed, and I flipped on the TV to entertain myself until I fell asleep.

At 7:30 Tuesday morning, my day nurse brought in a large Styrofoam cup of the chalky contrast solution I had to drink prior to my CT scan. I felt so nauseous and nervous that I was afraid to drink it. It sat on my table, waiting for me. A couple hours later my nurse brought my meds for digestion and saw that I still hadn't emptied the cup of contrast. I told her I was afraid it would make me throw up. I had come to seriously dread throwing up. She let me know that she understood, but there was no getting out of it. I had to have the CT scan before I could start chemo treatment, and I had to have the contrast solution for the CT scan to show anything.

After she left, I asked Mom if she could find a little something for me to eat, hoping it would help my stomach to feel less queasy. She came back from the nurses' kitchen with three small boxes of cereal for me to choose from, a half pint of milk, and a bowl and spoon. I chose Fruit Loops, and ate all of them. They actually did make my stomach feel a little better. When my nurse came in to check on me, I told her I felt a little better after eating the small bit of cereal, and she reminded me that I wasn't supposed to eat anything before the CT scan, although she thought that such a small amount of food might not be a problem. She left me with a strong order to drink the chalky substance in the cup.

At eleven o'clock, a transport came to wheel me downstairs to Radiation Oncology to have my MRI done. Mom waited in the room for me, and when I got back about 30 minutes later, the cup of contrast was still waiting for me. I sat on the edge of my bed, set my mind to swallow all of it, and told my stomach to be okay with it. Then I took one look at Mom, raised a toast to myself, and slammed it down. I wiped my mouth and lay back in bed, praying the nasty tasting substance would just keep moving downward, stay in there and do its work.

I rested in the quiet until Dr. Fleming came in about one o'clock that afternoon. He examined me and asked how I'd been feeling. He said the beta hCG level in my blood had risen to 4,000. He felt that was too high of a rise, that it shows the cancer is not responding to the current treatment, and that my treatment would most likely be changed, meaning different chemotherapy drugs would be used.

Shortly after he left, the transport came to give me another wheelchair ride to get my CT scan done, and from there I would be taken to Radiation Oncology to receive my daily dose of radiation. It was almost two o'clock when I returned to my room. I felt very hungry, but way too wiped out to eat. I laid my bed back, and slept.

Dr. Van Veldhuisen came in about 6:30 that evening. He confirmed that he would be changing my treatment because of the increase in tumor markers. He mentioned that sometimes smoking marijuana can cause a false increase in beta hCG counts. That in mind, he was still treating the rise in my count as if it was due to the cancer. I told him that I didn't think I smoked that much, only a couple of times each week when taking the Marinol wasn't enough, and he commented that I might want to keep that fact in mind, anyway. Once they had re-staged the cancer, he would let me know more about my new treatment plan.

By dinner time I was starving for something to eat. I called the cafeteria and ordered a peanut butter and jelly sandwich, two boxes of Captain Crunch cereal, a dish of pears, and a pint of milk. I ate it all and felt okay, which was a great relief. But I was feeling very anxious and nervous about the news from my doctors. Mom asked if I wanted to talk about it, but I didn't want to face it. I felt like my heart, my soul were mourning with fear. To think that the cancer growing in me was getting stronger despite the drugs... the drugs that were strong enough to kill me. I didn't want to think about it. I knew Mom was praying for me. I tried to sleep, saying silent little prayers in my head, asking God to help me. My sleep was pretty restless through the night. I woke up many times and just lay there thinking in anticipation of getting some answers in the morning.

By five o'clock the next morning, I was exhausted and very sleepy when the hospital staff started buzzing around. My breakfast was brought in about 8:00 a.m., but I was so tired I didn't want to eat. Mom encouraged me to eat something, even just a little eggs and potatoes if I could. I tried my best, but the nervousness in my stomach wouldn't allow me to eat much. I felt like throwing up, and I didn't want to go through that, so I drank a little of my apple juice and pushed my tray table to the side. I lay back and closed my eyes, drifting off into a light sleep.

About eleven o'clock that morning, the scary news started coming at me. Dr. Fleming came in to introduce Dr. Skikne from Hematology. He explained that the coming treatment would be more aggressive drugs. I would be receiving them as an outpatient, because the treatment regimen was different from the CEB treatments I'd been getting. Instead of receiving a four-hour treatment every day for five days, I would get a four-hour treatment only once a week. My recovery from treatment would be more difficult and longer in duration. It was planned that once my body recovered from this intense chemotherapy, my new stem cells would be harvested and kept to give back to me when my body had become completely unable to recover on its own. I had become a candidate for bone marrow transplant. I couldn't believe it. I never expected my news to get so much worse.

A resident doctor and another doctor from Hematology came to visit me later that afternoon and asked me plenty of questions. I told them I had recently had a nose bleed, and coughed up a little bit of blood. I also told them that my port was hurting, I had some head-aches, some nausea episodes, and that I couldn't breathe very deeply. I learned my exact beta hCG was already 4,255. That was an increase of over 3,000 in just one week. The hematologist talked to me about what they call "salvage chemotherapy," which is when they slam heavy amounts of chemo into the body to force it to replenish a larger sup-ply of white blood cells. At that point, they go in and take some of those stem cells in the bone marrow and freeze them for later use. They do this because the ongoing chemotherapy will gradually deplete the body's ability to do this on its own, and it will then need the saved stem cells put back into the bone marrow to help it rebuild itself. Once again, my head was spinning with fear of what was going to happen to me.

It was arranged that I be discharged from the hospital and return to the Cancer Center on Friday to start my new chemotherapy. I would get one dose of gemcitabine and paclitaxel once each week for three weeks, then one week off to allow my body to restore itself. After ten weeks of that routine, I would have some stem cells extracted, fol-lowed by larger doses of chemotherapy. I would not be reunited with my stem cells until chemotherapy treatment was completed in early spring.

While we were waiting for my discharge orders that afternoon, I told Mom and Mark that I couldn't believe I was being released from the hospital because I was too sick. It seemed bizarre and backwards. My cancer was worse, so they were sending me home. It was hard for me to come to grips with the fact that I had to change treatment because the cancer cells would not die. Dr. Van had said that I had most likely become platinum-resistant. That meant the cisplatin, the heavy metal, wasn't inhibiting the cancer growth at all anymore.

At home I thought about it, over and over. I thought so much that I got tired of thinking about it, because I grew more and more depressed. I did my best to accept what was happening to me, and I tried to keep a cool attitude about all of it, but the truth was my head was full of more fear, stress, and dread than anyone could have known. I looked for ways to help me forget the seriousness and escape the stress, and being with my friends and playing in our band were two things I missed most.

I still had my scheduled radiation treatments each day, and on the way home from my treatment on Thursday, I told Mom the news I'd received about the band I had been playing with before my diagnosis. Crimson would be playing its last show together that coming weekend. I shared with Mom that I hoped I would feel well enough to play with them. I had missed several shows in the past three months, and I was mentally preparing myself to play with them on their last gig, no matter how bad I felt. Mom, of course, was understanding, but had reservations about me in that potentially stressful and unhealthy environment. After all, the cancer was still getting worse. I didn't want to be concerned about that. I just wanted to be a part of the last show. She accepted my enthusiasm for it, though, and we put the conversation on hold until the day of the event.

The next day as Mom and I drove toward KU Cancer Center, my stomach grew more and more sick with the thought of a whole different set of chemotherapy drugs being injected into my body, and my uncertainty that they would kill the cancer. I stared out the window at the bare trees and brown grass along the cold gray highway, and wondered how in the world I was going to get through it all. My fears grew more intense the more I thought about it, and about how broken I already felt. It was definitely going to get worse.

We parked near the Cancer Center, entered through the main

lobby, and walked through the winding hospital corridors to Radiation Oncology for my regular appointment. When I was finished there, we walked back through the hospital again to the Cancer Center. I figured I wouldn't be able to do that all the time, but as long as I felt strong enough to walk the distance, I was willing to give it a try.

We went in through the back entrance to the Cancer Center, down to the other end of the long stretch of hallway, and around the corner to the nurses' desk in the treatment center. Michael recognized me and called the nurse who'd be taking care of me. She first took me into the lab to stand on the scale. I weighed 169 pounds. We then followed her through the grid of white-and-black tiled hallways to a private treatment room.

The private rooms were a 9-by-9 foot space. They each had a treatment chair, and most of them had a bed, along with a couple of other chairs for visitors. There was a TV in the wall above the sink and cabinets. Some rooms were separated by a thin wall, others by a glass wall covered with the green leaf print curtains. The entrance to each room was a wall of sliding glass doors to cut out the noise, and a floor-to-ceiling curtain for added privacy. There was at least one framed piece of art in every room. Some rooms had windows, but as always, I wanted the blinds tightly shut and the curtains closed to cut out as much light as possible. If there was a bed, I chose that over the chair, and I liked that we could close ourselves into my dark, quiet personal space.

I lay in the bed, and Mom pulled a chair up close to me. An aide came in to check my vitals, and after she left, my nurse came in carrying a syringe.

I was about to get a shot of epoetin. I couldn't stand the thought of it. Mom knew I'd need something to grip while the injection burned and stabbed its way through my veins. She stood near my head and offered me her left hand. We clasped hands, I mentally prepared myself... I thought, and told the nurse to go ahead.

The pain hammered into my arm, my bones, shooting through me like an electric current deeper into my shoulder, my arm, and fingers of my right hand. "Slower! Not so fast!" I ordered my nurse. I writhed and kicked my leg down hard on the bed. "FUCK!" I yelled out through clenched teeth, as I squeezed Mom's hand to deal with the pain. The nurse stood by until I visibly started to relax, then she quickly cleaned up and left the room. I let go of Mom's hand and looked up at her. Her eyes were filled with tears.

"I'm sorry, Mom... I didn't mean to hurt you." I breathed out heavily, feeling bad for her.

"No, no, Ian, it's okay... my tears are for you... I just didn't realize how bad that pain was for you... until you squeezed my hand so hard, and it makes me feel sad that you have to feel that much pain."

I didn't even realize how hard I had squeezed Mom's hand until later that afternoon, when Mark came to sit with us while I was receiving treatment. I saw her showing him the bruises on her fingers from my clenching hand, which was twice as big as hers. He was apologizing to her that he hadn't been here, then.

"What? You have bruises?" I was concerned.

"Oh, it's not bad, they're just little ones," she admitted.

"Let me see," I demanded.

She reluctantly offered her hand, spreading her fingers out to show me what she was talking about. "See? Just a little spot there on the knuckles of these two fingers." She pointed with her other hand, to the small bruises on her pinky, and middle finger. There was a tiny blood spot from a cut on the inside of her middle finger.

"Did I do that, too?" I asked, feeling like crap.

"It's just from my wedding ring, it cut into me a little bit, that's all. It doesn't hurt, honey... don't worry about it, I'm fine."

"I'm sorry, Mom. I didn't mean to hurt you."

"Ian, don't worry about it, please. I was glad I could be here with you... and I'm glad I was able to feel that, because now I have a better understanding of how horrible that pain is for you. I'm glad you squeezed my hand so hard."

Mark sat down in a chair near the head of my bed and patted me on the shoulder. "I'm sorry I wasn't here, Stretch. I didn't know you were going to have to do that before getting your chemo."

Dr. Van Veldhuisen's nurse, Kathy, came in to talk to us about Taxol and Gemzar. She took time to hear my concerns and answer my questions concerning the severity of side effects. I was mostly concerned about feeling worse than I already had in past months, and I looked for her confidence that these new drugs would set me free of cancer all together. Kathy was very kind in her way of telling me that these drugs were often very successful in killing cancer cells, even in lung cancer patients, but that it was very important that I follow doctors' orders and call her if I noticed any severe side effects. She pointed to all of them as she read them to me, making sure I was listening and understood her concern.

Taxol and Gemzar are drugs used to treat many other cancers, including lung cancer. To get me started with pre-meds, then hydration, then post-hydration, the total treatment time would be about five hours once each week.

Taxol, also known as paclitaxel, is among the plant alkaloids. An alkaloid is a plant compound that is toxic. Alkaloids can have physiological effects that make them useful in medicine and are used both in pharmaceuticals and were used in ancient medicinal practice. Caffeine, nicotine, codeine, and morphine are just a few common plant alkaloids. Taxol was originally derived from the bark of the rare Pacific Yew tree. The problem was that there were not enough of those trees in their native Pacific Northwest forests. The bark from a single tree yielded only enough Taxol for about one dose, so an alternative synthetically produced compound using the common Yew was developed. It works in a similar way as the other drugs I had been receiving, by interrupting cell division. To think, the ornamental shrub that grew outside my bedroom window could be a source of a drug to kill cancer.

Gemzar, also known as gemcitabine, is in the family of antimetabolites. Think molecules. A metabolite is required for normal biochemical reactions, like cell division and growth. An antimetabolite has a similar structure to a metabolite, yet it's different enough to interfere with normal functions of cells, including cell division. It screws up the DNA synthesis a cell needs in order to divide, causing cell death.

Just when I thought I had the cancer treatment game all figured out, this new line of treatment was bringing up a lot of new questions in my mind. I had heard of whole body radiation, and I felt good about the way it was working on my brain tumors. Dr. Van stopped in to see me while Kathy was still there, and I asked if radiation was an option to help get rid of the tumors in my stomach. The answer was no. The soft tissue in the lungs and other organs would not tolerate the high levels of radiation I would need. There was just too much cancer growing in me from the very beginning. I asked if I might be a candidate for the Cyber knife, or radiation injections, and the answer was also no, because there were too many lesions in my body. It would be impossible to target each of them individually, which is what those treatments are for. I was stuck with chemo and a stem cell transplant. And I knew it was going to be hell.

By the time Nurse Kathy left, my stomach felt like one big tied-up knot inside of me, and I felt I was going to throw up at any minute. Mom offered me some ginger and some peppermint, but I didn't want either of them. I was so mad at always needing something to make me feel better, and the fact that the results were always temporary. I lay quietly sulking, resigning myself to getting used to feeling like shit.

After about 20 minutes in silence, my nurse came in and gave me my pre-meds, accessed my port, and hooked me up to a bag of saline fluids before my chemotherapy was started. And for the next four and a half hours I just lay there, a nauseous, aching pile of bones and skin, with bags of seriously toxic drugs dripping into my veins, as my blood carried the drugs to every cell in my body. I felt like every sigh was a little prayer that God would get me through it, and every ache was a question if he even cared. I dozed, while Mom and Mark sat silently in the dark, waiting with me.

It was six that evening when my treatment was finished. Mark walked with us to the car. We drove him to pick up his truck parked in a distant parking lot, and started our long trip home. As always, I slept while Mom drove in the quiet. We arrived home about 7:00 p.m., and I was glad to be there. It had been a long day. You would think after lying around all day in the Cancer Center that I'd have some energy to sit up and do something, but I just wanted to lie down in my bed and be quiet. I had a headache and felt completely exhausted. I was bummed that it was Friday night, and friends were calling and texting me, but I didn't have it in me to get together with anyone at all. I was even too tired to talk on the phone. Mom gave me some acetaminophen for my headache, but the pain just seemed to get worse through the night. It even woke me up a couple of times.

The next evening, I talked to Mom and Mark about my playing with Crimson in their last show together that night. They both felt the same way. It was crazy, they agreed, to just think it was okay to go into a smoke filled bar in the city and play an entire set. It wouldn't be good for me. There were too many negatives, they said. I could contract a virus, or there could be a fight, or someone could throw something on stage, or something bad could happen on the street while we were loading or unloading our instruments. There were dozens of things that could happen to make my cancer worse. I laughed and told them they worried way too much. None of those things were going to happen.

"You didn't even have the energy to talk on the phone last night, Ian. How can you say you are well enough to do a show?"

"Mom, I want to do this more than anything else. This is my last opportunity to play with the band! This is going to be our last show together, forever... I have to be there! I can't miss it!"

She just looked at me, and thought for a long moment.

"What time do we have to be there?" Mom asked.

"I don't need a ride, the guys are picking me up." I started shuffling through my gig bag, making sure I had what I needed.

"Okay. Mark and I will be there," she said calmly.

"No, I don't really want you guys to be there. You've seen the set a dozen times, it's the same set list we always play."

"But I love watching you play! Don't we get to see you play in your last show? I want to be there too!"

I rolled my eyes. "No, Mom. No." I shook my head and looked at her. "I'll be fine. All the guys will watch out for me. You've been there.

You know it's a safe place, with a good crowd. Everything will be okay. And you know my white blood cell count is up, so I'm not going to get sick if someone sneezes on me. I don't feel as bad today... I feel okay to play, and I want to. I need to. Please let me have this, Mom. This will be good for me. I need to live my life. I need to be who I am without my parents always taking care of me wherever I go."

Mom stared at me. Her eyes looked very sad.

"Mom," I said with my best persuasive look and calm voice, "Please be okay with it. I'm going by myself. I need to do this." I had always been good at talking her into letting me have my way.

Mom still just looked at me, sadly.

"Promise me you won't go," I said.

She still just looked at me. I could see she was afraid.

"Mom... I'm 20 years old in two weeks. I have to feel like this is mine, my life... without my Mom and Dad watching over me."

"Please, Ian," she pleaded, "I would love to see you play your last show together... and I'll feel so much better if I know you're okay. I won't let anyone see me, I'll stay way in the back and I won't even try to talk to you after the show."

"Mom." My voice was a little stern. "No. If I know you're there, it's just going to upset me. It won't be mine... it will be like needing you in the hospital, Mom, and I don't want to feel that way. Don't go. I'll be fine, I promise. They're coming to pick me up in a little while, so I need to get my stuff together."

She heaved a heavy sigh and gave in with her one compromise. "Promise you'll call me after the show, Ian. Don't make me wonder. Keep in touch with me."

"I will." I extended my hand to her, and she stood up from my couch. I wrapped my arms around her and gave her a long reassuring hug. "Thank you, Mom. Everything's going to be okay."

The show did go well, and we had a lot of fun. After the show, I went with some friends to a party not too far from where we played. I stayed outside to smoke a little before going in. I didn't want to feel any pain or have any cares at all. I just wanted to have a good time. I didn't know anyone there except the guys I was with. I didn't call my Mom right away, either. I just wanted to be Ian without having to check in with anyone. I was so damned tired of being a cancer patient. I wanted to forget all about it and escape for a while. Sometime later, we went out to the car again, and I smoked a little more. I started coughing so bad that I had to open the car door, and I leaned out and threw up all over the pavement. At that point, my friends started to realize how sick I really was, and they suggested we call it a night and go home. I wouldn't have it. I insisted we stay. I didn't care how sick I was. I didn't want to be the cancer patient who had to go home because he couldn't handle it anymore.

I did send Mom a text message later, though, and told her I would not be home. I added that I'd had so much fun! I hoped that would put her mind at ease. I didn't want to go home and feel like a suffering cancer patient. I wanted to stay out, live life, and not worry about anything, and if I started to feel sick again, I could smoke a little more. She didn't want me staying out, of course, but there was nothing she could do. She reminded me to take my evening medications, and I sent a text back that I had.

I was home by eleven o'clock that next morning, and most of my Sunday was spent laying in my bed, feeling the familiar effects of nadir trying to creep in on me. We did have to drive to the Cancer Center so I could get another neupogen injection, but other than that, I had no will to go anywhere or do anything at all. Just the activity, the drive, being there in the Cancer Center, and the pain that followed that injection felt like it took way more energy than I had to spare. I slept the rest of the day recouping from my eventful Saturday.

I weighed in at 167 pounds in Radiation Oncology on Monday afternoon. Dr. Alvarez had good news for me. He told me I would not be needing the IMRT radiation boost after all, because there was a great tumor response to the ongoing radiation. He said he would add a few extra treatments to my current regimen in case there were any undetected lesions. He thought that would be enough, and I liked the idea. The report from the MRI done on my brain stated there was near complete resolution of the tumors, basically meaning that no old or new lesions were visible.

"Can I see? Will you show me the images?" I asked. It had been pretty scary looking at the cancer lesions in my brain less than a month earlier. Dr. Klish mentioned he had been impressed with my serious, concerned, and yet calm nature when I first viewed the increased number of tumors growing in my head a month before. It wasn't that I didn't believe they were gone, but I wanted to see it for myself... view the good news with my own eyes.

We followed both doctors to the conference room, and Dr. Alvarez pulled my brain images up on both screens. On the left was a past impression, and on the right, the latest image of what appeared to be my cancer-free brain. Dr. Alvarez explained that he felt there was no threat of the cancer continuing to grow. I would still be receiving extra radiation treatments to make sure that tiny lesions, if there were any, would be destroyed. Even after the treatments themselves were finished, the radiation would continue its effects for several weeks afterwards. I was okay with that, considering it meant being sure the cancer was truly gone. I would continue with a few more daily treatments, then radiation would be over.

Mom and I looked at each other. I felt relieved and happy at what I saw, but it was as if I was afraid to smile, afraid it might not be true. Then Mom's smile broke that fear away.

"You did it, Ian!" she celebrated.

I smiled at her, and then looked over at my doctors, who were both smiling, too. "Thank you," I said, very sincerely. I looked at the image on the right again, and nodded as I looked back at Mom and smiled.

I stood and extended my hand for her to stand with me. She wrapped her arms around my skinny rib cage, and I turned to her and wrapped my long arms around her, and just hugged her for the longest time. I felt so happy and relieved, and Mom was so happy she didn't want to let go of me.

Dr. Alvarez closed my file and turned off the monitors. He and Dr. Klish both stood, and each of them gave me a hearty handshake and sincere hug of congratulations.

All my suffering had finally paid off. I was so pleased about the news that the rise in tumor markers barely phased me. My tumor markers had risen and dropped before. I felt certain that could happen again. After all, my brain was going to be okay from now on, and I was almost done with radiation for good!

This was the greatest news yet, and for the first time in two months walking out after radiation treatment, I felt myself smile as I gave a wave to the nurses and admitting rep. As we walked to the car, I was feeling anxious to share my news. I thought maybe we could catch Mark at the office, which was only a couple of miles away.

"Hey, Mom... do you think we could stop by Total and see if Mark is there? I want to tell him in person, and I don't want to wait till he gets home."

"Sure we can," she smiled. "Call him and see where he is."

I pulled my cell phone out of my pocket and searched for Mark's number. I had him listed in my phone book as Mooky-Mook. "Do you think anyone else will be there, like Gary?" Gary was Mark's boss, the owner of the construction company, and a close family friend. It would be cool to be able to tell him the news myself, too." I dialed the number and Mark answered right away.

"Hey, Stretch! What's up?"

I didn't want to give it away on the phone. "Hey, where are you? Are you close to the office? Me and Mom want to stop by."

He said he actually was headed that way and would meet us there. He didn't ask, but I told him I had some good news.

Gary and a couple of other employees were there when we arrived, and we stood visiting until Mark walked in. After a little small talk among the guys, I announced I had some good news. They all turned their attention to me, and waited.

I looked at Mark, then glanced at Mom and the rest of them... "All my brain tumors are gone," I smiled. I glanced around at them again, and back at Mark. It felt great hearing those words coming out of my own mouth. I couldn't stop smiling as everyone smiled back at me, congratulating me with kudos, handshakes, and hearty pats on the back.

After visiting a little while longer, Gary invited me, Mark, and Mom to sit in his office, and we had some good laughs remembering stories about old times. Gary was also the head coach of all my Pop Warner league football teams for six years until I started playing for my school in seventh grade. Mark was the defensive coach, and together they made us a great team. We had a lot of fun, and some good memories to talk about for years to come. Mom was friends with his wife, Kathy, and over the years they had all shared a lot of good times, watching our football team and hanging out together.

Gary was happy for us, and for my good news. He suggested we go out to dinner on him to celebrate, and handed Mark enough money to buy dinner for the three of us. Mark didn't want to accept it, but Gary said he sincerely wanted to treat us to a special dinner. It was his gift to me for a victory well deserved. We asked him to come with us, but he insisted we go, just the three of us. There was only one place I wanted to go—my favorite Mexican food restaurant, called Manny's, just a few minutes from where we were.

We sat in a booth near the window, had nachos, iced tea, and my favorite, beef enchiladas with rice on the side. I loved putting the nacho cheese on my rice. We talked about this and that, taking some time off from what seemed to be our normal focus on my treatment and state of being. It was nice to just sit and talk, eat and drink, like all the other normal people in the restaurant. I felt pretty good for a change. I ate almost all my food, and didn't even feel nauseous when we were finished. As Mark paid the bill, Mom and I walked past the hostess desk and I picked up a toothpick and a piece of candy for each of us. And as soon as we got outside of the restaurant, I played my usual trick on Mom, dropping my candy wrapper in her purse when she wasn't looking. I made sure she always caught me, and we'd both laugh, pushing the wrapper back and forth at one another, stuffing it into any pocket we could reach. This particular time, she smiled at me and I grinned back. She picked the wrapper out of her purse, kissed it, and put it back in. I swung my right arm around her neck and pulled her close, as we three smiled and strolled through the parking lot. It was a good day.

That evening as I was in my room slathering my head with aloe vera, I commented to Mom that I was looking forward to getting the radiation over with. My scalp was peeling like a serious case of sunburn, and even the skin on the outside and inside of my ears was red, dry, and cracked. I'd been smearing aloe vera on my head two or three times a day, but it didn't feel like it was helping that much. The inside of my ears itched so often that I started keeping a small box of Q-tips on the floor next to my bed. I hoped that without the daily exposure to radiation, my skin could begin to heal a lot faster.

I was too exhausted to have a social life, and my activity in the week ahead consisted only of driving back and forth from my radiation treatments every day. I was just too damned tired and nauseous to care about doing anything else. At the end of the week I'd get my second dose of Taxol and Gemzar after my radiation treatment. I was hoping for good news about my tumor markers on that day.

10

Arsenic

On Friday I had to arrive at Radiation Oncology an extra 30 minutes ahead of my appointment, so someone could draw more of my blood for labs. That way the results would be ready when I went upstairs to the Cancer Center for chemotherapy after my radiation treatment. It was a cold, wintery day, and I did not want to go out in it. Mom stopped in front of the entrance to let me out before she parked the car in the small, registered patient parking lot. It was especially nice to be able to park so close on such a cold day in February. The frigid air followed me in and down the stairs to the waiting room. I sat on the couch shivering, and Mom soon ran downstairs as if the cold air was chasing her.

When the nurse called me in, she told Mom it was okay for her to come back with me while she drew my blood and took my vitals, if she wanted to. I was cool with it, and Mom liked to write down all of my vitals and anything the nurses said about me. After that, she waited for me on the couch near the receptionist while I had my radiation treatment. Mom always looked at me attentively as I walked out the double doors from the treatment area and offered a slight wave to the receptionist.

We opted to drive around to the Cancer Center instead of walking through the hospital. I felt too tired to make the trek. It took all my energy to walk up the stairs and out to the car. On our way around to the other side of the hospital, Mom asked me if I felt any different after a radiation treatment.

"Yeah, a little, but not that much." I laid my seat back and closed my eyes. "Why?"

"I don't know... it just seems like there's something different about you afterwards... I mean something in you, but I don't know what it is."

"Yeah..." I replied, still reclining with my eyes closed. "I can't describe it, but it's not that much." I shifted a little to get comfortable. I did feel different in some way, but I didn't even want to try to describe it. I didn't want to think about what radiation was doing to me outside of curing the cancer.

Mom had thought I looked as if something, a part of me, had been taken away from me, or altered in some not-so-good way. Not that I looked physically different, just that something about me was different than anything she had ever sensed in me before. It was very unsettling to her to see that in me, kind of eerie, she thought. Maybe it was that I threw up almost every time after the treatment, and she was just seeing the result in me from that, the way my face looked, and the way I carried myself after heaving whatever was in my stomach. It was so very routine, and I had gotten used to it and accepted it as part of the routine, but I still hated it... I still grew very tired of it, and disheartened by it. I'm sure my feelings affected the way I looked, and the overall energy about me.

We were starting our third month in visiting the Cancer Center, and Mom had just recently learned that cancer patients were allowed to park at the curbside directly in front of the Cancer Center. It was news we could have used long ago, but there were only about four spaces along that curb, and rarely was one available. On this very cold day, we were both glad to see a curb side space open just a few feet down from the Cancer Center entrance. The icy wind whipped around the concrete pillars and practically shoved us inside, as the glass doors of the entrance slid open. I walked past the large reception desk and waved to the three people working there. They all knew me by that time. I went straight to the bathroom adjacent to the waiting room and threw my guts up, again. They told Mom we could go back to the treatment waiting room when I came out, and she sat waiting for me in a nearby chair.

When I stepped out, I stood and waited for her to stand, then she followed me to the receptionist desk in the treatment area. Michael told me to go ahead and make myself comfortable in room 15 just around the corner. This was one of the private rooms, with three walls and a glass front with a sliding door and curtain. I was glad to have a bed to lie down in.

"I'll go and get you a warmed blanket and extra pillow," Mom said softly.

I just nodded. She turned off the light, and I heard the squeaky sound of the curtain being pulled shut, and the glass door sliding closed. I laid there in my silent space, just wanting to get it all over with. Dr. Van would be in to visit me before my chemo was started, and Mark would be joining us soon.

Mom returned with my blanket and pillow, and told me that my nurse would be Shari, one of my favorites. She was compassionate, friendly and mellow, and good with a needle. I had grown to greatly value anyone that could stick me in the arm or port in a way that I could barely feel it. Just knowing I would have a nurse I liked took my stress level down a couple of degrees.

An aide came in to check my vitals, and Shari came in to take more of my blood for beta hCG labs. They drew for tumor markers only in the Cancer Center. My blood that was drawn downstairs in Radiation was for all my other labs... a complete blood count of white and red blood cells, hemoglobin, platelets, and the like, including the counts of other elements in each cell. Plus they looked at the enzymes, and the chemistry, like potassium, glucose, calcium, magnesium, and a number of other things. Most of my counts were usually in the normal range, except for my blood cell counts, which were almost always on the low side until I'd had a few of those torturous shots. Shari told me that Dr.

Van would not be in to see me until he had seen the lab report on the beta hCG, and that it would be at least an hour. I resigned myself to nap away the time. Nothing more would be done until Dr. Van's visit.

Mark arrived at some point during my hour long nap, and I woke to see him and Mom sitting quietly beside me. Mark looked like he was napping, too. Mom looked at me and smiled slightly when I opened my eyes.

"Is Dr. Van here?" I asked, meaning had Mom seen him in the Cancer Center.

"I haven't seen him." Mom shook her head.

Mark opened his eyes and looked over at me. "What's up, brother-brother?" he asked as he reached out to take my hand.

I reached up to him and he leaned in to give me a hug.

"Just waiting for Dr. Van to get here," I said, feeling a little impatient and nervous.

"How are you feeling?" he asked.

"Really tired... and kind of sick to my stomach... but kind of hungry, too." I looked at Mom. "Hey, Mom, do you think you could find me something to eat?"

"Would you like a sandwich? They brought your sack lunch in while you were sleeping," she said. She stood and picked up the small brown paper sack from my bed table. Every cancer patient received a complimentary sack lunch during their treatment time, at the lunch or dinner hour. They were usually a meat and cheese sandwich, some chips and cookies.

"What kind of sandwich is it? Is it ham?" I was feeling hopeful. I didn't really have an appetite, but my stomach felt hungry, and that just added to my misery.

Mom opened the sack and pulled everything out. She unwrapped the sandwich and took a look between the pieces of bread. "It's turkey and cheese on wheat bread."

I thought about it. "Let me see it."

She held the sandwich toward me and showed me its contents. It had mayonnaise on it.

"Na." I shook my head with a look of dissatisfaction. "Will you go to the cafeteria or the gift shop and see what they have?"

"Sure," she smiled. "I'm taking my phone, so call me if Dr. Van comes in, okay?" She looked at Mark.

I didn't even know what kind of food sounded good, I just wanted something familiar, something I knew I liked. "You know what kind of stuff I like, okay? Just get me whatever you think I'll like..." I instructed her, as if she needed it.

While she was gone, I lamented to Mark about how I felt like I was spending my life in the Cancer Center and radiation treatment, and how much it sucked to be spending my entire day there. I was so tired of being sick, and sick of being tired. He looked at me and listened, and gave me a pat on the shoulder. I reached my hand up to touch his.

Mom returned, stepping into my room quiet as a mouse. I looked up at her, hopeful that she'd found something I felt I could eat. She smiled a happy smile at me.

"Well, I hope you like what I found." She set her paper sack down on my bed table, and pulled out a small one-serving box of Raisin Bran, a bowl, a spoon, and two half pints of skim milk.

"Mmmmm! Mom! That's perfect, thank you! I didn't even think about cereal." I slowly sat up on my bed, smiling at the thought of eating it. I eased my feet over the side of the bed to sit at the table.

Mom opened the box and poured the contents into the bowl while I opened the milk. I looked at the cereal, it looked good, and I felt a little bit of an appetite. "Thanks, Mom," I said again after taking a swig of milk, "You always know just what I want." I smiled up at her as I took the bowl. She looked happy to see me smiling and wanting to eat.

She sat down in her chair next to my bed, and the three of us talked while I ate... well, mostly I ate, nodding my head in agreement once in a while as I listened to the two of them talk. Mark didn't like mayonnaise either, so he ate the chips and Mom ate the sandwich, tucking the cookies in her purse in case I wanted them later. We were having a good moment, and they had both helped me to feel better.

I finished my bowl of cereal, drank some milk from the carton, and feeling full and satisfied, laid back with the head of my bed raised up a little. I asked Mom to turn the light down again, and closed my eyes. Mom and Mark sat quiet, and I felt okay for a little while, but it wasn't long before the feeling of nausea was starting to sneak up on me again. Shari came in to check on me and to let me know that Dr. Van was in the Cancer Center, so I could expect to see him within the hour. Mom took hold of my hand and we all sat still in the dark with our eyes closed, waiting.

About 45 minutes later, we heard a slight rap on the metal door frame, and heard the door slide open and the curtain pull back, letting in the light from the hallway. Dr. Van nodded and smiled hello to Mark and Mom, then turned to me.

"How are you feeling today?" he started.

I told him about my fatigue and nausea, and he nodded that he understood. He stood quietly looking at me for a moment, waiting or looking for more information.

"Can you sit up a little..." he reached for his stethoscope and moved a little closer to me. He listened through my back and my chest, and also my abdomen after I lay back down. He asked me the usual questions as to whether I'd been feeling any shortness of breath or chest pain at all, any coughing of blood, and inquiring about the degree of pain, fatigue, and nausea I'd been experiencing. He gently felt around on my abdomen and lymph node areas, then he stopped to look at me again.

I looked up at him, waiting for the good news.

"Your white blood cell count was too low today," he started. "I've put in orders for you to receive neupogen here at the Cancer Center every day for five days, starting tomorrow."

I closed my eyes in a long blink, and looked away briefly. When I looked back at him, I felt my disappointment showed clearly on my face. This meant we had to travel to the Cancer Center even on weekends when I didn't receive radiation treatments... over an hour on the road just to receive a ten-second injection.

He sat sideways on my bed next to my legs, and faced me, folding his hands in his lap. He silently looked at Mom and Mark, then back at me. Then he spoke softly. "Your tumor markers have shown an increase..." he said, looking at each of us again.

"How much?" I asked right away.

"Your beta hCG today is quite a bit higher... over 14,000." He delivered the not-so-pleasant news in his calm demeanor, but I could tell he was displeased. He paused, and we each sat quietly looking at him.

My beta hCG had shot up by almost 10,000. All I could think was, 'fuck.'

"It's too early into the new treatment to make any decisions based on the increase," he spoke slowly and quietly, looking directly at each of us, "so we're going to continue with the current treatment. I do expect that number to decrease by your next treatment, and we'll check your beta hCG again in a week." He paused again, allowing the space and silence to let the news sink in. There was a confidence in his mild manner, and I hoped he was right. "I also want to do a chest x-ray on Monday, so I'll have my nurse schedule that for you before your radiation treatment, if that works for you." He looked at me, then at Mom, and we both nodded in agreement.

I felt intense depression, but I tried holding on to what Dr. Van said about it being too early in the new treatment to know if it was working or not, that we have to give it time. I let his words stay in my head, that the tumor markers would decrease by the next treatment. I counted on it, and let myself believe that the chemotherapy would do its work. But after he left, I thought about the horrible news and couldn't stop my tears. I smashed my hands into my face to press the pain away. I didn't want to believe it could get worse. Mom and Mark both stayed strong for me, even though the news was hard on them, too. Mark stayed seated near me, and Mom sat on my bed next to me, holding my hand and looking down at the floor. I just laid there with my eyes closed, trying to keep my faith in my treatment. Neither one of us said a word for a long time, but their presence gave me a comforting strength.

The rattling sound of the rolling cart announced the aide arriving to take all my vitals, and so the all-too-familiar process began. Mom moved back to sit in her chair beside me. Shari came in with my pre-meds and fluids, and before long I was sleeping through the steady four-hour drip from the crystal clear bags filled with Taxol and Gemzar. Mom noticed my file sitting on the table near my bed, and discovered that the price of that one daily dose of Taxol was a little over 83,000 dollars. She couldn't believe it, and had to stare at it for a while to make sure she was reading it right. The insurance payments on my treatment were still in the processing stage, and even though we knew my treatment was very costly, those numbers were something we had not yet had to face. We had kept our focus on the treatment being successful. Mom had said she'd gladly spend the rest of her life paying for it, if it would save my life.

I slept most of that drive home, and once we were there, I fell into my bed and slept some more. That weekend, I didn't leave the house except for the ride to the Cancer Center to get my shot of neupogen. I was too nauseous and tired to care about doing anything but lying still or sleeping.

My appointment for the x-ray on Monday was at 12:30, with an-other injection of neupogen in the Cancer Center. I was not feeling very well at all after that injection, and I asked my nurse if I could just sit in the chair for a while until it was time for my radiation treatment. My ears had been hurting me a lot in the last couple of days, and I told my nurse that. She notified Dr. Van, and his nurse practitioner came in to take a look at my ears. She said they were very red inside with in-flammation, and there was fluid behind my right eardrum, most likely caused by sinus pressure and drainage. She prescribed an antibiotic, saying that there was probably some infection due to the drainage. I hoped it would work. I didn't know how long I could take that pain and pressure in my ears.

We drove around to Radiation Oncology, parked in our patients-only lot, and went down the stairs to my usual couch to wait for my name to be called. As it happened, the father of one of my friends from high school came into the waiting room and sat down in a chair nearby. He recognized us right away and said hello, asking if we remembered him. He told us that he also was being treated for testicular cancer. He had caught it early, and had only seven radiation treatments left. He was on his way to winning that fight, because he paid attention to his body, and he told his doctor when he found a lump in his testicle. We talked for a little while about our situations, then we wished each other well and shook hands goodbye when the nurse called my name.

Once I'd had my radiation treatment, I asked Dr. Alvarez if he would show my new x-ray images to me. When I'd seen them upstairs, I thought it had looked as if the cancer in my lungs had gotten worse, and that had me scared. He let us wait in one of the exam rooms while he had the images sent to him, then he took us into the conference room and pulled them up on his big screen. He explained to me that they did not look at all different to him. That, of course, was both good and bad news. On a second screen, he pulled up a previous image of my lungs taken just a month before, and with his cursor, showed me all the lesions, comparing the earlier image to the new one. They looked almost identical. The findings on all the radiology reports I'd seen never actually stated the number of lesions, only that there were multiple lesions, which, in my mind, meant "too many to count." I took a moment to count all the lesions that I could see. There were more than 22, scattered like tiny marshmallows throughout both lungs. At least it wasn't worse, as I had feared. One good thing was that the pneumothorax, or collapsed lung, had resolved itself, so that was something I could put behind me.

I rode home in the car feeling a mixture of emotions about the day's events. Radiation was burning my ears, and my infected sinuses were making it worse. My white blood cell count was always dropping too low, which made me feel like shit, and I was growing tired of those painful neupogen shots. The lesions in my lungs wouldn't go away, even with all the chemotherapy I'd had that made my whole body feel miserable and helpless. And then I thought about my friend's dad...

someone I actually knew who also was suffering from testicular cancer and treatment. I was glad for him that he was almost done with treatment, but I envied him. He had known what to do when he found a lump, and I had not. And after a little surgery and some radiation, he was almost cured, but not me. Even after the three months of what I'd been through, I felt I was not even close to being cured. He did not need whole brain radiation. He was being radiated just in his lower abdomen. The cancer had not spread into his entire body, because he had checked his testicles regularly, and got medical attention when he found a lump. He hadn't needed nearly the amount of treatment that I had, because he had been smart about it and caught the cancer in the early stage. He had not ignored the lump. He took care of it as soon as he noticed it. In fact, he had a different type of cancer in the past, and had overcome that, too. That was how he knew to check himself for testicular cancer. I was inspired and hopeful after talking to him, but at the same time, very weary that my situation was so much worse than his, and seemed it wasn't getting any better.

Tuesday night I had been suffering some serious back pain, and I coughed up a little bit of blood. It was almost noon when I woke up Wednesday, and I had a bad headache to go with the back pain, plus a little chest pain, too. Mom wanted to take me to the emergency room, but I didn't think it was bad enough for that. I hated going there. I was due for my radiation treatment shortly anyway, so I just laid in bed until time to leave.

Once we were in the Cancer Center after my radiation treatment, though, Mom made sure I told my nurse about all of it. Shari notified Dr. Van's nurse, Kathy, who came in to visit me in the treatment room. She said Dr. Van wanted to see me before I left the Cancer Center, but he would not be there until after 6:30 that evening. It was only about 1:45 in the afternoon. I would be lying in that No. 15 treatment room for the rest of the day. Mom called Mark to let him know, and he left work early to meet us there.

Shari came back in to give me the neupogen shot, bringing with her a warmed blanket. Then she accessed my port and started me on a saline drip, plus acetaminophen, morphine, and oxycodone for pain, and Zofran for nausea. About 30 minutes later, a nurse tech came into my treatment area to do an EKG on me, and just a few minutes after she left, a guy with a mobile x-ray machine came in to take pictures of my lungs. As usual, I removed my earring and my gold necklace and handed them to Mom.

I was getting sleepy from the drugs, but there was a fear in my mind that Dr. Van was concerned I wasn't doing very well. My thoughts began spinning around in my head, and my gut was starting to hurt. I was thinking about how the original ten weeks of bleomycin, etoposide, and platinum treatments failed on me... and since Friday, I faced a threat that these other drugs were not going to work either. Added to that, the pain and coughing a little blood...was I getting worse? What if my tumor markers wouldn't go down? Would there be other treatment drugs that worked better? What about the bone marrow transplant? I looked over at Mom sitting close to me and writing in her journal, and when she heard me move, she looked up at me. I held my hand out to her, and she took hold.

"Thank you, Mom." I said groggily.

"You're welcome..." she smiled, "for what?"

"Just for being here with me... I was just lying here, wondering what's going to happen to me, and I felt glad I wasn't here by myself." I told her about the questions haunting me as I got more and more drowsy. My eyes were feeling pretty heavy while she was telling me not to worry about anything until we hear what Dr. Van has to say, first.

I nodded my head slightly and let my eyes close to sleep.

Mom stayed next to me while I slept the time away, and Mark came in and sat in the darkened, quiet room with us. It was right about 6:15 when Dr. Van came in.

I woke when I heard the sound of the curtain being pulled open. He flipped on a light, then greeted each of us with a handshake, a kind smile and soft "hello." He asked how I was feeling, and the other usual questions, pulling me out of my sleepy state. He listened with his stethoscope to my lungs, heart, and abdomen, and said it all sounded fine. He said the EKG and chest x-rays both looked okay, so that meant my heart was all right, and my lungs didn't look any worse. My white blood cell count was okay, and he said the back pain could be caused by the neupogen. He also said he thought the pain in my ears could be due more to the radiation than to infection. He asked for more detail, concerning the blood I coughed up. It was basically mucus with a small speck of blood in it. He said a small amount would not suggest trouble, but to make sure to let him know if the amount of blood increased.

I asked him about the bone marrow transplant, if that was still going to happen if my tumor markers didn't go down as expected. He said the beta hCG needed to be down to 600 before the transplant would take place. Then I would be treated with higher doses of carboplatin and etoposide. I did the quick math in my head. My tumor markers had to drop more than 13,000 before we could move on to what I called "Phase 2" of my treatment. I had entered a calendar alert on my cell phone for March 20, with the note to myself saying "Phase 1 ends," in an effort to help prepare for the second phase of this line of treatment, my bone marrow transplant. I had one month to get my tumor markers down to 600. I had done it before. I remembered that it was close to my Mom's birthday in January that my beta hCG was down to 641. Mom had said that was the best birthday present ever. No one knew what had made the count jump back up into the thousands just three days later, but I hoped since the count dropped once, it could do it again.

I laid there in my bed and looked at Dr. Van, thinking about the question I wanted to ask. Fear brought on a sudden sense of queasiness to my stomach and heaviness in my heart. I looked at Mom, glanced at Mark, then back at Dr. Van. "What if this current treatment doesn't work?" I asked. I was afraid to hear the answer, but I wanted to know there was a Plan C—other cancer drugs that would work if this second line of treatment failed me.

Dr. Van looked at me silently for a moment, "We would most likely start treatment with drugs called methotrexate, and vincristine."

We were all silent.

He went on to explain a little bit about methotrexate and how it is currently being used. It's an anti-metabolite that interferes with DNA synthesis and cell division in a similar way to the other chemo drugs I was receiving. It is sometimes used in small doses to treat rheumatoid arthritis. In the high doses I would need to kill the masses of cancer still growing in me, methotrexate can be very toxic, much more toxic than the other five chemo drugs I'd taken so far. Dr. Van was willing to give my current treatment more time to work on me before resorting to that one.

"And if that didn't work?" I asked, imagining my fate on a flow-chart.

He paused to form his answer, "There are experimental treatments being done with arsenic," he said, "and there are other options with clinical trials... but I think there is still a good chance for tumor response with the current treatment. I'm willing to go one more round before changing the treatment, but I would like to see the beta hCG drop by next week."

The three of us were speechless. Mom usually had a dozen questions, but fear rose in all of us in hearing the words *arsenic,* and *experimental treatments*. This meant we were near the end of the line, with only one or two options left. I had thought there was an endless supply of cancer-killing drugs available to me, and that if one treatment didn't work, we'd try another... and then another, until the cancer was gone. I had known in the beginning that I had already been receiving the heavy hitters of chemotherapy drugs, but I hadn't realized that most of the others were not strong enough to help me in the first place... and especially not now at this stage.

Dr. Van was quiet with us, waiting for us to absorb the information. Then he glanced at each of us, "All right," he said softly. He patted me on the shin and stood up from my bed. "I'll see you again on Friday morning in my office," he affirmed. "I'm going to order a beta hCG count before you leave tonight, and I'll have my nurse call you with the count when we get it."

I nodded, "Thanks."

When he left the room, the three of us looked at one another quietly. I knew the fear showed in my eyes, and I could see that Mom was scared, too. Her eyes started to water, and I just lay there staring at the ceiling.

Mark heaved a heavy sigh and stressfully rubbed his face with one hand, his other arm still folded across his chest.

Mom pulled her chair up close to me again and took my hand. "We'll get through it, together, Ian. You'll get stronger, and everything will be all right."

I felt tears forming in my eyes as I thought about what Dr. Van had said. My fear of not knowing what might happen felt like it was eating a hole in my stomach. "I've never been so scared in my whole life," I admitted. "I'm so scared."

"Me too," Mom said softly, kissing my hand.

"Me too, Stretch," Mark offered, quietly.

The room was silent, and the fear and sadness that we all felt seemed to be settling on us like a thick heavy cloud of fog. We all had tears in our eyes.

I looked at Mom, then at Mark. Tears rolled out the outside corners of my eyes and down my cheeks into my ears. It was the worst news I had ever heard... that my options were running out. I had never felt so close to death before.

Mom's eyes flooded with tears, but she tried not to let herself cry. She kissed the back of my hand again, and held it to her cheek. "I love you so much, Ian."

"I love you too, Mom." I looked back toward Mark, "You too... thank you both for being here with me. I could never get through this without you." I knew they were trying to honor my fears and ease them at the same time.

Mark leaned up and put his hand on my shoulder, and Mom kept hold of my hand near her face. I closed my eyes, "I'm going to go to sleep, now..." I said weakly.

And I drifted off into the dream state as the three of us waited in the quiet, low-lit room for Shari to come in and draw some blood, and de-access my port so we could go home.

We all trudged into the house like a group of worn out soldiers. I went straight to my bed to lie down. Mom set her purse and journal in my room, and picked up my water mug to refill it with fresh ice and water. Mark grabbed a bite to eat and a shower, then came downstairs to say goodnight. I flipped through the channels on television, but after a couple of minutes turned it off. Mom sat beside me on the floor next to my bed.

"Let's pray," she offered.

"I'm too tired, Mom, and I'm tired of praying." I shook my head. "Will you pray for me?"

"Okay," she agreed with a little pout, "but promise you'll pray when you feel better, and visualize yourself being strong, and healthy," she added.

"I do that every day, Mom. I think about it all the time." I assured her. "I'm always picturing in my head how I'm going to be, what I'm going to do when I get through this."

"Okay," she nodded.

I closed my eyes, and she laid her head next to me on the bed. I knew she was praying, even though she was silent. As the night grew later, she eventually moved to sleep on my couch across from me. I was okay with her not being right next to me through the night anymore. The vertigo episodes had not happened in about a month and a half. I still had nightmares often, but I had come to know even in my sleep state that they were just nightmares, and I wasn't getting freaked out by them as much anymore. There was still a dim light in my room from my stereo and clock radio, and that helped, too. Mom still woke every time I did, and we'd exchange a few sentences before falling asleep again.

The next morning I woke when I heard Mom's voice answering her cell phone. I listened to the happy tone of her voice and opened my eyes to see her smiling at me. She thanked Kathy for calling, then she knelt down beside me to give me the good news.

"That was Kathy, she called to tell you that your beta hCG is down to 8,556!" Mom was jubilant.

"Really?!" I smiled, and opened my arms to her for a hug. She leaned over to embrace me as much as she could while I was lying down, and I wrapped my arms around her neck and squeezed as tight as I could. I felt excited and grateful. I sat up in my bed, rubbing my face with my hands to try to wake up. "Wow," I shook my head and looked up at her again, "that's great!"

I had my usual appointment for radiation a few hours later, so I moseyed into the shower while Mom fixed a little breakfast for me. I ate, even though I was still feeling pretty fatigued and a little nauseous. The radiation treatment of course added to the intensity of both, and I spent the rest of the day and evening in bed, sitting up only to eat a small bowl of pears and half a blueberry bagel for dinner.

I had been having nosebleeds lately, and it happened again about one in the morning. I woke from a light sleep to feel the blood dripping out my nose. I sat up in bed, one hand under my nose and the other hand fumbling for a tissue from the box on the floor. Mom woke up startled at the sight of blood dripping down the back of my hand, and rushed to help me with more tissues. I laid back down, and Mom brought me a cold damp washcloth to put on my head and nose. I kept the tissues to my nose to catch the blood, and after about ten minutes, the bleeding finally stopped. I stood up slowly and went into the bathroom to have a look at myself and wash my face. I started coughing, and I coughed a slight amount of blood. All of the activity and the taste of blood in my throat made me feel even more nauseous than I already had. I didn't sleep very well the rest of that night. Every time I moved, I felt like I was going to throw up. It was hard to lie still, because my body felt like it was being crushed with all the pain in my bones from the neupogen. Mom tried to keep me comfortable with fresh cold washcloths to keep on my head, but it was a pretty tough night, and I was very exhausted when she woke me at about ten o'clock the next morning.

Friday was a long day. I had an appointment with Dr. Van in his office at 11:20 in the morning, then a lab draw at 12:30. I had my radiation treatment at 1:15, then my chemotherapy treatment in the Cancer Center from 1:30 to 6:00 that evening.

I weighed in at 174 pounds, a small improvement. But I was feeling very, very sleepy and fatigued. I was having some intense hip and lower back pain, and my ears still hurt so bad they were giving me a headache. The nurse explained to me that as the neupogen stimulates the bone marrow to produce more white blood cells, the cells pack together tightly, causing pain mostly in the major areas of bone marrow production, mainly the hips, thigh bones, and sternum. There wasn't much I could do about it. The pain medications I was getting didn't help.

As for my ear pain, Dr. Van prescribed some cortisone eardrops. Just as he had told me a few days before, the nurse explained that my ears probably were hurting because of the radiation, not infection, so I would probably start to feel some relief after my last radiation treatment. That was just another thing on the long list of side effects I would have to put up with. But good news was just around the corner.

Mom and I strolled through the hospital to Radiation Oncology. I liked entering from the hospital side much better. I didn't have to go into the main waiting room at all. We walked to the nurses' station and checked in, and after my treatment, Dr. Alvarez met us there. He escorted us straight to an exam room and waited for me to sit down. His face looked happy. Dr. Klish came in to share in the news.

"Well," Dr. Alvarez said, "I am happy that we have seen a complete resolution of the tumors in your brain in the last MRI report." He went on to review why my radiation treatment continued past the report that there were no more visible lesions, and I let him know that I agreed it was good to make sure that no scars or tiny lesions would be left.

Of course there was a chance that other tumors could show up in the future, and Dr. Alvarez reminded me that the total amount of radiation I received was 4500 cGy, or "gray," which is how radiation is measured. I could only receive another 1500 gray if the cancer came back. I wasn't going to worry about that. As far as I was concerned, I was on the road to freedom from cancer. My brain was going to be okay, and the rest of my body would follow in line. I just knew it. I counted on it.

I had one more question... the bonus question. "Can I drive, now?" I asked with a smile.

Both doctors smiled, and Dr. Alvarez answered as he nodded his head, "Yes, I think it would be okay for you to drive."

There was a feeling of freedom in hearing those words. I had needed and wanted someone beside me for three long months, but not being allowed to drive, I craved autonomy like a 16-year-old without a license. I couldn't wait to get out and about on my own again.

Michelle and Leslie came in to congratulate me and give me my radiation mask to take home. Michelle told me to keep it, just in case I needed it again. It was like a trophy to me, signifying that I had successfully suffered through 30 treatments in 42 days of whole brain radiation, and triumphantly killed all the cancer in my brain. It felt good. Both doctors gave me heartfelt congratulations, and left to care for other patients. Mom and I stood up and hugged each other, and I started kidding around, putting my mask on backwards, upside down, and then forwards, and standing and acting as if I was running into the stretched net on my face. Mom was laughing and I was trying to find other ways of being silly to make her laugh some more. Even though I still felt like hell, it was good to also feel like kidding around. I was due in the Cancer Center for chemotherapy treatment, so we made a quick sweep through Radiation Oncology, making sure I got to say goodbye and thank you to all the nurses and my radiation therapists, Michelle and Leslie.

I wore my radiation mask on top of my head as we slowly made our way down the hospital corridors toward the Cancer Center, stopping occasionally so Mom could take a picture of me wearing my mask as a hat, or in some other funny way. We walked past the mailroom we'd passed dozens of times. There was a button near the postal window to call the clerk with a buzzing bell. I'd often noticed it and wanted to push it just to be mischievous, but I was always too tired and depressed to actually do anything like my old self would have done. Well, that day

I did. I had no resistance to reaching in the doorway and pushing that buzzer as we strolled past. Mom shook her head slightly and laughed. She had expected me to do that someday. It was fun to feel a little of my old mischievous self again.

We were so happy on that day. I almost didn't mind that I was going into four hours of chemotherapy. I walked into the main waiting room in the Cancer Center wearing my mask backwards, so it showed the shape of my face on the back of my head, and my face in front was framed by the large gray U-shaped bracket. Everyone at the desk waved at me and greeted me, some offering congratulations as the receptionist told me to go on through to the treatment area waiting room. They knew what having my mask with me meant. I felt so good and so positive. Nothing could bring me down. I was winning!

I chose the big comfortable chairs in the waiting room, and Mom and I sat talking about how great it was that I was finished with radiation. She took another picture of me wearing the mask backwards, and we looked at all the ones she had taken that day. I made up funny titles for her to list them on her cell phone, but as time ticked by, I was feeling more and more tired. I laid my head on the back of the chair and closed my eyes. I hated to admit it to myself, but the thrill of my good news was starting to be overshadowed by what I knew was coming next, and by the fatigue and nausea brought on by the radiation, and the intensifying pain in my gut and my bones. The longer I waited, the more sick I felt, as was usual after a radiation treatment and in dread of the chemo.

A nurse came and ushered us into a private treatment room with a glass door, and I went straight for the bed. She asked the usual questions as the aide checked all my vitals. Mom retrieved a warmed blanket and extra pillow for me, and before long, the nurse had accessed my port and hooked me up with pre-hydration and pre-meds to get my chemo regimen started. The clicking of the IV machine was a familiar sound that I was growing very sick of hearing, and I found myself beginning to feel very grouchy and irritable at my environment and situation. I lay there in my bed, quiet and barely tolerant. Mom had darkened the room and made it as quiet as possible by closing the doors and drawing the curtain closed.

Again, she sat with me in the dark silence for five straight hours. I didn't know how she could do that, but I sure appreciated it. I felt like a useless lump of bones, laying there with all that poison dripping into my body, trying to kill the cancer that was trying to kill me. No one understood. Not even Mom had any idea what that felt like. Before long, my whole body would hurt. Not just my muscles, like after a good hard workout, not just my bones and joints, like after playing a good, hard game of football, not just my gut, like after eating or drinking too much, and not just my skin, like after spending too much time outside in the sun. ALL of me hurt during nadir. All my bones felt like they were aching from the inside, the pain radiating all the way to the outside of my skin, my teeth, my eyes, and where my hair used to be. I'd had no hair on my head for two months, and now my eyelashes and eyebrows were starting to thin. I couldn't express how depressing that was. I couldn't eat or drink without throwing up. I couldn't move, I couldn't sleep, I couldn't get comfortable. And if all of that wasn't enough, when I had an IV pump, it seemed like it was always beeping for one thing or another. Those things sometimes drove me crazy. Mom would silence the alarm and then go to tell the nurse that it was beeping again. It meant one or more of several things, either one of the lines was clogged, or pinched somewhere, or one of the bags of meds was getting low, or the time had come to slow the dosage down or change it altogether. We never knew. Mom would just call the nurse.

This particular day was no different. Eventually though, I was able to drift off into a drug-induced sleep, and even when I woke from time to time from the IV machine beeping, I wasn't completely awake for very long. At around 6:30 it was time to go home again. I was unhooked, my port flushed and cleaned, and groggily I shuffled to the car with Mom, where I slept until we got home. I was much too tired and sick to even think about driving my car. I didn't care about anything but lying quietly in my room for the rest of the night. I had another neupogen shot to look forward to the next day, and the day after that, and the day after that, and into the middle of next week. I knew I was going to feel like shit for a while, both with nadir causing nausea and extreme fatigue, and neupogen causing the intense body pain.

My 20th birthday was the coming Monday. The effects of chemo had made me feel so horrible I didn't do much of anything that whole weekend. Friends and family called and sent cards, but I didn't even have the energy or the will to talk to anyone. I barely was able to open a card and read the whole thing. I felt like an empty shell... used and beaten up by the pounding waves of toxic chemicals and radiation flowing through me to kill the cancer. On Monday, my birthday, I felt so bad I couldn't even get out of bed by myself to take a piss. The bigger problem was that I had a bad case of diarrhea. All I had to say was "Mom," and she stood up, took my hands and pulled me up to a sitting position on my bed, then used her weight to pull and help me stand. She walked a foot or so with me until I had stabilized myself enough to walk quickly to the bathroom.

Once finished, I opened the door and shuffled back to my bed, fell into it, and laid there, wondering how I was ever going to make it through. My head was foggy, but full of fear of things to come, and dismay of all that I was feeling, emotionally and physically. My stomach was empty, my gut hurt, and I was thirsty, but my body felt ready to throw up or poop at any moment. My bones ached so bad, it felt like that was all that was left of me, a skeleton laying there, feeling too weak to lift even a finger. That was how I spent my birthday, and I felt too sick to care.

I even missed my appointment to receive neupogen on Tuesday because I was feeling so horrible. I could not get out of bed. Every time I moved, I thought I would throw up. I kept a trash can next to my bed just in case. The fatigue, the complete exhaustion, is something that there are no words to explain. I felt like there was no life left in my body. I barely had the energy to turn over in bed. My bones ached so bad, I thought I was dying a painful death. I wondered if death hurt so bad. I told Mom there was no way I could go in to receive that shot. I just could not do it. She had seen me push myself, and she had helped

me to continue forging through my treatment. And she knew by looking at me, and by the way I spoke, that I meant it with all that was left
of me. I couldn't go. I promised I would go the next day, no matter
how bad I felt. But I trusted that I would feel better by then.

Mom called the nurse at the Cancer Center to see if it was all right
if I missed that day's injection. The nurse made note of Mom's report
on the way I felt, and said it would be okay to miss one injection as
long as I would be sure to get there the next day.

By Thursday, I wasn't feeling quite as bad. I had an appointment
in the Cancer Center to consult with one of the hematologists about
my upcoming high-dose chemotherapy and bone marrow transplant.
The whole process was frightening. The plan was to give me one more
treatment dose of Taxol and Gemzar, then restage the cancer with a
CT scan on my entire torso, and MRI on my brain. If all tests showed
a good response to the therapy, they would then double-dose me in the
last week of March with neupogen to ultrastimulate my stem cells. I
would then be admitted into the bone marrow unit of the hospital to
start the frightening process of *Phase 2*.

I asked how the marrow would be extracted, and the doctor explained that a needle would be inserted into a bone in my lower back,
my hip. It would be very painful, and the pain would last weeks. In fact,
I would be in the hospital bone marrow unit for three weeks at the
very least after the transplant, unable to have visitors. It would take me
about six months to recover at home, where we had to practice serious
sanitation measures as well. My kitty would have to live somewhere
else. Mom and Mark made plans to have our house, the air ducts, and
my room professionally cleaned in detail, adding a new floor covering
and a hospital bed. Mom would have to clean and sterilize my environment every day, until my body was strong enough to fight off infection
on its own. Even visitors would have to be sterilized and wear masks,
so they wouldn't bring in any germs. In my imagination, it was going to
be like living in one of those Haz-Mat tents I'd seen in movies.

How could I have thought I'd had it so bad, just being exhausted
and nauseated? Throwing up for ten minutes didn't seem so bad when

I thought about what I was going to have to live through in the next six months. I was generally a pessimist. I usually planned for the worst, but hoped for the best, as people sometimes say. And I did fear the worst, but I hoped that I would be able to go through it all, that my body would respond to the ongoing treatment so that I could continue with the plan. Because if the Taxol and Gemzar didn't work as planned, the bone marrow transplant would be off the table, and I'd have to resort to the methotrexate, my last hopeful option.

Doctors use a rating scale to chart a cancer patient's overall health status, ability to perform ordinary tasks and to cope with treatment. It's called the KPS, or Karnofsky Performance Status. It's named after the guy who came up with it. The score ranges from 0-100, with 100 being "no complaints" and 0 being "deceased." I usually scored between 80 and 90, meaning that I was able to carry on normal activity, like dressing, bathing, and feeding myself, but with some symptoms and minor complaints, like pain, fatigue, and nausea. I had thought a higher score indicated a good overall prognosis. I guessed they would be using this scale of measure on me regularly in the next six months, and from what I understood about how the coming treatment would affect me, my performance status score would probably drop lower than it had ever been.

A couple of days later, I woke up with my new song that had been in my head for the last month or two. As I lay there thinking about how I felt as a cancer patient and how it had changed me, the song began to write itself. I started hearing chords in my mind that would go with the words forming into whole thoughts about my experience. I got up and grabbed my pen and notebook to record the words as they flowed out of me. Then I took my guitar out of its case, sat down on my couch with it, and tuned it to the key I was hearing in my mind. I played around with the chords a little bit, then I reached for my notebook to go over the lyrics again, as I thumped the rhythm with my thumb on the body of my guitar. When I had the rhythm worked out, I started strumming the chords and singing softly to myself.

I always thought it was funny that whenever my cat heard the sound of my guitar, he ran off to hide, while my Mom came running down-stairs to hear me play. I heard a thump in the stairway, then Mom came limping into my room, saying she'd just tripped over the cat as they passed each other on the steps. She was smiling, though, and happy to see me sitting up with my guitar and smiling back at her.

"I almost got it, Mom," I said, gleaming up at her. "You want to hear?"

She smiled and skip-hopped closer to me, planting herself cross-legged on the floor in front of me. She sat waiting, smiling with bright eyes of anticipation.

"It's not polished yet..." I always prefaced, "but tell me what you think of it so far."

As I played and sang, her smiling, proud face began to soften into an expression of wonder, and tears filled her eyes as they often did when she heard any of my songs for the first time. The lyrics were tender and sad, but with chords that expressed feelings of hope for a better day.

"That is beautiful, Ian," Mom softly spoke, still looking as if she was in awe. "It's so beautiful!"

"Thanks," I said, smiling and looking at her, then glancing down at my guitar. "You know how I've told you that cancer feels like a cage..." I looked back at her.

"Yeah... and I love the way you have turned it around. It's very cool. And I love the chords you chose, especially the part about cancer waiting outside the cage."

"Which one? This one?" I strummed the one I thought she was referring to, the last chord in that line of the song. I liked it, too.

"Yeah! That one. It's so pretty, the sound of your voice with it."

"Thanks," I laid my guitar down in its case. "I want to work on it some more, but I'm really tired now. I'm going to lie down for a while."

"Okay," she said as she slowly stood up. "I'll get you some fresh ice water."

I moved over to my bed and lay on my side, thinking about the song, and my situation. I slept most of the afternoon, and if it weren't for feeling hungry, I probably would have slept longer.

I hadn't been feeling as bad in the last couple of days, so I made some plans to get out with friends. I didn't understand it all. I was feeling pretty good, other than fatigue and a little nausea, so that should mean that my health was getting better. How could it be that my lungs still had so many little tumors in them, yet I felt fine? Those kinds of thoughts depressed me. It was just what I needed, I thought, hanging with friends to divert my thoughts from my bleak future.

Mom tried to be cool about my going out alone. She worried that I would not be putting myself in the best environments to help fight the cancer in me. Even though she trusted me to take good care of myself, she felt no one else would be watching out for me the way she did. Still, she found ways to take care of me while I was out, by cleaning my bathroom and bedroom, changing my bed sheets, and washing all my clothes. I knew she hated those nights when I stayed out until morning, but she didn't hound me about it. As long as I sent her a text message to let her know I was not coming home and that I was okay, she tried her best to be okay with it. She saw that my spirits were lifted by being able to go out on my own. She always looked so relieved when she greeted me coming in late at night. She occasionally reminded me of her opinion that partying with friends was not exactly good for my health. She thought my energy would be better spent at the gym, getting the exercise that the doctors prescribed. Truth was, I was too weak to give it a chance. And even though she was trying to push me as I had asked her to do early in my treatment, I wasn't really hearing the importance of it. I hadn't realized it, but my enthusiastic attitude for kicking cancer's ass had been greatly diminished with all the bad news, and what was left was going up in puffs of marijuana smoke. Even though I disagreed with her that my actions were going to affect the outcome, I really appreciated that she respected my wishes and tried to understand.

I did come home fairly early that night, though, and the next day she and I were sitting in the living room, talking about heaven and earth, spirit, and all the events that can happen in one person's life.

"I can see that cancer has been, is a blessing in my life," I reflected, "because it's opened my eyes to living..."

Mom looked thoughtful, and nodded as she looked at me and kept listening.

"You know, like I was saying before?" I went on, "It's like I didn't even know I was alive, until cancer. Like I was living in a cage all my life, not realizing what living was all about, then I stepped out of the cage and cancer was waiting for me, and it made me realize how alive I am."

Mom listened for more, then she said, "God has a plan for you, Ian, just like for the rest of us, and I have faith that you can live on and tell people about it."

"Yeah... I hope you're right." I didn't feel sure about anything. "I hope it won't be as bad as it all sounds, the treatment, I mean. I hope I can get through it. I keep praying I will."

"Me too, honey," she replied.

"And I can see now how important it is to have people who really care... like you and Mark, and our whole family," I was feeling very appreciative.

She smiled. "We love you so much, Ian."

"Mom, you know what? You're one of my very best friends. I don't know how I would get through cancer without you helping me and being with me every day."

She gave me a big smile. "You're my favorite person in the whole world, Ian. I would never choose to be anywhere else but with you."

"Actually, you are my best friend," I added. "If a best friend is someone you spend most of your time with, and you can talk to about anything, you know you can trust them, and you always have fun together, well, that's you... because I've been with you more than I've been with anyone else in my life, and we never fight...I mean, yeah, we've had disagreements, but we've always made it all good... we're always okay."

Mom nodded, thoughtfully, "Yeah..."

"And you know what? Even if you weren't my mom, you would still be my best friend." I smiled at her. I meant it. I thought about it for a moment... "I wish I had a best friend just like you, now, only a guy... you know... because then we could do more stuff together... two guys... because you know, a guy... a grown man can't always hang out with his mom. It's just... nobody does that."

"Yeah," she said. "That's the only bad part about being a mom. But I'll always love you, more than anyone else in the world... because you're my son."

We sat quietly for a moment.

"Do you think we'll be together in Heaven?" I pondered, looking at her.

"Yes. I do. I believe we will always be together," she smiled. "Forever."

"Yeah, me too." I smiled.

11

How Bad Can It Get?

I flipped off the television and laid in the dark for a moment. Mom had fallen asleep on my couch after watching Late Night with Conan O'Brien with me. I was bored with television, but I couldn't sleep. I started thinking about my song, which led me to thinking about the past week, and what was to come in the next month.

The hematologist had told me to get an appointment with my dentist to make sure all my cavities were filled, including even the tiniest holes in my teeth that would normally pose no problem. The reason was that bacteria can grow in those places in the mouth, which the average healthy person would not even notice. With very few white blood cells once I had started bone marrow treatment, I would have no ability to fight off anything like that. I would be so weak that the normal bacteria living in my own mouth could lead to an infection that could kill me.

The appointment for my bone marrow biopsy was getting closer. It would be done on the morning of the first Monday in March. I would get a test dose of chemotherapy at nine o'clock to make sure my body would handle it, followed by the biopsy in my spine. I'd get my first full chemo treatment for *Phase 1* of the bone marrow transplant after that.

Just thinking about that one day scared me a lot. But the rest of the treatment scared me so much more. Once I'd made it through the month-long chemo treatments that were pretty much going to kill every cell I had left, I still had the stem cell harvesting to look forward to. That was when they would fill me with huge doses of neupogen for a few days, then jab the needle that looked like it was made for a gorilla into my lower spine or my hip to draw out the stem cells from my bone marrow. I would endure that every day for four days in a row. My imagination was telling me I wouldn't be able to take it. It would be the worst pain, the worst hell that I had ever been through in my life, and it would last for a long, long time.

I tried to imagine what it would be like, lying in that bed in the bone marrow unit, near death and unable to move. I thought of the pain, the nausea, all the agonies that I had already experienced. This would be so much worse. I wondered how bad the pain and nausea could get before I couldn't take it anymore. The thought that I couldn't have a single visitor in my room with me, not even Mom, terrified the shit out of me. How could I take it? She couldn't stay with me anymore. Would I go crazy being alone for so long? No one to look at, or talk to. No one to hold my hand and help me keep fighting. I had been in that bone marrow unit once, during my first round of chemotherapy back in December, when all the rooms in Unit 42 were full. At that time, it was not as big a deal, because I could have visitors. I remembered there was a visitor's viewing window next to the door in every room. It was sealed, tempered glass. You couldn't hear a normal voice through it. That is how everyone would visit me this time, for at least three weeks, standing at that window and waving at me, mouthing and signing "I love you," and holding up signs for me to read. Nothing from the outside world would be allowed in my room. No human contact, except for my nurses and doctors. I didn't even know if I would be allowed to talk on the phone, or if I would even have the strength.

I remembered how small the room was. All the windows were air tight. There were four large red UV lamps in the ceiling above the bed, used to stimulate bone marrow production. The room was stuffy and hot. I hated it then, and I could imagine how much I would hate it the second time.

I had never liked being alone, even as a little kid. 'What if I die, alone in that room?' This thought was so loud in my head that I wondered if I had actually spoken it. I lay quietly and thought about it. Three weeks, all alone. The thought of loneliness itself sounded painful enough to kill me.

To top off all the fear I was feeling, I had a frightening question that loomed around me from time to time, and it found its way into my conscious thought more and more often. 'What if I live through all this, but the cancer comes back and I have to do it all over again?'

My doctors told me I would need frequent checkups for the next five years, before I could actually be considered a cancer survivor. And since my testicular cancer was at such a late stage and spread throughout my body even before diagnosis, the chance of finding more cancer later in life was very likely. I had read that people diagnosed with late-stage cancer usually don't live very long, even if they survive their original treatment. I also read somewhere that cancer patients are rarely given whole brain radiation unless the odds are that they will not live more than two or three years longer. I didn't know if that was true, but the idea of it made me feel extremely depressed. Whole brain radiation was some serious shit. It can really foul up the central nervous system. My doctors told me I would probably experience memory loss, difficulty learning, confusion, and other side effects of mild brain damage for the rest of my life, probably worsening with age. Chemotherapy also causes these side effects. Some cancer patients call it "chemo-brain." I had a hard time thinking clearly already. The fear of what whole brain radiation and heavy doses of six different chemotherapy drugs in the last three months had done to my brain and central nervous system brought on a dreadful feeling.

I thought I was damaged goods at only 20 years old. All my muscular strength and tone were gone. The color had gone out of my skin, and my face was marked with the dark spots of what they call "chemo-burn." My hair was gone, and I was looking at a future with progressing brain damage. I felt like I already looked like death walking. Would I ever be the strong, energetic, fun-loving person I used to be? I wouldn't be able to father children, so would any woman want me? What would I be able to do for a living if I had trouble learning and remembering things? Gina had told me I could be looking at an assistant manager's position at work, but could I handle it? What if I couldn't handle life on my own? Would I be able to figure things out for myself? What if I lost my creativity and couldn't write songs anymore? I had already experienced that, and I felt like I was losing myself. The song I wrote a week ago was the first song I'd written in more than three months. What if I live with all of this, and the cancer still comes back? I was so very tired of the pain, and the constant pity that I felt coming from others. Fear of my future was pulling my hope under, like a sinking rock. And the fear of dying all by myself in a small, stuffy white room, was the worst pain of all.

I couldn't take my own thoughts anymore, and I felt like I was about to throw up. I turned the television back on and got out of bed. I pulled my pipe, a lighter, and small bit of weed out of a cabinet, and took them with me to the laundry room. I'd found a clever way to keep the smell out of the house. I filled the pipe, lit it and took a long, deep hit. When I couldn't hold it in any longer, I opened the empty clothes dryer, blew the smoke in, quickly closed the door and turned the dryer on to pull the smoke outside through the vent. It worked great. Even Mom had said it was a pretty ingenious idea. I took a couple of more hits off the pipe, crouched in front of the dryer like that. When I returned to my room, Mom woke up and looked at the clock.

"You're still up?" she asked. It was almost two in the morning.

"Yeah," I mumbled. "I can't sleep."

I sat down on my bed, and looked at her. "Mom, I hate smoking by myself."

"Don't worry, Ian, I can't even tell. You look the same to me."

I breathed a heavy sigh. "Yeah, but it's not the same, being the only stoned person in the room. I wish you would smoke with me." She and I'd had this conversation a couple of times before in the last month. I kept trying to get her to join me so I'd feel better about being stoned.

She sat up and came over to sit beside me on my bed. "Ian, you know I've thought about it, but it doesn't feel right. It isn't the responsible thing to do. And what if I had to take you to the emergency room for some reason, like we do now and then? I'm afraid I couldn't handle it." She smiled. "And what would your doctors think of your stoner mom driving her son to the hospital, being all smoked up with red eyes...."

I smiled at the thought of her in that scenario. "You worry too much." I shook my head and lay down in bed. "It's just... it would be nice to have somebody to share it with." I rolled onto my back and scooted over to make room for her beside me.

"I'm sorry, Ian. I'm doing the best I can. I still think you shouldn't be smoking anyway. I can't imagine that it doesn't affect the cancer in your lungs."

"Yeah-yeah, okay, okay..." I stopped her. "Here." I patted to fluff a pillow for her, and stretched my arm out just below it for her to lay her head down next to me. "I don't want to talk."

She looked at me thoughtfully, and with a surrendering smile, lay down along the edge of my bed, her head on my arm. I wrapped my arm around her neck, and she hugged me around my stomach.

"I just want to lay here." I had my eyes closed. "Let's just lay here and forget about the world for a while."

We were both quiet for a moment.

"I love you, Ian," she whispered.

"I love you, too, Mom," I said, eyes still closed. "Thank you."

The truth was, she was probably right. I may not have been taking care of myself as well as I should have, though I didn't consciously realize that at the time. I had been doing my best, trying to do what the doctors said, but the cancer kept getting worse, and that was beating my fighting attitude to the ground. I was so tired of thinking and worrying about my situation and my future that lately I had been spending more evenings away from home, where I could try to distance myself from my painful life. It was a place where no one cared about me the way Mom and Mark did, where I didn't have to smoke by myself. I could smoke without having to cover the smell, and no one would be concerned about me. Getting stoned was like an escape, taking a break from all of it. I wanted it to take me away from the constant mental pain of my troubles, so that I wouldn't care about any of it: the cancer, the horrors of treatment, and my future living with cancer as a constant threat to my life.

When Mom asked me where I was going on those particular nights, I lied to her. I knew she wouldn't be okay with where I was going. Then later, I sent her a text message to tell her I wouldn't be home for the night. She was so worried about me when I stayed out, and in the mornings when I came home, she voiced her concern that I was being nonchalant about my health and well being. My argument was that I was 20 years old, and I needed to get out and live my life. She had seen how depressed I would get after lying around the house for so many days, and getting out with other people did make me feel better, and she saw that in me, too. I knew she didn't want me smoking, although I didn't really think I smoked all that much. And it did help me to feel better, sleep better, and eat more food without throwing up all the time. And she worried even more about me breathing in secondhand cigarette smoke when I was out. But I never thought that was anything to be concerned about, and the people at this particular place I stayed once in a while didn't care anyway, so there was no pressure on me there. Besides, I only stayed the night maybe a half-dozen times or so. It didn't seem all that serious to me, and I wrote off Mom's concern each time she expressed it.

I slept until about two o'clock the next day. Mom woke me earlier in the morning to make sure I took my morning medications, but I had gone right back to sleep. She tried to keep the house as quiet as possible for my benefit, but we lived in a small, older home, and I could always hear the floors creaking above me as people walked upstairs. It was annoying when I was trying to sleep, so I'd usually give up and get out of bed, when all I really wanted to do was sleep my day away.

My appetite was much better, though, and Mom was happy to fix me a hot meal. I worked on my song for a little bit, but after being up for a few hours, my back and chest started to hurt on the left side, similar to the way it felt when I'd had the pneumothorax. I didn't want to tell Mom right away, because I didn't want her to make a fuss and call the Cancer Center. I knew this kind of pain was one of the reasons that we should make a call, but the other times I had been referred to the ER only made me feel worse. Everything had always checked out all right, so it seemed I had gone through all that misery for nothing. Even though it never was, in my case I knew that chest pain could be serious, but I thought I'd wait and see if the pain got worse before telling Mom.

It didn't get worse, but it didn't go away either, even after taking a little extra pain reliever. It was about seven o'clock that night when I finally told Mom about the pain. It wasn't bad pain, just constant.

Of course the Cancer Center wanted to do a chest x-ray on me. I had already made plans for the evening. Sitting in a hospital waiting room wasn't part of the plan.

"Mom, I can drive myself down there. There's a party I want to go to later, and I'll have the x-ray done, then I'll go to the party after that."

"Are you kidding me?" Mom asked in disbelief. "Chest pain could be very serious, Ian. It could be your heart! It could be a problem with your lungs... I can't let you drive yourself! That would be irresponsible of me as a parent."

I rolled my eyes at her drama. "Mom... I'm not a kid. I know how the pain feels, you don't, and I can tell you for sure, it's nothing. You know every time we drive down there and sit for eight hours, it's never anything. They always send me home with more pain reliever, and tell me to call if it gets worse. I'm so sick of that."

"Ian. I'll drive you, then you can go out when we get home."

"Mom, no. It's just a freaking chest x-ray. They'll tell me everything looks fine, and I'll leave. That's the way it always happens. I don't want to come all the way back home again."

"Ian, please don't take your situation so lightly... you're still fighting cancer. You asked me to help you, and now I'm telling you, I think it's not a good idea to drive yourself all that way."

I busied myself with getting ready to go, while she continued.

"What if the pain gets worse along the way and you can't get there? You could have a car accident if your pain gets so bad you can't take it. What then?" She paused to let me think about it, but I didn't. I felt she was taking it all too seriously.

"Ian, I'm worried about you. I'm going to drive you there. If they tell us that everything is all right, then you go out to the party, but let me drive you to the hospital, at least. I'm ready to go." She had her purse on her shoulder and her keys in her hand.

I didn't answer her. My mind was made up. She wasn't going to get her way. I was almost a foot taller than her, and nearly 40 pounds heavier, even in my skinny, unhealthy state. She wasn't strong enough to force me even if she had wanted to, and she didn't want the stress of an argument, either. What was she going to do, get Mark to force me into the car and strap me in?

She stood across from me as I sat on my bed and put my shoes on. I stood up and held her face in my hands. "Mom," I said in my most consoling voice, "Thank you for taking such good care of me, but I'm fine. It's just an x-ray, not a heart attack. Okay? It's just an x-ray. I'll call you from the hospital, and you can talk to the nurse if you want. Let me take care of it myself. It's no big deal. It's not my heart, it's not my lungs, it's just like when my port hurt a little, before." I turned and grabbed my coat.

"Ian!" she started.

I left her standing in my room as I headed upstairs, and picked up my keys from the shelf near the door. "Bye, Mom... I love you... bye Mook!" I yelled to him as I opened the front door. Mom was standing on the stairs behind me, looking up at me as I turned around to close the door from outside.

"I love you Ian. Please call me."

"I will... Love you..." I closed the door. The way I saw it, I had just a few days left until my bone marrow treatment was started. I intended to live my life the best I could until then. And I wasn't going to live it cooped up in my room, and being carted back and forth to the hospital.

Part of me didn't even want to go to the Cancer Center, but I knew that I should, just to be sure. It wasn't hard to find a parking space in front of the Cancer Center that late at night, but the main front doors were locked after hours, so I had to enter through the hospital. The walk from the car, through the hospital lobby, and down the two long corridors to the treatment center made me feel pretty short of breath. They drew some blood, took a urine sample, and did the x-ray. Once all the reports were in, a doctor came in to see me, asked me a bunch of questions, and examined me as usual. About an hour later, I was pronounced to be okay, and sent home with instructions to take extra oxycodone for the pain if I needed it.

I called Mom as soon as I got out to the car. I told her that everything checked out all right. I told her about the blood and urine tests and the x-ray, and what I could remember of what the doctor said. The one detail I left out was that my urine sample showed a trace of blood. I didn't want Mom to get all worked up with worry again. The doctor apparently wasn't very concerned about it, so I wasn't either. He had told me to watch for blood, and if I saw any, to call the Cancer Center. I told Mom not to worry about me, and that I'd call her later. I didn't call later, though. I sent her a text message in the early morning hours, telling her I wouldn't be home. She hated it when I did that, but appreciated that I at least let her know.

A sad fact of the matter was that just two nights later, I forgot that I had sent Mom a text to tell her I wouldn't be home, but she had received the same message from me three times that night. She asked me about it the next day when I came home around noon. As soon as I walked in the door, I apologized for not letting her know I wouldn't be home. I had no memory of ever sending her a text at all, but discovered I had a few identical replies from her on my cell. It was as if our cell phones were sending the same messages over and over again. Mom was more worried than ever, and told me she didn't want me staying out at all anymore. I told her as usual, to not worry about it, that everything was fine. In fact, everything was not fine.

During the party a few nights earlier, some fighting broke out in the front yard between some of the people there, a few who were strangers to me, and another couple of guys who were friends from school. As the tension escalated, it felt like my whole world was spinning out of control. To me, it sounded like everyone was screaming, and I knew someone was about to get seriously hurt. I felt I needed to take control of the situation, and looked for the quickest way to break up the altercation. I grabbed an unloaded shot gun from inside the house, stepped outside to where the fighting was, aimed at the sky, and cocked the gun, making the sound of a shell loading into the chamber. The strangers scattered to their car, peeling away and leaving smoke from their tires behind them. I stood there, holding the shotgun, looking at the surreal world around me. I felt as if I wasn't even a part of it, but in the center of it, and I could feel my heart pounding in my chest. I just stood there, staring. I felt like I was about to throw my guts up right there on the front patio. A good friend was standing behind me. I stumbled past him and into the house, laid the gun on the floor and fell into the nearest chair. He and a few other friends gathered around me. I was pale white with cold sweat. I felt I was about to throw up, and I started coughing. My heart was beating at what felt like twice the normal rate. My chest hurt, and I couldn't breathe very deeply. All my doctors had told me that stress was the No. 1 thing that would be detrimental to my health and overcoming cancer. That event was probably like pouring gasoline on the cancer fire growing in me. I told everyone to just leave me alone, that I'd be fine, and the party thinned out pretty quickly. I was too weak to give a shit. I felt drained of all desire and promise that life would one day get better. And when it was all said and done, no one, including me, even gave one thought that getting medical attention for me that night might have meant saving my life. Most of us were under age, and the house was full of alcohol. No one wanted to risk getting caught with that, especially the one adult who was responsible for it all.

By Friday, my stomach was hurting more than usual, and I was feeling pretty nauseous, too. I was also feeling very sluggish and exhausted, and lay in bed, sleeping off and on through the day and night.

When I woke up about eleven o'clock Saturday morning, I didn't feel well at all. Mom thought I looked very pale. When I sat up in bed, my head hurt even worse than it did just lying there, so I lay back down. Mom asked me to rate my headache pain, and I told her it was at a seven when I sat upright, and about a four while lying down. I also had a temperature of 100.2.

She called the Cancer Center to ask for advice. Dr. Van's nurse, Kathy, asked Mom if I had noticed any blood in my stool, my urine, or in what I coughed up. I told her I had only coughed up a little bit of blood in the last couple of days, but not much, but my urine was yellow, my poop was dark brown, and I hardly ever coughed up anything at all. Kathy suggested Mom take me to the emergency room.

Again, I faced the grueling chauffeured drive down the long stretch of highways, full of bumps, noises and movement that made me feel even worse. Mark loaded my duffle and Mom's in the trunk of the car so we'd have them in case I was admitted, and off we went.

I lay down in the back seat while Mark drove. Mom kept a close watch on me, and laid her front seat back a little to be closer to me. It was a quiet, nauseous ride. My head pounded, throbbing with each heartbeat. I rated my back pain a six. My stomach started to ache worse than before, and I was feeling pretty short of breath. Mark pulled up to the entrance, and Mom got out and jogged inside to get a wheelchair for me. I didn't feel I had it in me to walk, my head was hurting so bad, and I felt I could throw up any minute. The triage nurse met us as Mom wheeled me in. She took me directly into her office and checked all my vitals, and I had to wait there for about 15 minutes while they got an exam room ready for me. Mom tried to massage my neck and head a little, hoping to ease the pain, but I felt very nauseous and asked her to stop and pull the wastebasket close to me. I just knew I was going to hurl. I sat leaning on the arm of the wheelchair, resting my throbbing head on my hand, my back aching, and my body feeling like the last bit of energy had been sucked right out of me. Mark stood restlessly behind me, and Mom pulled a chair up to sit close to me.

The ER was full that day, and the only room they had for me felt like a stuffy closet with a heavy wooden door. Still, I was relieved when I finally had a bed to lie down in. I stood from the wheelchair and went to sit on the bed, but in an instant, lunged toward the tall trash basket near the door, and threw up. The nurse handed me a few tissues, then she and Mark helped me onto the bed to lie down. When she left to let the doctor know I was there, Mom helped to cover me with the blanket. Limp and exhausted, I welcomed the cool, damp cloth she made for my head. That always felt good.

The nurse came in again and started me on IV fluids, drew some of my blood, and gave me some medication for pain and nausea. After about 30 minutes, the ER doctor came in to examine me, and told me he had ordered a CT scan with contrast to check for bleeding in my brain, and that Dr. Van had been notified. He also said they might check my urine.

The room was so small, there was barely enough room on either side of the bed for a person to stand. I was feeling claustrophobic and completely miserable. I was impatient, very irritable, and crabby. My head felt like it was being crushed in a vice, and my lower back wouldn't let me get comfortable. The stale, hot air in the room was making me feel very nauseous. I was thirsty as hell, but they wouldn't let me have any water before they did the CT scan on me. Two hours passed, and nothing had been done. I just wanted something for my dried-up throat. Mom got tired of waiting and went to the nurses' station to get a cup of ice for me. She spoon fed it to me one little crumble at a time. It was not enough, but it helped.

Eventually, someone did come to take me to Radiology for a CT on my head. I was glad to get out of that room for a while. Fortunately for me, they gave me contrast intravenously, so I didn't have to drink any of that crap. But once my short jaunt to Radiology was over, I was back to waiting in the stuffy little room again.

The clock ticked off the hours while I had more fluids, and more pain reliever for my back and headache. The doctor had reminded me that Taxol can cause headaches, but I hadn't thought the pain could get as bad as this.

Hours passed, and we were getting very impatient and upset with what felt like a low level of care I was getting that day. I grew more and more cranky. We were feeling ignored. In actuality, it was taking time for the CT scan report to be sent to the doctor, who then had to figure out what to do from there, before he came to talk to me. We weren't sure of anything, so Mark stood in the doorway of my room, making sure that we weren't being forgotten in that little closet in the corner, while Mom stood near me and held my hand, feeding me chunks of crushed ice from time to time. I was in torment, with the hot stuffy room, the pain, the uncomfortable waiting, and the not knowing.

Four hours later, the doctor came in to tell us that the CT scan showed there was no sign of hemorrhage or fluid in my brain. That was a relief, but why did my head still hurt like hell, I asked him. He said he didn't know, but that it may be just a chemotherapy-induced migraine.

Mom asked what they learned from the blood work, and he told us that they had not sent my blood to the lab. He had felt it was not necessary, since I had just had lab work done four days ago. Mom wanted to say, send his blood to the lab anyway, but she didn't let herself speak. She listened to the doctor's excuse for not doing it, but didn't listen to her inner voice.

By 6:45 that night, I rated my decreased headache pain at a two, but my back pain still hurt at near a five. I was so fatigued my body felt full of lead. The doctor asked me to stand up, but I didn't even have the energy to do that. I wanted more morphine for the pain in my back, but that request was denied. I'd already received my limit. An alternative pain reliever was prescribed for me, and that turned out to help, after a while.

After more than seven hours in ER, I was released to go home. The nurse gave me a list of symptoms to watch for that would indicate bleeding in my brain, and suggested acetaminophen and oxycodone for my headache.

"See, Mom?" I said as I slowly sat up. "It's just like I was saying, I lay here for hours in misery, then he sends me home telling me to take two Tylenol and call him in the morning."

Mark chuckled. "Yeah, but now we know it's not something more serious." He offered me a hand to help me stand.

My head was still throbbing and nausea was still hanging on, but the pain in my back wasn't quite as bad. We slowly filed out of the little room, and walked to the car just outside the ER entrance. I lay down in the back seat all the way home. I still rated my headache at a four lying horizontal. I hoped I could just fall asleep to escape the pain once we were home. As we were pulling into the driveway, Mom realized that they never did check my urine as the doctor had mentioned.

Mark opened the garage door so I could walk straight into my room without having to navigate two sets of stairs. He carried our duffle bags into the house, while Mom followed me into my room to help me get settled and comfortable. She straightened my blankets and fluffed my bed pillows before I lay down, and when I dropped into my bed, she slid my shoes off for me. She filled my water mug with fresh ice water and sat down on the floor next to me.

"Are you hungry?" she asked.

"No thanks, my head hurts too bad," I said.

I rolled a little onto my side to look at her. I held my hand out for her to take hold of it, and when she did, I lightly kissed her knuckles. "Thank you for being my Mom," I said sincerely.

She smiled. "Thank you for being my son."

We looked at each other eye to eye. I was feeling very grateful for her.

"Mom, I would never want to go through all this without you. You're the best mom in the whole world."

"You're the best son in the whole world," she said with her loving smile. I knew she meant it. She had told me that a lot through my life.

She leaned in to hug me, and I wrapped my arms around her and squeezed her as hard as I could. I held on to her for a long time. "I feel so lucky that you're my mom. I don't know how I would do this without you. Thank you, Mom, for everything you do for me."

She sat back a little.

I took hold of her hand again and squeezed it, holding it close to my face and kissing it with several little pecks on her knuckles.

"Mom, you take such good care of me, you always have... and I love you, so much... I just love you so much...you're the best mom ever, and I'm so lucky that you're my mom... but sometimes I feel like I'm mean to you, and I don't spend enough time with you... but you still love me and take good care of me anyway...you've always been here for me.... thank you so much, Mom... you don't know how thankful I am that I have you."

I wrapped my arms around her again, and hugged her as close to my heart as I could. "I love you, Mom," I whispered. I gave her a loving peck on the cheek. She loved it when I did that.

"I love you, too, Ian," she whispered back. I released my hold on her, and she sat back on the floor. "I love you more than anyone else in the world. You're the best son a mom could ever ask for, and I'm proud and happy to be your mom." She smiled.

"Thank you, Momma," I said, still looking at her.

She kissed my hand a few times and held it close to her face as we looked at each other for a moment.

She sat still, looking thoughtfully at me. "You know, Ian...I know I've said this before," she began, "but I just want you to know how sorry I am, for anything I've ever said or done that might have hurt you."

I nodded and gave her a knowing, grateful smile. "... Me too."

"You've always been my reason," she continued, "I never made any decision without thinking of you first, and what I thought would be best for you...and I know I've made decisions that ended up hurting you, but at the time, I thought it was the right thing to do, and I'm sorry if I messed things up and you got hurt."

"Mom, it's okay. It's all good, you and me, we're good. I know you love me, you show me that every day... you really are the best mom in the world." I pulled her in for another of my long-armed hugs, and I squeezed her as hard as I could. "I've done some things that I know hurt you, too."

She sat back, and we looked at each other eye to eye again, smiling. We were quiet for a few minutes, then she thought of something.

"I'll be right back," she said with a twinkle in her eye.

"No! Where are you going?" I asked, playfully pulling on her hand.

"I bought something for you yesterday, when I went to the store." She smiled. "You'll like it."

And she dashed up the stairs.

She came back with three small plastic bags, one with dried banana chips, one with dried pineapple chunks, and one with raisins.

"Mmmmm!" I smiled and licked my lips. Banana chips were my favorite.

She opened the bag and offered them to me. Still lying down, I stuck my fingers in the bag and pulled out a few. "Thank you, Mom!"

"You're welcome, Ian. You can keep them here by your bed, for whenever you want a little something." She smiled.

We munched on the fruit and I flipped through the channels on television.

"Hey, Mom, want to watch a movie with me?"

"Sure! Do you have one in mind?"

I didn't, but she read me the ones I had filed in my entertainment center, and I chose Fight Club.

"Ask Mark if he wants to come down and watch with us," I

suggested. "We can make some popcorn in my microwave."

"Actually, he's already watching TV with his eyes closed," Mom remarked, jokingly.

Mark was an early-to-bed, early-to-rise kind of guy, but Mom and I had always been more of the night owl type, even though she could rarely hang with me into the wee hours of the mornings much anymore. Mark often said he needed his beauty sleep. Mom and I always laughed about that.

After the movie was over, Mom and I stayed awake for a while talking about it, and about life. We pondered over why humans like to fight, and watch others fight. I had always been somewhat of a peacemaker with the people around me, even as a little kid. I hated it when people I cared about didn't get along or even had a disagreement of some kind, and I often found myself in the middle, trying to put out the fire. But still, I liked to watch a good fight scene in a movie.

Eventually our conversation wound down, and I turned the television back on. We watched a couple of funny shows, then Mom fell asleep on my couch. All the pain medication I'd been given in the ER and taken at home that night made me pretty drowsy, but still I had a hard time sleeping through the night. I tossed and turned with the pain and nausea, and was tormented with thoughts and fear of my new treatment getting started on Monday. I had one more day, and I prayed I would feel well enough to get out of the house for a while.

I was sound asleep until about one o'clock Sunday afternoon. Mom checked with me as soon as I woke up, asking me to rate my pain. My temperature was only slightly up, at 99.2, but other than that, nothing had changed since the day before. I didn't know how long I could stand that headache. She gave me some extra morphine with my first meds of the day, including extra pain relievers for my headache, but it wasn't enough to stop the pain. I felt like the pain was beating me down, and the occasional nausea and vomiting were keeping me there. I was completely fatigued, even though, with the exception of taking a short shower, I hadn't been out of my bed since nine o'clock the night before. I did manage to eat a little bit of the food that Mom brought me, but my appetite was overpowered by my aching head and unsettling feeling in my stomach.

Mom tried all kinds of things in an effort to relieve my pain. She made ice packs for my head and back, which helped only a little. She tried giving me herbal tea, but the taste made me throw up, which then made me cough up a little blood. She tried massaging my lower back and my head, but that didn't help either. The only thing I could do was lay still and suffer the pain, try to get used to it. Mark came downstairs to hang out with us for a while, but the constant pain kept me from having much conversation, or even keeping my eyes open for very long. I felt like all my energy had drained out of me. Mom stayed with me into the night, helping to adjust my pillows when I struggled to get comfortable, urging me to take at least small sips of ice water, and holding my hand when I talked about my fears of starting my bone marrow treatment in the morning.

12

We Never Thought It Would Happen to Me

Mom woke me at 7:15 a.m. We had to leave for the Cancer Center in half an hour. The dreadful day had arrived. My head felt like it was exploding with intense pain, and my lower back hurt even worse than days before. I felt lightheaded and dizzy as I stood to pull on my jeans and a clean t-shirt. Mom had made some toast for me, but I felt too nauseous to eat.

Mark had the car warming up and waited in the doorway of my room to take us out through the garage. I slid my feet into my shoes, pulled on my favorite blue hoodie, and grabbed the bag of raisins from beside my bed. I thought it would be good to have them in case I got hungry. Mark walked next to me as I hobbled my way to the car. Mom followed us out and sat in the back seat so I could be more comfortable in the front. I laid the seat all the way back, and propped the green pillow between my head and the door. I set the bag of raisins next to me in the seat. I felt cold, so Mom took the afghan from the back seat and helped to drape it over me, and I tried to lay still and suffer the drive in silence.

Mark dropped Mom and me off at the Cancer Center at 8:30, and parked the car in the garage across the street. Mom stayed close to me as we walked in through the two glass doors. I was still feeling dizzy and very nauseous. I hoped I could control it until I was inside the bathroom near the waiting room. I didn't even look at anyone at the desk as I walked past. I kept my eyes down and walked straight to the bathroom, and I barely made it before I started vomiting some really nasty-tasting bile and stomach acid. I had come to think that a lot of that nasty-tasting and foul-smelling stuff that I threw up also contained some of the chemicals from chemotherapy. I had remembered that the body would flush the residual chemicals out through bodily fluids, and I figured vomit was in that category.

When I came out, Mom stood to walk behind me to the desk inside the treatment center. They already had a room ready for me, and that bed was a welcome sight. I eased myself slowly down into it, with the crushing pain pounding in my head and back, and my stomach feeling like it was going to throw up again. My vitals were taken right away, and showed that I was orthostatic, which is when the blood pressure is inconsistent. Mom noted also that my complexion was very pale.

A nurse came in and accessed my port, started me on fluids, morphine, and medications for nausea. My blood was drawn for labs. A hematology nurse came in to see me in the treatment room, and said my bone marrow biopsy would be rescheduled because I was feeling so bad. She would get in touch with us after Dr. Van came to visit me, and we had a better idea of my condition. The pain was more than I could take, and my nurse gave me two more milligrams of morphine at my request.

It was an all-to-familiar picture. Mom had turned off the light, pulled the door and curtain closed, and drawn the blinds shut. She pulled her chair close to my bed and sat holding my hand. Mark was sitting in the treatment chair at the head of my bed, with his hand resting near my head. I laid still and quiet, grateful for their comforting presence, but suffering the unending pain in my head and my body. The three of us waited in silence, neither of us knowing what was happening to me, and feeling anxious for things to get better.

My nurse came in and told us I would be receiving two units of blood right away. My labs had shown I was anemic. I instantly felt more nauseous, and pain intensified in my stomach with that news.

Having someone else's blood mixing in with mine gave me a creepy feeling. It made me feel dirty. I expressed my disheartenment to Mom and Mark about it, and Mom gave me the same speech as before, saying that God makes the blood of life, so it can't be unclean. Her words didn't help me. I was still repulsed by the thought of that blood in me. I suspected she would have felt the same way if she needed a blood transfusion, but I knew she was trying to help me. I had no choice, and after all, knowing the transfusion would probably make my headache go away was enough to get me through it.

I was still getting my second unit of blood when Dr. Van came in to see me. He quietly rapped on the door and walked in unassumingly. He greeted each of us with a slight nod of his head. Mom stood up to move her chair away from my bed so he would have room next to me, but he told her it was okay to stay where she was. He walked around to the foot of my bed and sat down next to my legs. He asked me how I was feeling, and I expressed myself by shrugging my shoulders and raising my hand slightly toward the bag of blood hanging above me. He nodded that he understood.

He asked me a few more questions about how I felt and the intensity of my pain. He listened to my lungs and heart, then he sat still for a moment. He took a deep, quiet sigh, and pursed his lips together, thinking of the words he had to say. He looked at me, then at Mom and Mark. Looking back at me, again, he spoke softly. "Your beta hCG is very high today."

We three sat quiet, frozen in alarm of the news.

"How high?" I asked."

"It's over 53,000, up from 8,000 just two weeks ago."

My heart sank into my stomach. Fear filled my lungs as I breathed in small short breaths.

"What now?" I asked, lying very still, afraid to hear the answer.

Dr. Van chose his words carefully. "This means that the cancer is completely resistant to current treatment."

"It's not working at all?" My heart felt empty and lost.

Mom was biting her lower lip.

Mark was very still.

"No," he shook his head slightly. "A rise in that degree shows that the cancer is not responding to the treatment." He paused, allowing me to think about what he'd just said, then he continued. "We won't be scheduling the bone marrow transplant for now." Another pause, looking at each of us, and allowing me the time to emotionally process the horrible news. "We can start you on methotrexate, but we have to wait until your body is stronger. Your resistance is very weak right now, because you've lost quite a bit of blood."

I covered my face with my hands. I couldn't believe what I was hearing. I dropped my hands to my sides again. "What if that doesn't work?" I looked at Mom. She took hold of my hand.

"If the methotrexate doesn't cause a tumor response," he paused, as if making room for the pain of bad news, "we're looking at a situation that would be fatal... within... two or three months' time." His expression was very solemn.

Fatal...fatal....fatal... the word echoed in my head.

He looked compassionately at me, then glanced at Mom and Mark, and back at me, "The cancer is resisting treatment, and it's growing very fast now."

"What are my chances that the new treatment will work, the methotrexate?" I wanted to know.

"I would say, fifty-fifty," he said, "given what your tumor response has been to this date."

"Well... how soon can I get that new treatment started?" I asked, trying to feel calm.

"We first have to find out where the bleeding is, internally," he said. "We're going to admit you today. You'll be receiving more blood. We may be able to start treatment in a day or two."

He sat with us for a few moments, waiting for any questions.

The shock was still running through me.

"All right," he said, "I'll be here, call me if you need anything or have any other questions... and I'll see you after you've been admitted." He nodded to me, then he gave me a pat on the leg and stood up and nodded goodbye to Mom and Mark. He closed the glass sliding doors as he left.

As soon as he stepped out, the nurse came in to check my vitals. They had been doing that every half hour. We were all silent while she recorded my statistics, checked my IV unit and bag of blood, and left the room.

Mark, Mom, and I then looked at each other as our eyes filled with tears. I felt like the whole room was full of our sorrow and dread. Mom moved from her chair to sit on the bed next to me. She leaned over and held me, and I wrapped my arms around her so tight, I squeezed her with all of my strength. We didn't sob, but we both had tears on our face. We all three were trying to be strong for one another. I loosened my hug, and she sat up to look at me.

"Mom, can I have a minute by myself?"

"You want to be alone?" She was surprised. She had never before seen that look in my eyes, on my face. She saw fear, but it was mixed with wisdom and courage.

"Yeah, I just need some time... a few minutes, okay?" I needed to be with my fate... to face it alone... to have a good cry, and pray to God in my heart.

She and Mark honored my request, and stepped out into the hall.

"We'll be just out here in the hall," Mom assured me, closing my curtain and glass door behind them.

After a while, I heard a gentle tapping on the metal door frame, and Mom spoke through the closed curtain. "Do you want some more time?" she asked.

"No, come in," I said.

Mark walked in behind Mom, and she walked slowly over to me. Her eyes were red from crying, just like mine. She sat down gently on my bed, and we just looked at each other. She looked so sad as she reached to touch my face. Then she took my hand and kissed my knuckles. Mark sat down in the guest chair that Mom had pulled close to me earlier. I could tell he had been crying, too. He leaned over to me and gave me one of his huge hugs. Then he sat up and put his hand on top of mine and Mom's. The three of us sat there like that, just look-ing at each other for a moment or two, in the quiet room with only the clock ticking, my IV pump clicking, and the faint sound of televisions chattering in other patient rooms.

There was another rap on the metal door frame, and Dr. Fleming walked in with a resident doctor. Mom and Mark moved to make room for them near my bed. Dr. Fleming introduced the other doctor, and then sat in the chair next to my bed and talked to me about what was planned for me in the next few days upstairs in Unit 42. He basically expanded on what Dr. Van told us, and the whole conversation wore me out, and made the pain in my head, back, and stomach more in-tense. Then he gave me a pat on the leg and said he'd see me upstairs, and he was gone. Again, the room seemed full of dismay and uncer-tainty, as the clock ticked and the televisions chattered on.

When my nurse came back at 4:30 to check my vitals, I asked for more pain medication. After recording my vitals and taking care of my IV unit, she left and came back with two milligrams of morphine for me. I thanked her as she left, and the room was quiet once more.

Mom sat next to me in the chair. "Do you want to pray?" she asked me.

"No." I closed my eyes. "I just want to lay here and rest."

I lay still and thought about my fate. I couldn't believe what was happening. We were all so optimistic in the beginning. I didn't ever really believe that I would lose the battle. I never expected to hear a doctor tell me I might not live, after all I'd been through. I thought I was going to live on, to do some public speaking about testicular can-cer, teaching other guys about it like Mom and I had planned. None of this would ever have happened, if I had known what to do about the lump in my testicle a year ago. I wondered if the world would notice if guys like me kept dying of this curable disease. I opened my eyes and looked at Mom. She was writing in her journal, the events of the day.

"Hey, Mom?"

She looked up, ready to get me what ever I needed. "Yes, Ian?"

"Mom... if I die... will you write a book about me?... So other guys will know?... and they won't have to go through what I've been through?"

She looked very sad to hear me say such a thing, but I knew she saw the sincerity and trust in my eyes. She knew I was serious, and that I trusted her to do it, if she said she would. But she couldn't let herself say anything to make herself believe that I might die. She didn't want to give up hope, so she said, "Well, I have another idea... how about you survive the cancer and live, and we write the book together?"

"Yeah, we will... but seriously, Mom. I really mean it. If I die, will you write the book?"

She nodded. "Yes, Ian," she said sincerely, "I promise you, I will write a book about you. I will make sure people know your story." She took hold of my hand.

"Thank you," I whispered. I looked at her for a moment, then turned my head toward the window slightly, and closed my eyes. I knew Mom could write my story as if I were telling it myself, all the way to the end. She would know that's what I wanted.

At 5:00 p.m., I was admitted to room 4214 upstairs, and I didn't even have to leave my bed. Two people came to transport me and my IV machine by taking the whole bed, with me in it. That was good, because I didn't know if I could have made the trip to the fourth floor sitting up in a wheelchair. When we passed the nurses station in Unit 42, my nurse followed us into the room. There was an empty space already prepared for my bed to be wheeled into place. The transport people left, and my nurses and aides immediately were busy getting things set up for me, checking my vitals, and asking me the routine questions.

Mom noticed right away that there was no chair that folds out into a bed in the room, and asked the nurse if one might be available. The nurse said she'd check, but later came back to say they were all being used. She told Mom it was okay if she slept in the other patient bed next to me. Mom wasn't too sure about it, because she didn't want to be that far away from me. I didn't want her that far away, either. With all the bad news I'd had in the last eight hours, I wanted her close enough that I could reach her if I needed to get her attention.

"Is it okay if I move this bed closer to Ian?" she asked.

The nurse said it was okay, but that the staff would need room to get in between the beds to check my IV unit and vitals. Mom thought about it, then put the decision off until later. Maybe a chair-bed would become available in time. She made herself comfortable in the regular chair next to me, and Mark leaned on the bench style air vent next to the window.

My back, stomach, and head were still hurting, although my headache wasn't as bad. There was no time wasted in taking care of me. Only 30 minutes later, the mobile x-ray unit was wheeled into my room to take a picture of my lungs. I took off my gold necklace and earring, and handed them to Mom, and put them back on after the x-ray was finished.

Dr. Fleming came in about an hour later. He talked to me about the procedures that would be used to determine where I was losing blood. They would be collecting my stool to test for blood in it. They would also do a rectal exam. If that didn't show proof of any bleeding, I would get an endoscopy, and possibly a colonoscopy. They had to find the leak in me, so it could be stopped, and we could move forward with treatment.

I asked him what his thoughts were on why the tumors have been resisting treatment. He reminded me of the two types of cancer cells that were seen in my biopsy in November, embryonal carcinoma and coriocarcinoma. The corio cells are the most aggressive and most difficult to treat, and those were the cells that were growing fastest and resisting treatment.

"So, knowing the way it's gone, do you think you would have done anything differently, if you were sitting here instead of me?" I asked him pointedly.

"No, not at all." He didn't even hesitate. "We have treated this cancer as aggressively as we were able. The risks are always there. Sometimes the treatment doesn't have the effects we know are possible... but no, I would not have done anything differently. I would have made the same decisions as you did with your treatment."

"Is there any way that surgery is possible now, to get the cancer all out of me, since the chemo isn't working?" I couldn't let myself believe I was out of options.

Dr. Fleming was patient with my questions. "No, there are too many lesions in too many of your organs. Surgery has not ever been a viable option to treat this cancer, because of this reason alone."

It seemed these painful answers were manifesting as pain in my chest and my back, and I asked if I could get more medication for the pain. I was rating the chest pain at a seven or an eight. It took a while, but at about eight o'clock that evening, I was given six milligrams of morphine to knock the pain out. Dr. Fleming had approved up to ten milligrams in one hour if I needed it. As it turned out, I did, and half an hour later I received two milligrams more.

Forty-five minutes later, I was given my usual eight medications before they got me started on receiving another unit of blood. At 10:30, the blood transfusion was started, and I received four more milligrams of morphine.

Mark was getting ready to go home for the night. Mom wrote a short list of things for him to bring back with him the next day. She already had our duffle bags packed and ready for any emergency. There were a few more items we wanted him to bring, including my own pillow and green Mexican blanket. I also had the idea that we needed some board games to play, or "Games of the Board," as I liked to call them. I wrote down all my favorites, then chose four of them and gave the list to Mark. Back in February, we had gotten together with Mark's brother and his wife to play Risk at our house. We'd had a lot of laughs, and I was looking to get some of that fun in the hospital to break the monotony. While Mark and I were going over the list, Mom went down the hall to get three more blankets to add to her bed, and mine. When she returned, he hugged us both goodnight, and headed for home.

I was lying quietly, and music was playing in my head, as it often did. I had been trying to remember a certain chord progression, and I thought I had it right then.

"Hey, Mom," I looked over at her, trying to figure out how to move the other bed, "can I have some paper and a pen? I want to write something down before I forget."

She handed me her journal, opened to a blank page, with the pen attached to its spiral binder. I sat up slightly in my bed and propped the book on my bent leg so I could write. I drew the neck of my guitar, with the six frets where the chords should be played. I labeled the strings, then closed my eyes to envision the chord finger placements I'd just had in my mind. I drew them as I saw them and heard them in my head, and labeled my notes, "John Meyer 'E'" without B. I studied it to make sure I hadn't forgotten anything, then I set the book down on my bed and laid back on my pillow.

"Thanks, Mom." It had made me feel very tired to sit up and do that, but it felt good to be able to remember the chord long enough to write it down. "I've been trying to figure that chord out for a long time. Now when I get home, I can try it out on the guitar and see if I got it right." I smiled a sleepy smile at her.

She walked around to the far side of my bed and sat down in the chair. She picked up the book and looking at my drawing, nodded, and smiled back at me. Then she propped a pillow between the chair and my bed, and laid her head on my bed next to me.

"Are you going to be able to pull that bed close enough?" I asked her.

"I think I can get it close enough that I'll be near enough to touch you. Is that going to be okay?"

"Yeah." I reached for her hand. "I need you close, Mom. I'm kind of feeling scared again, of what's going to happen."

She kissed my hand and looked up at me.

"I love you, Mom, so much." I gave her hand a squeeze. "Thank you so much for being my mom. You really are my best friend.

"I love you more than everything, Wonderful You," she said with a smile.

I looked at her for a moment. "I don't know what I would have done all this time, without you. You and Mark have been so good to me. You guys have always been there for me."

She hugged my hand to her face. "Ian, you are the best son a mom could ever ask for. I'm so lucky to be your mom.

I pulled her hand up to my face and gave it a little peck kiss. "You're the best mom in the whole world," I said, smiling at her.

It was midnight, and I was about to be hooked up with my fourth unit of blood. I couldn't believe all the blood I needed. I wondered if it was just leaking out of me as they were putting it in. I asked my nurse if she knew anything about it. She said she couldn't be sure about the bleeding until they had run the tests, but that according to my medical records of the day, I had been dangerously low on blood when I arrived at the Cancer Center that morning. I was just getting a replacement of what had already been lost in the past week.

I woke at some time in the early morning hours, and Mom was holding my hand, asleep in the chair next to me, still resting her head on my bed. I had to let go of her hand to turn onto my side, and when I did, she woke up. I had my back to her, and she softly patted me on the side. I reached back with my left hand and took hold of her fingers, just to let her know I appreciated her being there, and we slept like that until the aide came in to check my vitals, and I had to turn onto my back again.

The sun was barely up that morning when my nurse woke me to say it was time for my rectal exam. What a way to start the day, but best to get it over with, I thought. The resident doctor came in, and I could actually tell him that I slept okay, and I didn't feel as bad as the day before. My headache felt better, even though it was still a problem, but I wasn't nearly as nauseous. I had to get out of bed, and it was difficult for me to move around because of weakness, pain and stiffness, but I managed while the doctor observed my status.

No sooner had he left than a transport came to take me downstairs for an MRI on my head. I was so hungry, I couldn't wait to get back to my room for breakfast. Mark was there with Mom when I returned, and he looked happy to see me up and feeling a little better. We talked for a while about my morning's events, and how all the activity had knocked my pain level up a few notches. I asked for morphine, and my nurse gave me six milligrams just after I finished ordering my breakfast. By the time my food arrived, my pain wasn't as bad, so I could enjoy eating. I had pancakes, bacon, eggs, and a fruit cup. I ate almost all of it, though I suffered a stomach ache afterward. But it felt so good to have an appetite, and the food tasted great. Another good thing about being able to eat is that I was also able to poop. It wasn't much, but enough that the nurse could tell me that there was blood in it. That was at least an answer closer to finding the source of my bleeding.

Dr. Fleming came to see me about 11:30. He started off with the not-so-good news. The MRI revealed several new scattered lesions in my brain. That news sent me sinking down very fast. I thought I had won that part of the fight. I couldn't help but feel defeated with that news. Dr. Fleming didn't dwell on it, though. He continued, saying they would be re-staging my cancer that day, using a CT scan, labs, and the MRI results of that morning. He wanted to keep a close watch on the blood in my stools and my red blood cell count for the next couple of days, also. He said that sometimes bleeding can subside unaided.

I liked Dr. Fleming's attitude in treatment. He told me that the priority was re-staging and base-line treatment, taking an aggressive action toward the tumors, and that the bleeding, while important, was secondary to treating the cancer. That was the way I felt about it, too.

I asked him what could have caused the internal bleeding. He said it could have been chemotherapy-induced, because the drugs I was receiving can cause bleeding. He said that sometimes a tumor will get large enough to tear away like a scab, and that can also cause bleeding. The only place he suspected that could happen would be in the largest of tumors in my abdomen, and if that was the case, they would soon find out with the endoscopy. He made sure I hadn't been in any accidents or the like that would have caused me injury, and I told him I hadn't. He reminded me that I'd be getting a trip downstairs for a CT scan very soon, and they would begin staging as soon as possible, and just as he was finishing up, my nurse came in to put an IV in my hand to receive contrast for the CT. The doctor and I shook hands, and he quickly stepped out my door to finish his rounds.

In addition to the IV contrast, I had to drink a cup of that contrast nectar. I managed to choke it down, and right after that, my nurse brought me six milligrams of morphine for the constant pain in my back.

Mark stepped out of the room and down the hall to the visitor's lounge, where a few members of his family were waiting to come in and visit with us.

Mom and I were sitting quietly, and I was thinking about what may have happened to cause me to bleed internally. I thought about that party a week or so ago. I was trying to remember if there was anything about the night's events that could have triggered the downturn in my health.

Mom looked up at me from her journal momentarily, and noticed the serious expression on my face.

"What's the matter?" she asked with a concerned look.

I just shook my head and looked away.

Mom took my hand in both of hers, and leaned up a little closer to me. She looked at me with a compassionate but sorrowful smile.

I heaved a sigh, and looked over at her again. She just stayed quiet... listening.

I told her about the party, and the fight, and how sick I had felt with the stress of it all.

"And you didn't think it might be a good idea to tell your doctor?... or someone who cares about you?" she quizzed.

"I figured there wasn't any point. I didn't get hurt or anything." I stared straight ahead of me, thinking about the event.

Mom stayed quietly listening. She was disappointed in my nonchalant, passive attitude in view of my health.

"I'm sorry I didn't tell you about it," I said, looking over at her again.

"Yeah," she said softly. "Maybe that's not when the bleeding started... it's probably what Dr. Fleming thinks it is, so don't worry about it, okay? That's just more stress that you don't need."

"Yeah..." I closed my eyes.

It was good when Mark's family came in to my room. It broke my mind away from my pain-filled thoughts. They always had something funny to say, and we often batted jokes back and forth. Mark showed them all the board games he brought in earlier, and we talked about which one I wanted to play after I got back from my CT scan, if I was up for it.

I think they could tell I was in a lot of pain, because they kept their visit short, but they stayed nearby to visit with Mark and Mom once I had gone downstairs for my CT.

My nurse came in with six milligrams of morphine for me, and just then, the transport showed up to haul me downstairs for the CT. Once again, I took off my earring and gold necklace and handed them to Mom for safekeeping. The process took quite a while, and while I was sitting in the wheelchair waiting for my transport afterwards, I felt a very sharp, painful muscle spasm along my ribs on the right side. It was almost unbearable. The stabbing pain lasted almost all the way to my room, and continued to hurt even after the original pain, which I had rated at an eight to a nine.

I climbed into my bed and called my nurse to see if I could get some morphine. While we were waiting, Mom offered my jewelry back to me, and helped me put the gold chain back on. It was getting to be more of a hassle to keep doing that. I'd had to take them off before every procedure, MRI and CT, including the endoscopy. I thought about not putting them back on, but I had worn them for so long, it felt weird to be without them. I'd been wearing that gold chain for three and a half years, since Carrie gave it to me for Christmas, my junior year in high school.

Mom asked if I wanted to play one of the board games. I thought maybe I could do that. Mark pulled them all out of the bag and set them on my bed. I looked at the boxes, thinking about the games inside. I didn't want to play one that required a lot of thought, or that would take a long time to play. It had been a long time since we had played some of them, and we talked about each game to help me decide. I chose Scrabble. I raised the head of my bed to a sitting position, and we set the game up on my bed. Mark pulled the chair up to one side, and Mom sat on the foot of the bed. Setting it up was fun, because we talked about the rules of the game, one of which I made up: If you can use the word in a sentence, then you can use the word in the game. We laughed at the possibilities of that one.

Just as we were getting started, my nurse came in with my morphine. It was more than an hour since my last dose, so she gave me eight milligrams to get rid of the lasting pain from the spasm.

"Okay," I said after she left, "Let's get this game going before that morphine kicks in. I'm not sure how well I'll be able to think after that."

We each took several turns, and then I had only one word option that I could see. It was time to apply my special rule. I laid it out on the board, "S H A T."

Mom grinned up at me. "What?"

Mark laughed.

"Shat," I pronounced, "past tense... as in, I just shat myself."

Mom chuckled as she reached for the bag of tiles, and we joked around with each other as she and Mark took their turns.

Mark handed the bag to me, I pulled out four tiles and set them on my tile rack.

"I'm starting to feel that morphine," I confessed. "I don't know how long I can last."

I stared at my tile board for a minute, rearranging the tiles to try and spell anything at all. I couldn't think clearly enough to spell even one word on that board, not even when using my funny rule. The tiles looked just like a bunch of letters to me, and my ability to concentrate had faded. "I'm sorry," I shook my head. "I can't think anymore... I just can't even think."

They looked at me, waiting for my decision.

"We'll have to call it a game." I looked at them, and then leaned back against my bed, clasping my hands behind my un-thinking head and stretching my legs out to straddle the bed.

"Well, let's say you won that one, for your creative use of the word *shat*," Mark chuckled.

"You guys can keep playing, and I'll lay here and listen. You can leave the board there." I folded my legs on the bed, and drifted off to a light sleep while they played a couple of turns longer.

The rest of the evening was pretty uneventful, except I was having some really severe pain in my abdomen that felt like my muscles were tightening up, and my head was starting to hurt with the same intensity as when I'd been admitted Monday evening. I was using my hourly quota in meds for anxiety and nausea, and extra doses of morphine throughout the night when I couldn't take the pain.

The next morning I was visited by a resident, an intern, and a group of students who came in to stare at me. I felt like they had been told to visit this young cancer specimen, to see what someone in my condition looks like. I didn't like that at all, but that was just part of the package when being treated in a university hospital. He examined me and asked me the usual questions about my level of pain, fatigue, nausea, coughing, bowel movements, all that stuff. I tried to be polite, and I knew he was there to help me, but all of that just irritated me. I didn't like having to answer the same questions to so many doctors. It made me feel even more sick.

I learned Margo was my nurse, and I was glad to see her. After I ate a little breakfast, she hooked me up with a PCA, which is the Patient Controlled Analgesia using the IV machine for morphine. Instead of getting the doses separately each hour, I would receive a continuous four milligrams as a basal rate, and I could give myself an extra two milligrams every 15 minutes using the button if I needed it. The bag of liquid morphine hanging above me was no bigger than the foil juice packs Mom used to buy for me when I was a kid.

My stool that day was very dark and hard, and I told my mom it hurt bad. She made a note of it so I would remember to tell Dr. Fleming when he came in.

He was there about noon. He told me I would be getting another blood transfusion soon, that Dr. Van would be in to see me later that evening, and that I would be starting the new chemo treatment on the following day. We talked about the treatment, and I tried to understand how it works. It was interesting to me that all the chemotherapy drugs worked by interrupting the process of cell division and growth, but they each did that in a different way. Dr. Fleming told me that metho-trexate works by inhibiting dihydrofolic acid reductose to incapacitate the thymidilate synthetase. When he told me that, I just grinned at him.

"I have no idea what you just said." I laughed.

Dr. Fleming chuckled, and broke it down into simpler terms. Mom gave him her journal, and he drew his explanation for us to try to grasp what he was talking about. I gave him a smile as an idea came to my head.

"Will you write that down for me? When Dr. Van comes in, I want to pretend that I know what he's talking about." I grinned.

He laughed, "I'll tell you what, when he comes in, tell him you think this treatment will work, and tell him why, using this description."

He had a sly smile on his face as he scribbled my lines down for me in Mom's journal. This was his way of teasing Dr. Van, and I was in on it. It would be fun. I had developed a good relationship with the two of them over the last three months, I thought. I liked to make them laugh. I told Dr. Fleming about one time when Mark, Mom and I were walking in the hallway down on the first floor and ran into Dr. Van on his way to his office. He walked and visited with us, and I told him that since I was spending so much time at the hospital, he should look into getting a ping-pong table set up for me in the basement, so I would have something to do. I told him we could have tournaments with the other departments. He had laughed about that, and Dr. Fleming chuckled at the story, too.

He showed me the statement and went over it with me to make sure I had the pronunciation right. I rehearsed the lines a couple of times, and Dr. Fleming chuckled at the thought of seeing me say that to Dr. Van. He said he would be in to see me the next morning, and he wanted to hear about Dr. Van's reaction to my statements about treatment. We shook hands and he left the room smiling.

In the meantime, I had an appointment at 1:30 for the upper endoscopy, or EGD. I knew that procedure. It was the one that those other gastroenterologists tried on me before my cancer diagnosis. I trusted that things would go a lot better than they did back then.

It was almost two hours later when I was returned to my room, and I was very, very sleepy. When the aide checked my vitals, it showed that the oxygen level in my blood was low. It's supposed to be at ninety or above, and mine registered at seventy-nine. I lowered the head of my bed so I could lie almost flat, as Margo came in to hook me up to the oxygen while I slept. She told me to be sure the nasal cannula, the oxygen tubes in my nose, stayed put, to make sure I got the oxygen I needed to raise my saturation level, meaning the amount of oxygen in my blood.

The resident doctor came in and Mom woke me to hear what he had to say. The results of the EGD revealed an ulcer on the duodenum, near my stomach. This was where the largest tumor was, just as Dr. Fleming had suspected. It was scabbed over, and the scab had pealed away, causing the bleed. Dr. Fleming had explained earlier that when cancer cells grow very fast, the new cells starve off the older cells, causing them to die quickly, which is what the resident was referring to as the scab. They had treated it with epinephrine to stop the bleeding, and cauterized the site to seal it. They scheduled a biopsy on the site after it healed in two weeks to make sure there was no more tumor growth. I would also be given a fifth unit of blood later that day.

I was starting to feel worse than I did earlier in the day, more weak, more tired, just over all more sick. I was weary from being in the hospital for so long, and needing so much attention and care. It seemed like I had been away from home for weeks, and it had only been three days. I missed my cat, my car, and my own room. Friends were calling and sending texts on my cell, but I didn't have the life in me to respond. I wished Carrie would call. I wondered if the cancer was still getting worse. Mom and Mark tried their best to be the comforting presence I needed, but the uncertainty that loomed over me was slowly chipping away at the last bit of hope I had left in me.

"I wish I could see Carrie," I mentioned to Mom. "I don't care how bad I look."

When I drifted back into sleep, Mom slipped out into the hallway with her cell phone, and called Carrie. Mom would not admit even to herself that my condition was deteriorating. She just told Carrie that I wasn't doing well at all, and hoped that Carrie would visit as soon as she could.

It was 5:00 p.m. when Margo brought in my fifth bag of blood. I had the blood transfusing through the port in my chest, and fluids and morphine through the IV in my arm. My oxygen saturation level was a little higher, too, and that helped me to feel better. She told me that Dr. Van would be in to see me within the hour. I was looking forward to seeing him.

I raised the head of my bed so I could sit up a little more and feel awake to talk to him. I hoped he would have good news for me about my condition and treatment.

"Mom, can I see your notebook? I want to read over my lines for Dr. Van." I smiled at the thought of it. I read it aloud a couple of times to recall the pronunciation. I shook my head and grinned. "I hope I can do this without smiling," I said, looking at Mom and Mark. "I don't know if I can."

"Practice on us," Mom suggested. She stood beside me as if she were Dr. Van.

I read the lines, smiling the whole time. "Hey, I should tear off a little piece of paper for me to read from, so he can't see it. He's going to see this notebook and that will ruin it." I tore off a corner of the last page in the book and started to copy what Dr. Fleming had written. My hands were shaky and my writing wasn't very good, so I asked Mom to write it out for me. "That's perfect," I smiled. I tucked the small piece of paper just under my blanket near my leg, so I'd be ready when Dr. Van came in.

13

The Cancer Lottery Grand Prize

Dr. Van Veldhuisen knocked lightly on the door and entered my room, closing the door gently behind him. I greeted him as he walked toward me, and we shook his hand as he greeted us. He asked how I was feeling and examined me, as usual. He stood beside me and told me that the results of the CT were not in yet, but he believed my lungs to be worse than before. The chest x-ray I'd had on Monday showed that the masses in my lungs appeared to be slightly increased in size when compared to the chest x-ray that had been done six days before that.

I would be getting a second IV in my left arm in order to receive higher doses of a medication like Prevacid to speed the healing of the ulcer. Dr. Van first wanted to get that healed and my blood under control before starting me on treatment. He estimated it would be two or more days before treatment would be started. There was my cue.

I leaned back a little, propping my right leg up to hide the small piece of paper with my script written on it. I took the paper in my right hand and looked at Dr. Van at my left, trying to keep a serious expression on my face. "Yeah, I was going to tell you..." I started with a studious frown, "I think the methotrexate will work... because," I glanced down at my note, "it will inhibit my dehydrofolic acid reductose to incapacitate my thymidilate synthetase." I tried to stifle my smile, but it shown in my eyes.

I saw a very subtle moment of curiosity in his eyes, but other than that, there was no change in his expression at all and he didn't flinch one muscle. He was looking right at me. "I agree," he said calmly.

"Yeah," I nodded. I tried to keep a serious face, but I couldn't do it.

The corners of his mouth turned up a little.

"Man! I didn't get you..." I smiled. "Did you think I knew what I was talking about?"

He gave me a big smile that lit up his face and stepped closer to the bed. "Who told you to say that?" he asked, still smiling.

"Dr. Fleming set you up," I grinned. "He told me to say all that." I showed him my notes.

Dr. Van looked at the paper and chuckled, nodding his head. "You did pretty good!"

"Yeah, well I figured I couldn't get through it without smiling." We were all laughing.

"Well," Dr. Van smiled and said in his quiet manner, "You can tell Dr. Fleming that I told you he's the one who can hook you up with a prime suite that has a hot tub and a ping-pong table, because he has the connections."

"Okay!" I smiled, "I'll tell him that!" We all laughed.

Dr. Van looked at each of us for a moment, as if making sure our conversation was finished. "All right," he said with a polite smile, "I'll see you later." He reached out to shake my hand, nodded goodbye, and turned to leave the room.

"Thanks... later," I replied. I laid the head of my bed back a little. I looked at Mark and Mom, and smiled. "That was fun."

As the door of my room closed, I caught a whiff of the dinner cart. I hadn't been hungry when I ordered dinner earlier in the day and couldn't remember what I was having.

Dr. Fleming came in to check on me as I was picking at my dinner. He laughed when I told him about Dr. Van's reaction, and joked he'd see what he could do about the suite.

My vitals later that night showed that my oxygen saturation level in my blood was all right again, so I didn't need the oxygen tubes stuck in my nose. I was glad about that. It was just one less thing to be troubled with, especially when I had to get up to go to the bathroom to pee. Having to haul my IV machine back and forth was bad enough. The IV Prevacid was started a little bit later, and I thought the night was going to be okay. About two hours later, though, my nurse said I had to drink some Milk of Magnesia to help me have a bowel movement. I hated that stuff, because it always made me vomit. And sure enough, 30 minutes later, I had to throw up. I didn't have time or the energy to jump out of bed and run to the bathroom with my IV unit and all the tubes and heavy cords dangling from me. I only had to say, "Mom..." and when she looked at me, she knew what I needed. There was a three-foot tall trash basket next to my sink, and she had that thing next to me in a matter of seconds. I sat on the edge of my bed and hurled my stomach up. It hurt like someone had reached in through my throat and tried to pull my stomach out on a meat hook. After the vomiting had subsided, Mark helped me to amble to the sink to brush my teeth and wash my face. While I was doing that, I started having these horrible, intense pains in my back. They felt like muscle spasms, and I could hardly take the pain. I reached for my PCA button and gave it a push. After several minutes, the pain was still torturing me, so I called my nurse, and she gave me a bolus shot. Once I was feeling better and falling asleep, Mark gave me a hug and headed for home. He had to be up at four in the morning for work. Mom had been sleeping nights, sitting in the chair next to my bed, with a pillow across the arm so she could lay her head on my bed and keep her hand holding mine. She thought it was better than trying to keep the other bed close to me and in the nurses' way, with my IV machine between us.

Mom woke and sat up when a strange man came into my darkened room and quietly walked over toward my bed. She watched him as he plugged a device into the oxygen port in the wall by my bed.

"Excuse me," Mom whispered. "What are you doing?"

He explained to her that he came in to check the oxygen hookup in my room. As it happened, I had awakened Mom earlier, telling her I was feeling short of breath and breathing was painful. Mom had asked my evening nurse about it, who told her that my blood oxygen level was over ninety, so I would be okay without the extra oxygen. Of course, since I didn't like wearing the nasal cannula, I was okay with that.

Mom mentioned my breathing trouble to this technician, and asked if he thought I should be using the oxygen. He had a moment to check my blood oxygen level, and he was kind enough to do that for me. It was down to eighty, "dangerously low," he said. He pressed the button to call my nurse.

"Two more hours like that, and you would be in ICU," he told me. Then he said in amazement that it was purely by accident that he came into my room. The equipment is checked randomly, and he doesn't check every room, but he just happened to choose my room on that particular night.

"It was no accident," Mom said to him. "You are an angel sent by God." She thanked him and wished him a blessed night, and he left the room. We never even learned his name, but Mom thanked God for him out loud.

Trying to sleep with that oxygen blowing into my nose was not easy. It was almost impossible for me. The oxygen felt cold, and it hurt the inside of my nose, and I was always fussing with it to try and get more comfortable. Between that and the pain in my stomach, my back and my chest, I was using that PCA button pretty regularly.

The next morning, my nurse said I had to take some more Milk of Magnesia, so she first brought me some medication to help prevent nausea. Mom had noticed that I was now breathing in short gasps, and it scared her. She asked my nurse about it, and the nurse told her it was because I was on so much pain medication. My lung muscles were so relaxed that I wasn't breathing very deep or in very long breaths. Mom didn't like that, and mentioned to me that if I could stand the pain a little more, to try to hold off on the PCA button if I could. I wasn't sure if I wanted to. I was getting so groggy from the nausea medication, Benadryl, and morphine, I didn't even care about anything but being comfortable.

When the resident doctor came to see me, I was so sedated and delirious that I couldn't communicate with him very well. It was difficult for me to sit up or move around, and I couldn't talk or think well, either. Mom mentioned to him that I had been groggy since the endoscopy the day before, and she was concerned about it. I told him as well as I could of my new complaint of chest tightness and pain.

He said I'd be getting another transfusion of two more units of blood during the morning sometime, because my counts were still low. He said also that my low blood cell counts suggested that I was still bleeding somewhere. I was also restricted from eating or drinking anything because they wanted to do another GI scope to look for more bleeding. On top of that, my oxygen intake had to be raised from two liters up to five liters, because my oxygen saturation level was still low.

My doctors also had another procedure planned for me, called an arteriogram with emolization. A doctor from Radiology came in to explain that one to me. This procedure is where they would shoot dye into my artery to find the bleed, then block off where the bleeding is located. If they found more than one bleeding location, they would address that when they came to it.

So by 11:00 that morning, I had started receiving my sixth unit of blood. I would receive two more units by late that afternoon. All my vitals checked out okay, including my oxygen level. I still had a bad headache, and my chest still hurt at what I rated a seven, with shortness of breath. I was feeling worse than the day before. My mouth was so dry I could hardly swallow. Margo brought me a cup with a tiny bit of ice water, and a package of plastic sticks with small foam sponges on the end of each stick. The only thing I could do to soothe my dry mouth was to dip the sponge end of the stick into the water and rub the sponge around inside my mouth. It helped a little. I was so drugged up that I would ask Mom to help me with it. She took hold of my hand and placed the stick in my palm, holding it there until my fingers wrapped around it. Sometimes she had to raise my hand up to my face until the sponge touched my lips, and other times she helped me brush the sponge along my gum line. Margo caught me once trying to chew on the sponge and swallow the water, and she told me I wasn't supposed to do that.

I hadn't been coughing all that much, but once when I had to get out of bed, the effort caused me to start coughing, and I coughed up about a tablespoon's worth of bright red blood. It felt like it came straight out of my lungs. I told Margo, and she notified my doctors.

It was three hours before I was back in my room after the arteriogram procedure. The procedure was done through an artery in my upper thigh, in the groin, and afterwards it hurt like hell. I rated that pain an eight. I couldn't even move my leg, it hurt so bad. That was almost unbearable. Margo gave me a bolus four milligrams of morphine, but my PCA was inactivated for the time being.

It was good news, though, that they had stopped the bleeding at the ulcer on my duodenum again, and there was no visible bleeding from any of my arteries. Dr. Fleming said I was good to go ahead with the chemotherapy as soon as possible. I would have my blood drawn for labs every six hours to keep an eye on things. I still couldn't have anything to eat or drink, except small amounts of ice cream or sips of water for the next 24 hours.

My vitals were still good, as was my blood oxygen level, and I managed through the evening, although I was miserable with pain and tightness in my chest. A respiratory therapist came to my room with some kind of breathing treatments. I had to breathe in some medication that was supposed to help me breathe easier, but it was very hard for me to do. I couldn't breathe in very deeply or hold it in very long. The medication made me cough, and the coughing was very painful in my chest.

I didn't sleep long through the night, because I would wake up coughing. It was horribly painful, and I felt a growing anxiety in my lack of ability to breathe on my own.

Again, my vitals looked fine the next morning, including my oxygen. I asked my nurse for something for the anxiety, and for anything she could give me to help with shortness of breath. I never knew it could be so frightening, not being able to take in a good deep breath of air.

At 7:30 that morning, the x-ray machine was rolled into my room. I took off my gold necklace and handed it to Mom. "You still have my earring?" I asked her.

She nodded, "It's in my rosary purse."

"Put this with it. Just keep them for me, okay? I'm getting tired of taking them off all the time."

She put it away, gave me a kiss on the cheek, and left the room for the x-ray.

It was only 15 minutes after the x-ray guy had left that Dr. Van came in to see me. He said the x-ray they had just taken showed that the lesions in my lungs were quickly growing larger. The CT showed there was also a tumor now in my spleen, measuring two by three centimeters. That's close to one square inch. He wanted to start me on the methotrexate as soon as possible. There was concern over the ulcer in my duodenum, and they wanted to do another endoscopy to check on it, but there was worry about my difficulty breathing and my inability to sustain a healthy oxygen level. I was already in real danger of lung failure. Dr. Van felt there was no time to waste in treating the growing cancer in my lungs, and I was all for it, if there was even the smallest chance that it could kill the cancer that was now causing more pain than ever before.

I'd had a few very painful coughing spells, causing me to spit out small amounts of blood. The pain in my lungs felt like it was crushing me. I rated it at an eight, and Margo gave me a four milligram bolus dose of morphine. I continued to breathe in short, quick gasps while I was awake. Mom said when I was asleep, she could hardly tell that I was breathing at all. She called Mark and gave him the latest news, and he made arrangements to leave work and come to be with us. Mostly my day was spent trying to breathe, trying not to cough, and trying to stay without pain. It was Friday, and each day I had been in the hospital, my health had deteriorated a little bit more.

Dr. Fleming came in to discuss my critical status with me, Mom, and Mark. He told me I may be in possible need of respiratory support, and that he had already notified the staff in ICU to be prepared in case of my pulmonary failure. The resident doctor and my nurses were all checking with me to make sure of my full code status, meaning did I want all measures to be taken in an effort to keep me alive. My answer was yes, if there was a possibility that I could live beyond this disease, I wanted them to do everything possible to save me.

Every day, more people had learned about my situation. My room was full of greeting cards, gifts, flowers, and food. Mom had been taping the cards up on the wall at the foot of my bed for me to see all the support. All the other things were lined up along the air register and on one of the bed tables in the room.

Visitors came, but I was too out of it to have a conversation with anyone. I was too jacked up on medication to even care who was there. I still had my dignity, though, and I often reminded Mom to not let people stand in my room and talk about me or around me like I wasn't there. She knew the look on my face when I wanted others to take their conversation somewhere else. I was in obvious discontent, and I felt that anyone who cared would see that it took a great deal of effort for me just to breathe.

At about six o'clock that night, Margo started me on the medications I needed to support my body during the chemotherapy, and around 9:00 p.m., my first dose of methotrexate had begun. We were all praying it would work to start killing the cancer right away. I couldn't breathe very deeply, and the pain in my chest wouldn't go away. I was getting as much morphine as my body would handle without inhibiting my respiratory rate. The cold oxygen was blowing so hard, it made the inside of my nose hurt. I felt more and more miserable and depressed at my state. I wasn't sure how much more I could take, but I kept thinking that I was going to get through it.

Mark planned to stay the night, so he went looking for a fold-down chair to put next to me. He slept with his hand on my bed, so I'd know both my parents were with me. Mom pulled the other bed as close to mine as she could. We were less than a foot apart, with the end of her bed touching mine. She lay with her head and torso on my bed next to me, with her hips and feet supported on the other bed. She held my hand through the night, and when I had to get up to go to the bathroom, or the aide or nurse came in to check on me, my vitals or my IV machine each hour, Mom sat up and moved her bed away from mine so I could get out, or they could get to me. She sat on her bed, waiting and watching as they attended to me, then moved her bed back in the same position, and laid down next to me again.

I woke often with coughing and pain in my chest. My oxygen level had to be increased again during the night, and I was feeling more and more anxiety at not being able to take in a deep breath. In the early morning, my nurse gave me a new oxygen mask that covered my nose and mouth because I was not sustaining a healthy blood oxygen level. The amount of oxygen I would receive from the port in my room was raised to 15 liters per minute, more than twice the amount I could receive with the nasal cannula. The oxygen supply level was also increased to 75 percent. That meant I was receiving almost the highest possible amount of oxygen that wall outlet was capable of giving me.

That mask made me feel better at first, because it was easier to breathe, but after I wore it for a while, I started to feel a little claustrophobic. I kept fussing with it, constantly trying to readjust it to get comfortable. I told Mom that the plastic was very cold on my skin, and my whole nose was cold inside of the mask. The cold oxygen blew out from the top of the mask into my eyes. She tried to find ways to help me. She cut a small strip of gauze to place along the bridge of my nose between my skin and the plastic mask, hoping that would block the air from flowing out. That didn't work. She tried placing small pieces of tissue next to my skin, but that didn't work either. She even tried holding it herself, slightly raised from my skin so it wouldn't bother me, but she couldn't hold it for hours, and we tried other ways of making me comfortable with it. Nothing worked. I was so doped up, and I didn't like the way it felt on my nose, near my eyes, but it was just one more thing I had to put up with. I also had started getting the hiccoughs now and then, and they were annoying and painful. I tried everything we could think of to get rid of them, but nothing worked. Sometimes they went away on their own, but they always came back.

Two or three different doctors came in at different times to examine me that morning. I told each of them about my anxieties, and I asked if I could have more pain medication, mostly because of the constant pain in the right side of my chest. If I tried to breathe in a deep breath, the pain got worse and I would start coughing. I also had been feeling something like heartburn, a burning pain radiating from my abdomen to my throat and making me feel like I had to burp. I was given some Maalox for that. Another thing I had noticed was that my vision had gotten worse over the last four or five days, and that was scaring me. Over all, though, it appeared that I had tolerated the methotrexate well, and I would be receiving the rescue dose of leucovorin later in the day.

My blood counts had remained stable, but were still low, so there was ongoing concern about that. My white blood cell count was high, and that brought concern of possible infection or continued tumor progression. Neither one was good news.

Dr. Fleming said the pain I felt when I hiccoughed was possibly caused by inflammation of the lesions in my lungs and liver rubbing together. He said he could hear it while listening to my breathing in my back and rib cage. As he talked about it, I laid there hiccoughing at him. He showed me a trick to get rid of them. He said if you stimulate the gag reflex, the hiccoughs will go away. He demonstrated on me with a tongue depressor, pressing lightly on the back of my tongue when I opened my mouth. In an instant, I gagged, and my hiccoughs were gone. It was a great relief.

He also said the acid reflux feeling in my chest was probably a tumor instead of heartburn, and that it could possibly be a good sign of tumor response to the chemotherapy. I told him about my trouble sleeping and breathing with the claustrophobic and uncomfortable feeling of the oxygen mask, but unfortunately, there was no remedy for that. I had to use it if I wanted to breathe.

After he left, it wasn't long before I started hiccoughing again. I asked Mom to hand me my toothbrush so I could try the gag reflex remedy myself. I was glad to see that it worked instantly. Mom put my toothbrush back with my things, and I laid back to rest.

My blood counts were too low again, so I received another unit of blood. Other than that, I tried to stay asleep all day and all that night, with Mom and Mark sitting quietly on each side of me. I woke often with pain in my chest, or coughing blood, needing more medication for the pain, a return of the hiccoughs, or having to go to the bathroom. It was getting more difficult for me to get to the bathroom on my own, because I was very medicated and short of breath. The oxygen line was long enough that it would reach, but with the effort of walking, I felt desperate for air by the time I got back to my bed, even with Mom and Mark helping me. I had to pee in a bottle anyway, because they were checking the ph levels in my urine often, because of the chemotherapy. I preferred to use it in the bathroom, but as I grew more sick and short of breath, I reduced myself to just standing beside my bed. When I had to go, Mom and Mark got up and closed the curtain around my bed and left my side, so I could have privacy. When I was finished, they took the bottle away and pulled the curtain open to stay beside me again while I slept. It was kind of humiliating, but I had no option, and at least I was still able to stand up and take care of things.

Through the night I woke up coughing frequently. Sometimes I coughed for 15 minutes or more. My cough was a deep rumble, intensely painful, and it made my eyes water because it hurt so bad. Each time, Mom and Mark got up and sat with me until the coughing stopped and I fell back into my bed, racked with chest pain. When I woke with hiccoughs, Mom got my toothbrush, and they waited nearby while I sat on the edge of my bed and tried to gag them away. It didn't always work, after having to do it so many times. Sometimes I sat there brushing my tongue at the back of my throat for several minutes before giving up. I was so drugged up even my gag reflex wasn't working anymore. And so my night went, lightly sleeping, coughing my lungs up, spitting blood, gasping for breath, hiccoughing, gagging, and peeing in a bottle. I was suffering a terrible, torturous hell, and it was killing all three of us. It was about three o'clock that morning when Mom noticed my toothbrush had become tinged pink with blood, and her heart broke for me. She stood at the sink and cried for me as she put my toothbrush away. The hiccoughs kept coming back. The intense, brutally painful coughing continued. And the pain kept me reaching for more medication.

Even with the mask, I had become unable to sustain a good oxygen saturation level in my blood, and my oxygen supply level was raised to 100 percent. My nurse told me I was getting the maximum output available from the oxygen port in the wall. If my condition worsened, that would not be enough oxygen for me. I would probably be transferred to ICU very soon, so that I could receive a stronger oxygen supply. There would be nothing more they could do for me in Unit 42.

The next morning, I was still out of it, very sedated and sleepy when the first doctor came in to see me at 6:00 a.m. I did manage to tell him how I felt, though. My shortness of breath, painful coughing of blood, and worsening fatigue would not go away. And at some point, I had accidentally disconnected the line to my oxygen, and I suddenly became very short of breath. I started coughing and coughing, deep, painful, rumbling coughs, and they brought up more blood.

I had another chest x-ray in my room. I had lost count of how many chest x-rays I'd had in the last week. Several doctors, aides, and nurses were checking on me throughout the morning, but all I could do was sleep and try to breathe. Plans were being made to transfer me to ICU. They didn't want to wait until I got to the point where the oxygen I was getting wasn't enough. They wanted to get me there before then.

My nurse came in with two other nurses, one who was male, and a male oxygen technician. She introduced us and said they would be helping in my move to ICU. She explained that as a team, they would lift me to a transport bed, which would have all the equipment on it needed for my transport. I was much too weak and drugged up to move from one bed to the other on my own very quickly, and they needed to move me fast. She explained that I would be transferred from my oxygen on the wall to the oxygen in the tank attached to the transport bed, and that it would be only a few seconds that I would be without the oxygen. I wasn't able to take in a breath and hold it or breathe deeply on my own at all. It would be as if they were taking my breath away from me. She warned me that it would be a little scary, but assured me that they all understood that I needed that oxygen right away, and would not waste one second in getting me the air I needed. She told us not to be alarmed that the team would be moving my bed very fast through the hallways to get me upstairs as quickly as possible. The oxygen tank on the bed was not going to sustain me for very long. It was not an ample oxygen output for me, I needed more pressure than it was capable of giving. They had only a few minutes to get me from my room on the fourth floor to ICU on the sixth. It was important that I was moved fast, and it would be a stressful, hurried transport. I had to be prepared for that.

Fear was growing inside me, and I looked at Mom and Mark. Mom was holding my hand, and they both reassured me that they would be right with me, and that everything would be all right. Mark already had our duffle bags packed up, and the bag of board games ready to move. He would carry them while Mom stayed with me. A couple of the nurses rolled Mom's bed away from mine to make room for the transfer. There was a knock on my door, and a transport person wheeled a bed into my room. They lined the bed up with mine, and the three nurses and the transport person took their places, two at my head and two at my feet. The oxygen tech stood ready at the head of the transport bed holding my IV lines. I felt terrified of what was about to happen. They counted, one, two, three, and lifted me to the transport bed, and my hand slipped out of Mom's, and that made me feel even more terror. She came to stand near my side and touch me as soon as there was room for her. Then it was time to switch my oxygen. The tech readied the oxygen tank on the bed, and calmly told me he was going to make the switch in oxygen masks. As soon as the mask was removed from my face, I felt as if I couldn't breathe in any air. Within seconds, the tech placed the other mask over my face, and I reached for it like I was starving for it, and I held it to my face until I felt I was breathing again.

The transport person was talking on his radio to relay the news we were on our way to Medical Intensive Care Unit 65.

I was consumed with intense fear, and it shown in my eyes. I reached for Mom and gripped her hand in both of mine as the team started to roll my bed out of my room. "Mom, don't leave me, don't leave me, stay with me, stay with me..."

"I will, Ian, I promise, I promise, I'll be right here with you."

I held onto her hand until I had to let go as my bed was rolled out the door.

She kept talking to me as she followed us out of the room. "I will not leave you, Ian, I promise. I'll be right here with you." She was trying to keep from crying. There was not room for her to walk beside me, but she ran to keep pace with my transport team.

She and Mark followed us down the hall as we hurried past the other patient rooms, down the long corridors toward the elevators. The nurses and oxygen tech were talking to each other about my status. They had a heart monitor on me, a blood pressure monitor, and an oxygen monitor on my finger. I could hear my IV machine rolling behind me. I kept calling for Mom, to make sure she was there. She still couldn't walk beside me and hold my hand, but she was right behind me, talking to me, and telling me that she would be on the elevator with me very soon. She was still running to keep up with me. Mark was keeping pace with us behind Mom, and when we got near the elevators, the transport person stepped ahead of us and pushed the button. Everyone was talking about me and coordinating their efforts, and I was looking for Mom. I could hear her talking to me from behind as they wheeled me onto the elevator. There was barely enough room for my transport team to stand around me. Mom squeezed in on my right side, and right away I reached for her hand. There wasn't room for Mark and all the gear he was hauling for us, and it was a sad and tense moment as the closing doors separated us and he was forced to take the next elevator by himself. I didn't want to take my eyes off of Mom. Looking into her eyes and holding on to her hand eased my fear. The elevator began to move, and suddenly I had to remove my oxygen mask and lean over to throw up on the bed and my shirt. What came out of me was a very dark green, nasty-smelling bile. I was deeply embarrassed and looked at Mom remorsefully, saying I was sorry. She shook her head sorrowfully, telling me it was okay. She covered the green liquid, folding the sheet up a little and wiping my shirt with it.

I wiped my mouth on my sleeve, laid back down with my oxygen and took hold of Mom's hand again. I looked up at her and we held our gaze at one another, eye to eye.

"Don't leave me, Momma."

She had tears in her eyes. "I will never leave you, Ian. I will always be right here."

The doors of the elevator opened to the sixth floor, and I was quickly taken down the long stretch of corridors to Unit 65. Mark was right behind us again. The nurse on my right made room for Mom to walk next to me. Mom held my hand and kept eye contact with me the whole way. She was trying to help me focus on her love and support for me, instead of the terrifying event that was taking place all about me. The tension seemed to relax slightly as my bed was wheeled into the unit and toward my room. I was quickly transported to my new bed, where my new source of oxygen was waiting for me. Mom and Mark stood near as my new nursing staff buzzed around me, hooking me up to all the equipment in my new room. I was exhausted from the stress, and I just kept looking at Mom and Mark. The ICU was a whole new world. There was a monitor above my head that would constantly display all my vital information, beeping in separate tones with the colored lines on the monitor that signaled my heart and respiratory rates.

I stayed awake for a long time that day, even though I was still very drugged up. My entire bed was elevated so that I was about three feet up from the floor, about waist high so the staff was better able to attend to me, and I was also closer to Mom and Mark as they stood next to me. We exchanged I love you's, and I thanked them again for being with me, and for helping me through all of it, reminding them that I felt I would never have been able to handle what I'd been through without them by my side. We talked about all kinds of things, short little conversations in between my moments of drifting off into light, short naps throughout the day.

It wasn't long before a catheter was placed in an artery in my arm to monitor my blood pressure, and another one inserted into my bladder. The one in my arm didn't hurt much more than having an IV put in, because they numbed my arm a little. But I was convinced the nurse who placed the catheter in my bladder was a sadistic bitch. She assured me there would be no need for anesthesia, even though she had to stick the catheter up through my penis. The thought of it sent chills of horrors through me. I asked Mom if she would please stay and hold my hand through the procedure. The nurse said, right before she skewered me, that it would be unpleasant for me and for Mom. Of course Mom didn't watch. She held my hand and tried to be as comforting to me as she could be. The pain was more than I could take. I yelled out, screamed and cursed so loud that people could hear me at the end of the hall. It was the worst pain I thought I had ever felt. And I hated that nurse.

I was NPO, meaning I could not have any food in my stomach, but I was getting some nutritives in my IV with needed fluids. I had three IV pumps to support all the drugs and fluids I was getting, because I couldn't take anything by mouth anymore. There were five or six lines coming from each pump. I was still breathing okay with just the mask on my face, and I could be awake and talk a little bit, but mostly I was very doped up and slept a lot because of it. Mom noticed that the nurses' notes described me as being "mildly sedated but arousable." Mom stayed right next to me. At night she slept sitting up with her head on my bed and holding my hand. During the day she either stood or sat beside me and prayed or talked to me, or just stayed silently with me, her head on my bed, her hand holding mine. Every day she washed my face, my hands and my feet, fluffed my pillows and straightened my blankets. When my mouth was dry, she dipped a sponge swab into some ice water and gently swabbed inside my mouth for me. Mark slept in the waiting room during the night, but he mostly stayed with me during the day, and he told me he loved me each time he had to leave my side.

"I love you too, Mooky," I'd look up at him and reply.

Another chest x-ray showed the cancer in my lungs was still getting worse, my new ICU doctor told me. I was still coherent enough to tell him that I was feeling some mild back pain. I was still receiving the usual 15 different drugs, all through my IV, for pain, nausea, and all the other side effects of chemotherapy. The methotrexate levels in my body, and the ph in my urine were still being checked daily. My oxygen supply level had been raised a couple of times as my lungs grew gradually weaker with the spreading cancer. The extra oxygen I was getting was also helping me to feel a tiny bit better, at least better enough to stay partially awake to have small amounts of conversation.

Dr. Alvarez and Dr. Klish came in to visit me. I hadn't seen either of them since my last visit to Radiation Oncology in February. They each told me that it had been an honor to know me and to treat me, and that they thought of me not only as a patient, but as a friend. I returned the compliment and told them that when I got better, I would stop in for a visit with them someday.

By that afternoon, there were lots of people coming in to see me, and I was barely awake enough to engage in the visit. Mark and Carol, two of my favorite nurses, came from Unit 42. I managed to lift my hand off the bed to wave hello, and open my eyes to look at them. They each told me that they were glad they had gotten to know me and my family during the last four months, and Mark even thanked me and said he would always remember me. They both agreed I was one of their favorite patients.

Mook's family and some close family friends had been pretty much camped out in the waiting room since I had arrived in ICU, so they were popping in occasionally to sit with us and visit a little. I usually wasn't very coherent, but I was able to establish an occasional physical response by moving my hands or trying to open my eyes, or attempting without success to sit up in my bed.

My grandpa and his wife flew up from Florida and were at the hospital each day. My grandma came with friends, and they visited with others in the waiting room while she sat with me for a while. Mark's boss Gary, and his family brought a basket full of snacks for all my family and friends staying in the waiting room, and an extra rosary and a small bottle of holy water for Mom and me.

As time passed, I received more and more medication for the pain in my chest and my back, to the point where I was always in a dream state. I did talk in my sleep some, thinking I was having conversation. I would open my eyes many times and look at the people who loved me, and I tried to communicate with them, but the truth is, I was way too out of it to focus my vision or to speak the words that were in my head. I wanted to reach out and to talk, but I had sunken into a deep sedation of morphine and fentanyl. The only communicative motions that came from me were slurred speech and acting out of the comical and serious dream state that was going on inside my head, while those closest to me stayed near, tearfully watching me and chuckling at the funny things I said and did. I could still squeeze Mom's hand when she was holding mine, though, and my fingers sometimes wrapped around hers when she kissed the back of my hand. And I always opened my eyes when she spoke my name.

Mom and Mark could tell when I was playing my guitar, or holding a pen and writing a song, and a couple of times I even made a comment about my music that caused them to laugh. Mark commented that I was still a comedian, even in my sleep.

My nurse came in to check on me and mentioned to Mom and Mark that eventually I would have to be intubated. That meant I would need a breathing tube inserted into my lungs through my throat, because of my deteriorating ability to breathe from the mask alone.

My doctors were telling us that my prognosis was poor, but Mom wouldn't have it. She insisted that God was in control, and that I was soon going to be living proof of the miracle of life and faith. It would happen, because she believed it would, and had been praying about it since November.

Only a few hours later, my oxygen supply level was increased again, and my doctor told Mom and Mark that I would have to be placed on the ventilator as soon as possible. He made it very clear that I needed the ventilator in order to breathe. I was quickly losing the ability to inhale the amount of oxygen I needed on my own. The ventilator would push the air into and out of my lungs, and they could continue to adjust the amount of oxygen as I needed it.

In order to be intubated, I would have to be completely sedated from that point on to keep me from instinctively trying to pull the tube out of my throat. Mom wanted to stay with me. She didn't want to let go of my hand during the procedure. My doctor and nurse stood on the other side of my bed and talked to her about the process, as Mark stood beside her, holding her other hand and listening to them.

My nurse stressed to Mom that she would find it a very disturbing process and would be a very unpleasant and emotionally painful experience for her to observe, even if she didn't watch. She strongly suggested that Mom not be present. They both assured her and Mark that I would be completely sedated, and would not suffer or struggle at any point in the process. They said the procedure would take about an hour and a half, and they would notify Mom and Mark as soon as it was time to return to my room. There were some papers Mom had to sign before they could start the procedure. While she did that, Mark talked to me in my sleep state. He said they would not be far away, and that it was all going to be all right, and that he loved me, and would see me again soon.

My doctor and nurse left, and Mark went out to the waiting room to share the news with everyone else. Mom stayed close to me, holding my hand and softly stroking my face, talking to me and telling me how much she loved me. She said she was only going out of the room because she had to, and that she was not leaving me, but just stepping away while my doctors took care of me. She leaned over my bed and held me and kissed my face, whispering that she loved me more than everything. I was too sedated to even open my eyes. Mark came back to the room to get her, and she stood up, still talking to me. She kissed my hand and held it close to her face, and told me she was not leaving the hospital, that she would still be with me, just not in my room. I couldn't respond to her with anything more than lightly squeezing her hand.

It was almost 5:00 p.m. The doctors were ready to start, and Mom didn't want to leave me. She knew that when she came back, I would be different. She was afraid of that, of coming back into my room to see me completely sedated with a tube sticking out of my mouth. She stood and cried at the thought of walking away, as the doctors stood waiting at my door with expressions of urgency on their faces. Mom finally kissed me once more and told me she would be right back.

She and Mark decided to go to the cafeteria, because people had been bringing crackers and fruit into my room, trying to get Mom to eat. She hadn't wanted to leave my room for a meal. While they were eating, they realized that the guys in the band might not know I'd been moved to ICU. Mom called Pat. He thanked her for calling, and asked Mom if she had called Carrie. Mom told him she had. Pat and Carrie were friends, and Pat said he would call her, too.

When they had returned from the cafeteria, Mom stood in the doorway of a small waiting room inside Unit 65. She could see my room from there, and she was waiting for the okay to go back in. My bed linens were being changed and I was being cleaned up, but as soon as my nurse opened my door and looked at her, Mom started walking toward my room. She said hi to me as soon as she walked in, and talked to me as she walked around my bed to stand by my right side and hold my hand. She wanted to make sure I knew she was there. My hand did squeeze hers, and that made her feel better. She kissed my face and stood looking at me and telling me how much she loved me, and how wonderful I was, and how lucky she was to be my mom. Tears rolled down her cheeks, and she bit her lower lip to keep from crying. She pulled her chair up next to me. Her blankets were folded and stacked so that she could sit up higher to my bed. She positioned a pillow to lean on, and laid her head on my bed next to mine and held my hand. She stayed like that for hours and hours, no matter who came into my room.

The ventilation machine was about five feet tall, with a monitor on the front of it and a long blue tube that reached to the one in my mouth that went down my throat. The machine made a loud, rhythmic breathing sound, as it pumped oxygen into me. I was given a feeding tube for better nutritional support, which required a fourth IV pump, and another tube in my mouth that went all the way down into my stomach. I was still receiving doses of leucovorin and lots of fluids to help my body survive the methotrexate. I was also still getting Decadron to treat the swelling caused by the new lesions that had shown up in my brain, and I received another unit of blood. I had tubes coming out of me from everywhere, from the veins in both my arms, two from my mouth for my stomach and bronchial tubes, one from my bladder, and one for the blood flowing into the port in my chest. The monitor above me beeped in steady, rhythmic tones, while my four IV machines clicked and ticked, each one to a different beat. Every 20 minutes the pump at the end of my bed would hum as it pumped air into the pads around my calves to keep my blood from clotting there. It was called an Intermittent Pneumatic Compression Device, and I needed the long, thigh-length pads because my legs were so long. I had a pillow under each knee, a pillow under each arm, two under my head, and pillows on both sides of me for body support. The head of my bed was always raised about ten degrees, so I was never lying completely flat. My wrists were lightly restrained, not all the way to the mattress, but just enough so I couldn't raise my hands all the way up to my mouth. I had already tried to pull the tube out of my mouth a couple of times when not restrained. My nurse told me how important it was that I leave the tube in my mouth, and in a kind but firm voice, explained to me why I needed the restraints. I was sedated and didn't open my eyes to her, but she knew I was awake enough to understand at some level. They had already had to change the mouth tube a couple of times, because I had bitten down on it, so they gave me a sturdier one. I had an extra blanket just for my feet, because they were always cold. It was so chilly in my room that Mom had started wearing both of my hoodies at once to try and stay warm.

Pat and the rest of the band came in together to visit me. Mom wasn't emotionally able to tell anyone what the doctors were saying about me. She tried to relay to the guys, though, that it wasn't good. She knew I would have been happy to see them, and said she was sure that I would hear their voices and understand what they were saying, even though I couldn't respond. They sat and talked with me, telling me about their latest events, who was doing what, things that had happened since we had last been together. They were great. They all talked to me as if I was sitting up looking at them. Mom was sure that I appreciated that. She knew how I hated being pitied and treated differently just because I was sick.

Jennie, the hospital chaplain, stopped in to see us. She said a nice prayer for me with Mom and Mark, and offered to call our ministers for us. She, and both Reverends Connors and Jones from our church, had been visiting me regularly in the four months of my treatment, sitting with us and praying for me often, and I had once joked that Jennie had to keep their numbers on speed dial because of all the unplanned trips we made to the ER.

The next morning we were told I had developed a pulmonary hemorrhage...bleeding in my lung, and there was now a pneumothorax. A tube was inserted just above my eighth rib and into my lung to relieve the pheumorthorax and drain the fluid. The fluid was a watery red color and drained down through the long tube the length of my bed into a bag hanging off the side near my feet. I also had an ECG to check my heart, which apparently was doing fine. I had a low grade fever, too, and that was noted on the report. On my nurse's report, she had written that I was sedated and appeared comfortable, and she explained to Mom and Mark that if I was uncomfortable or feeling pain, I might have a grimace on my face, or a frown, or body tension. She talked to me, checking my pupils and holding my hand, checking for neurological changes. When she spoke my name, I opened my eyes briefly. On her report she wrote, "responds to voice." One of my doctors came in and did the same thing to test for neurological changes during his examination. His way of expressing the same response from me was, "follows commands." They said that it was a good sign, that sedation and oxygen levels were still okay. They would be checking on me like that every four hours, reducing my sedation level temporarily, just enough so that I could respond. And every two hours, two nurses came in to turn and adjust my body into different positions, stuffing pillows around me for comfort, and Mom helped with that, too.

Mark was doing everything he could to take care of others and at the same time be with me and Mom. He was trying to take care of everyone. He tried to give equal time to my two stepsisters and his own family, and be with me and Mom as much as he could. My Aunt Denise was arriving from Spain with my cousins, and they were going to stay at our house. Mark drove an hour to the airport to pick them up, and then took them to a car rental agency near our house so they would have their own transportation. He then took them to our house to get them quickly settled in, so he could drive back to the hospital. He was gone for about four hours. All he wanted to do was be in my room, but he made sure that everyone else was being taken care of, too. When he got back to the hospital, he was exhausted, and after he held my hand and stood with me for a while, he fell down asleep in the fold-out chair-bed that was in the corner of my room.

Aunt Denise had rented a car, and she and my cousins arrived to see me shortly after that, and stayed at the hospital day and night. When Denise first walked up to me and spoke, I opened my eyes to her. I tried very hard to keep them open, but I couldn't do it. A tear rolled down my face, and it made my little cousin, Christian, feel sad for me. He was just twelve years old. He had bought a tiger marionette puppet for me in the hospital gift shop, and was excited to give it to me. His mom explained to him that I was sedated and would not be able to respond. He understood, but was still a little disappointed that I didn't wake up to look at him when he tried to show it to me.

Mom had given my cell phone to Kristen and Traccy, and asked them to call all my friends in my phone book, especially Carrie. They called as many as they could. Within 24 hours, the waiting room and hallways were packed with people. They came in small groups to stand with me for a few minutes.

Two of my other favorite nurses from Unit 42, Tracy and Angela, made the trip upstairs to see me and visit with Mom and Mark. They had each said it was a pleasure to have been able to take care of me, and that they never expected the cancer to get so bad. Angela said she was always impressed at the love and support that I was surrounded with, and how Mom and Mark were always in the hospital with me.

When Carrie walked in, a hush fell over the crowded waiting area. Everyone knew who she was, and Carrie's tall, confident, and naturally beautiful appearance commanded attention everywhere she went. Kristen came in to announce Carrie's arrival and to make sure it was a good time to send her in. Mom waited for her in my room, so she could tell Carrie a little bit about what was going on with me. Carrie was the only person that Mom felt without question that I would prefer to be alone with. Still, Mom talked to me about it, stating that she was not leaving me, but just going outside my room so Carrie and I could be alone. I was not able to respond to Mom about that, but she trusted that it was what I wanted.

Carrie walked into the room, and Mom said, "Ian, Carrie's here."

Carrie said "Hi" to Mom, and as soon as she said that, I sat straight up and opened my eyes. I tried very hard to stay that way, but I was too sedated to do it. My eyes were wide open, but weren't focusing, and my body was too weak to do what my heart wanted to do. Carrie was standing beside me. I tried as hard as I could to be awake for her, and at first it startled Carrie a little.

"He loves you so much, Carrie," Mom told her. Mark and Mom both remarked that I had reacted like that only to Mom's voice several times, and once to a cousin. Mom told Carrie that it meant I was glad Carrie was there, and that I was trying to communicate. She explained to Carrie that I was completely sedated, and even if I did not respond to her, I knew she was there, and her presence with me was very important. She assured Carrie that even if we couldn't talk as we used to, our spirits knew we were together, and communication would take place on that level. Mom left the room and went to my nurse standing at her desk next to my room. Mom asked her to go into my room and tell Carrie everything in detail about my status, so Carrie would know what was happening to me, and Mom wouldn't have to speak the words that she would not even allow herself to believe.

After my nurse had been in to talk to Carrie, she left me with slightly less sedation for a while, so I could better respond to Carrie. Whenever Carrie asked me to squeeze her hand, I did. And when she spoke to me, she could see on my monitor that my heart rate would speed up while I was hearing her voice. My eyes leaked a lot of tears when Carrie was there, and my pain was causing a grimace on my face, but my Carrie was with me, and that was what I had wished for.

A little over half an hour later, Carrie opened the door of my room and Mom went to her. Mom thanked her for being there, and invited her to stay as long as she wanted, or to come back the next day. We were both glad that Carrie was there to see me.

The next day a priest came in to visit me. He prayed beautiful prayers for me, as he anointed my head with oil and holy water. Reverend Jones came in that day, too, visiting and praying with Mom. The cards and gifts that people sent were stacking up along the counter area near the cabinet space in my room. Mom had taped an eight-by-ten photo of me up high on the cabinet, so we could all see me in perfect health and hold that vision for me. She had also taped a prayer card with a picture of the Sacred Heart of Jesus on a hook at the head of my bed when I had first arrived in the ICU, just as she had always done in my other hospital rooms, and prayer cards lined the nurses' viewing window at my feet. Aunt Denise and Christian had visited a cathedral while in Portugal after Mark had called them about me. A native woman had walked up to Denise and saw her crying, and gave her a prayer card of Saint Jude, the patron saint of desperate cases. Aunt Denise added it to the collection in my window.

Mom stayed next to me, holding my hand, resting her head on my bed, and talking to me as if she knew I was listening. Once in a while, I wrapped my fingers around hers for as long as I could hold it. My doctor told her it was just a reflex in my hand, but she didn't want to believe that. Sometimes my eyes would move when she spoke, as if I was looking toward the sound of her voice, and I even opened my eyes completely a couple of times for just a few seconds when Mom kissed my hand and said "I love you, Ian." She sang to me, and sometimes placed her headphones near my ears so I could listen to music CDs. She kept my face clean with washcloths ready by the sink in my room. She kissed away the tears that leaked out of my eyes, and gently wiped the saliva that collected in the corners of my dry mouth. She kept my lip balm in her pocket, so she could easily find it to put on my lips when I needed it, to keep them from getting dry and cracked. And twice each day, she unwrapped the air pads from my calves and washed the sweat from my legs with a cool washcloth. She put the pads back on after giving my skin a few minutes in the open air.

I had another chest x-ray that morning, and all three of my ICU doctors had been in to have a look at me. The medical reports were not good, and they would be discussing my status with Dr. Van Veldhuisen that morning.

Dr. Van and Dr. Fleming came into my room together. At first, Mom and Mark were happy to see them. They stood and shook hands as they each greeted each other, and Dr. Van stepped to my side and looked at my face for a moment. He looked up at my monitors and studied them briefly, then he looked across my bed to Mark and Mom. Dr. Fleming stood quietly at my feet.

"Ian's beta hCG has almost doubled," Dr. Van said, stifling his emotion. "The cancer is progressing quickly."

Ironic, isn't it... the very hormone that protected me from infection inside my mother's womb was evidence in my own blood 20 years later that I was dying of cancer. My beta hCG was almost up where it had been when I came into the hospital on that first weekend in November. The difference was that my lungs were now full of cancer lesions to the point that they could no longer function on their own to keep me alive, and the hope of seeing a positive response to any other type of chemotherapy was very minimal. Dr. Van suspected there was no tumor response in my brain lesions as well. He felt the continuation of chemotherapy treatment would be futile. Mom and Mark had a choice. They could allow treatment to continue, or they could stop treatment and continue keeping me comfortable on the ventilator. He was suggesting the later.

Mark and Mom were reluctant to give up hope. Dr. Fleming tried to help by explaining that continued chemotherapy would just make my sick body even weaker than it already was. He concurred with Dr.

Van that there would be no use in giving me more chemotherapy to treat the cancer, because the cancer was resisting all treatment and the chemotherapy was killing what good cells I had left. They both stayed nearby, and gave Mom and Mark some time to think it over. Mom cried and cried, and asked Dr. Van if he was sure there was nothing else that could be done. He told her he was very sorry, and that he wished there was something else, and his emotions showed as tears flooded his eyes. It was more than two hours before they reluctantly agreed to stop my chemotherapy treatment, and Mom cried for the rest of the day.

Later that day, my ICU doctor came into my room with my nurse to talk to my parents. There was one more thing to consider. I was on record as being full code for all life saving measures to be applied in the event I needed CPR. He discussed the idea that there was no reason to give CPR to a patient on ventilation if the heart stopped, especially since chemotherapy treatment had been discontinued for the reason that it was. The cancer would continue growing, and eventually my living body would succumb to the cancer.

Mom just looked at him. She didn't want to believe what she was hearing and insisted to the doctor that I still had a chance. Anything could happen, with God, she said, and she resented his lack of faith.

My nurse stood quietly beside me, and the doctor explained very calmly to Mom and Mark my current situation. I was already receiving near the maximum amount of oxygen the ventilator could give me. My oxygen supply level could still be increased a little, but eventually that would not be enough, and my heart would continue working harder and harder to try to keep my blood oxygen level circulating. That would put a heavy strain on my heart, and what would follow would most likely be a cardiac arrest. CPR would be very stressful to my weak body, and trying to start my tired heart beating again would probably only result in bruising my chest and possibly cracking my ribs. Even if they did get my heart beating on its own, it would only be a short while before it would wear itself out and stop beating again. Again they would use CPR measures, with the same potential results. This would be a traumatic way for me to die, he told them. It would be better for me, he strongly suggested, to change my code to DNR, meaning "Do Not Resuscitate." In that case, whatever happened, I would be allowed a more peaceful transition.

Every sentence he spoke brought my parents more tears. He was sensitive to their painful position, and told them to talk it over and let him or my nurse know when they had made a decision.

When he left, my nurse stayed to talk with my parents. She explained in more detail what happens to someone in my state during CPR, confirming what the doctor had said. "It's just not a good thing, when the patient is so weak," she said. "It's very sad, and it's so traumatic for the body."

Mark and Mom cried about it for hours, and when my nurse came into my room, they told her through tears that it was okay to change my status to DNR. After that, they had to tell the news to everyone else.

When my friend Jared and his girlfriend came to visit, Mom sat with them for a while in the small waiting room inside ICU. Jared was having a real hard time seeing me so sick, sedated, and hooked up to all that equipment. He couldn't get himself to walk into my room to see me the way I was. When Jared asked Mom how I was doing, she told him that my doctors were saying I was dying. She still couldn't state the fact outright. She wouldn't let herself believe it. But she told him if he would go in and stand near me, I would feel the connection we always had with one another. She told him to talk to me, that it was important to do that. When he was ready, Mom walked to my room with him. She leaned down and kissed me on the cheek, and told me Jared was there, then she stepped out of the room so he could be alone with me for a while.

Keaton was not able to get leave from the Air Force, because he was still in his first year, and I was not immediate family. But his mom and younger sister were there, and brought Keaton with them in spirit.

My good friend, Karl, had called our high school football coach to tell him that I was in ICU, and Coach and his wife came with Karl and his family to see me. Karl came in first, and laid my No.9 football jersey over my feet. He told me it was a gift from Coach. They all came and stood around me for a long time, while a CD of my own music was playing on small speakers in my room.

Reverend Connors came that evening, and invited all my family and friends in the waiting area to come in to my room and pray with her. Mark and Mom of course were at my side, and Mom held my hand and kept her head on my pillow next to mine. My room was packed wall to wall with people. They surrounded my bed as the reverend stood at my feet and prayed a long, lovely prayer for peace in my transition into Heaven.

It was getting to be about ten o'clock that night, and my room was again becoming quiet after a long 12 hours of visitors coming and going. My nurse told Mom and Mark that she had never seen a patient so well loved, to have had so many visitors for as many days as I'd had. She cried as she told them that she knew I must be a really wonderful guy, to be so well loved by so many people. Her name was Kristy. She had been my nurse when I had first arrived in ICU, and for most of my time there. She was very nice, and I at least had been able to talk to her in those first few days.

Aaron, another good friend, drove straight to the hospital all the way from Chicago that night. He couldn't get a flight any faster, and his good friend Dan came with him and insisted on doing the driving. Aaron was in such a hurry to get to me that Dan felt Aaron would be a danger on the road. Aaron came into my room with his parents, and they stayed with me and my parents for a long time. Aaron gave my mom a clear acrylic stone with a purple heart in the center. He told her he had prayed for me every day while holding that stone.

My oxygen supply level had been raised again in the night. It was up to 100 percent. The ventilator was now giving me the maximum amount of oxygen it could. My mom barely slept that night, sitting in the chair next to me with her head resting on my bed next to mine. Both she and Mark were awake at 3:30 that morning, and my nurse explained to them that I would be getting worse by the hour as the oxygen saturation levels in my blood continued to drop.

At 5:00 a.m., my nurse walked quietly into the room again. She recorded all my vitals, held my hand and spoke to me, and checked the pupils in my eyes for dilation. Then she checked all my IV needle sites, and emptied the plastic reservoirs of blood and urine at the end of my bed. "He's doing okay," she whispered to Mom. She was keeping a close watch on me all morning, coming into my room frequently to look me over.

It was eight o'clock that morning when my doctor came into my room. He examined me, and he too held my hand and spoke to me, and checked for dilation in my pupils. He stood thoughtfully at my head, and looked at Mom and Mark.

He had been telling them through the past several days that I was not going to live. He hadn't minced words, he hadn't given them a fluffy version of the truth. He had said it outright, and Mom still wouldn't hear it. She felt that he just didn't understand. She gripped onto her faith that God's miracles show up when the outcome seems most bleak. The doctors were wrong, she had thought. They are allowing themselves to be influenced by their own medical instruments, and so many years of experience with other dying people, other cancer patients, that they can't expect miracles any more. I was not just any cancer patient, she felt sure of it. I was Ian, and God was taking care of me, and tomorrow the doctors and nurses would gather around us and say they don't understand what happened, but somehow, this guy Ian appears to be breathing on his own again and his blood oxygen levels are back to normal. She couldn't let go of that faith. My doctor had been frustrated with her because of this. He saw it as denial.

But this time he was different. His face was firm, not frustrated. His expression was definite, but not stern, and his dark brown eyes looked at her with a physician's kind of detached compassion. With a new and gentle voice, he began to explain my health situation to them. My respiration levels were weakening by the hour. He reminded them that the ventilator was already set at giving me 100 percent, and soon, that would not be enough. My lungs were still leaking bloody secretions, and my respiratory situation was what they call agonal. That meant my breath could not sustain life, because my low respiratory rate and low oxygen saturation level was causing a buildup of carbon dioxide in my body. It was likely that some small amount of brain damage had already occurred. As a result of all of these factors, my organs were showing signs of lack of blood support. Diminished bowel sounds were the first signal that organs were beginning to stop working. My heart rate was already very high, a state they called tachicardia. As my blood oxygen level became lower, and it would, my heart would keep working harder, and the eventual result would likely be heart failure. He was strongly suggesting that my parents may not want to put me through that. They could have my ventilator removed to let me die a more peaceful, natural death.

Mom admitted to him that she didn't think she could make such a decision, to give up on her son.

He told them to take their time and think about it. Ask questions. "Ian might live on life support for a day or two, maybe even a week in a best-case scenario, but he will never be without the medication that keeps him asleep. Ian will not ever wake up. He will never leave this room in ICU. He will live completely sedated like this until his heart can't do it anymore." He left Mom and Mark with those thoughts, and reminded them that my heart rate was already very high.

In the sleepy quiet of my darkened room, they couldn't believe what was being asked of them. They talked about it, and cried about it for hours and hours. Giving up was unthinkable. Mom laid quiet with her head next to me, her hand holding mine. Mark sat quietly by our side. Mom thought about what the doctor had said. It couldn't be true that she had to decide to give up. It seemed the only option was to keep me on ventilation, and wait for me to get better. She only cared what I wanted, and she had been praying for my highest good all my life. She had always prayed that she would be everything I needed my mom to be, and trusted that God was guiding her in every aspect of that, if she could keep herself open to it. But now, she did not feel that the answers were being given to her. It was too emotionally painful to be able to make a decision like the one she was being asked to make.

Every now and then she would ask me aloud, "Ian, please tell me, what do you want me to do?"

Minutes ticked away into more hours. She never moved from my side, thinking, crying, holding and kissing my hand. Mark stayed right there with us, sitting beside Mom, resting his hand on her back, being the pillar of strength and acceptance that he always had been. Mom talked to me over and over about it. She asked me to tell her what I wanted her to do. She begged me, saying that she could not make such a decision. She held my hand, and asked me to please give her a sign to let her know what I wanted.

She was crying when the doctor came into my room to check on us all. She admitted to him that she did not know what was the right thing to do.

He looked at her compassionately, and asked if she thought it would help if she saw what my lungs looked like on the inside. She kissed my cheek, and told me she'd be right back. She went with him to the desk across from my room. His computer showed my medical records, and he clicked on my latest chest x-rays. Mom read my name at the top of each screen he showed her. On a monitor next to him, he clicked onto an x-ray image of the normal lungs of another patient. He showed Mom that the normal lungs were clear, and all black in the image. The all-white images on my x-rays showed that my lungs were 90 percent full of cancer. My doctor explained to her that I would never have the ability to breathe again. Never.

Mom came back into my room and told Mark what she had seen. My nurse came in to check on me, and asked them if they had any questions. Mom told her that she'd seen my lung images, and my nurse understood that Mom and Mark were now trying to process the emotions brought on with that information. She noted my blood oxygen level, and said that I probably didn't have much time. She held my hand and talked to me a lot, trying to get me to respond. She checked the dilation of my pupils, and talked to me some more, saying my name repeatedly, with no response from me. Even at 100 percent oxygen supply, I was not sustaining enough oxygen to support life in my body. She told Mom and Mark that I was showing small signs of brain damage.

Mom started crying again. She thought it would just be horrible for me to be stuck inside my body the way it was, and started to feel that this was my way of telling her that I wanted her to let me go. She and Mark stayed quiet together, looking at each other and looking at me. They talked and tried to decide together what I would want them to do for me, then they sat quietly with me again. Mom held my hand close to her face and kissed it over and over. She didn't want to let go. She sat quietly looking at my face for the longest time, as hundreds of little memories of me in our life together flashed through her mind. She was thinking about how much she loved me, how lucky she felt to be my mom, and wondered what was the right thing to do for her son now. Time ticked away, and she just sat there, holding my hand against her cheek, looking at my face, as if waiting for me to look over at her.

"What do you want me to do, Ian?" she asked, with tears on her face.

"Let me go..." in an instant, she thought she heard me whisper.

She looked over at Mark, his head laying on my bed.

When he sat up to look at her, they both knew in that moment, as if suddenly my peaceful answer was theirs. Mom cried and sobbed at the thought of it. When my nurse came in a while later, Mark told her they had an answer for the doctor. Their one request was that they be left alone with me during my transition, once all the medical devices had been removed. They told my doctor they would let him know when they were ready. They still wanted time with me alone.

Mom blessed me with holy water again, and prayed the rosary for me, hoping I was able in spirit to pray with her. She and Mark sat quietly holding my hands, crying, and loving me. Mom kissed my hand over and over, and laid her head next to my face, kissing my face, and my head, my eyes, my nose, and the corner of my mouth. She whispered in my ear, "I love you, Ian." Mark laid his hands and his head on my legs, and quietly loved me. Mom cried and wailed, and said, "I love you, Ian," over and over, kissing my face and my hand, and holding it close to her face. And she lay quiet, with her face next to mine and her arm resting on my chest, holding my face in her hand and listening to my breath.

My pain meds were increased slightly to make sure I stayed without pain, then all my IV's were removed. Mom and Mark stayed with me while the staff removed everything attached to me. Mom and Mark hid their eyes in my bed while the vent and feeding tubes were gently pulled out of my mouth. Once my body was free of all of the life supporting devices, I breathed shallow breaths on my own for only ten minutes. Mark laid his head and arm across my legs. Mom lay still next to me, with her face right up to mine, listening and catching the scent of my breath and my skin, kissing my face now and then, and holding my hand close to her heart. After my last breath, she laid her head on my chest and listened until my heart beat for the last time. The last beat was a little slower than the rest, as if to say "Good - bye."

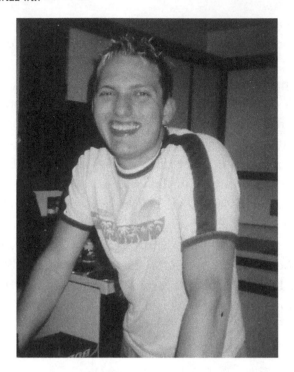

Me in better days, laughing with friends.

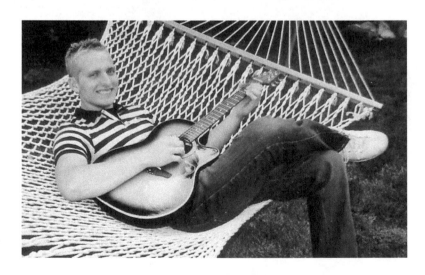

Me in my backyard, writing a song

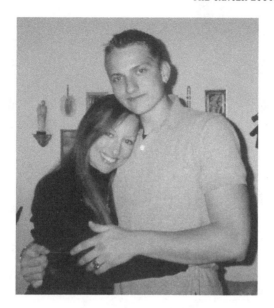

With my mom, before cancer

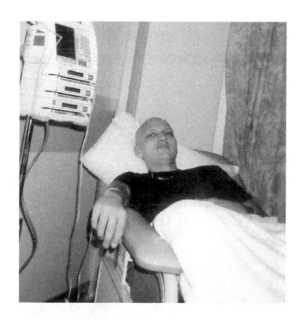

Getting ready for chemo in KU Cancer Center

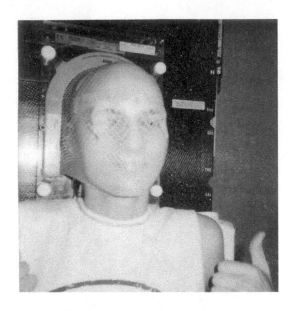

Wearing my radiation mask, bolted down for treatment

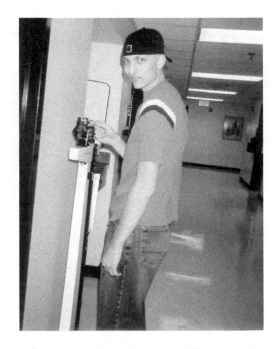

On the scale weighing 158 pounds

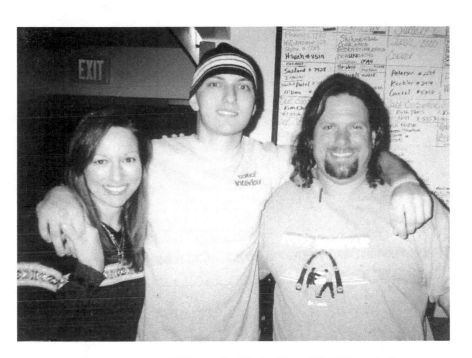

Mom, me, and Mook in Unit 42 at KU Hospital

14

Testicular Cancer Information You Can Live With

Ian's story did not have to end the way it did. Testicular cancer is curable if it is treated in early stages, and there is no reason any other young man should have to go through what my son went through. Awareness of testicular cancer will hopefully lead to monthly self examinations of the testicles. Monthly self examination is the key to finding this cancer in the early stages. This, and getting medical help as soon as a lump is noticed, are the best things a guy can do to protect himself from testicular cancer. As a guy reaches puberty, it is a good idea to find a family doctor who will take the time to talk to him about testicular cancer.

Learn about testicular cancer, and talk to others about it.

Doctors, talk to your young male patients about testicular cancer, and give them literature on it.

Patients, ask your doctor to talk to you about testicular cancer. Ask for information.

Teachers, tell your students. Youth group leaders, tell your members and hand out information about it.

Parents, talk to your sons and daughters about testicular cancer. Girls can help spread awareness, too.

Testicular Cancer Facts:

- Testicular cancer, although considered to be a rare cancer in the realm of all cancers, is still the most common cancer in young men, ages 14-45
- A growing number of testicular cancer diagnoses are in boys as young as 12 years old, or just after the age of puberty.
- An undescended testicle, or family history of testicular cancer, appear to be the only risk factors, but do not necessarily indicate that a young man will develop testicular cancer.
- Many young men who have been diagnosed with testicular cancer have had no risk factors in their health history.
- Most commonly affected are white males between the age of 14 and 45, but testicular cancer does affect all races.
- Testicular cancer can grow quickly, often with no symptoms except one or more lumps in a testicle.
- There usually is no pain in early stages.
- Testicular cancer is curable with early detection and early treatment.
- Monthly self testicular examination is the key to early detection and survival of testicular cancer.

Please teach young men about testicular cancer and its symptoms!

- The first sign of testicular cancer is usually a small lump in one of the testicles. Often, a testicle lump is nothing to worry about, but only a doctor can make that determination.
- A young man should take note of the size of the lump, and size of both testicles. He should then check often for changes in the size of the lump and testicles, or for an increase in the number of lumps.
- If a young man feels something is not right with his body, it is very important for him to find a good doctor who will check him for testicular cancer, and talk with him about it.
- A test for testicular cancer is not painful. Testing is done with one or more of the following: ultrasound, CT scan, X-ray, MRI, and blood testing.

Symptoms to look for:

- One or more lumps in either testicle.
- Changes or enlargement of a testicle.
- Any feeling of "heaviness" in the scrotum, or sudden collection of fluid in the scrotum.
- Pain or a dull ache in the testes, or groin area.
- Enlargement, lump, or tenderness of one or both nipples, especially if combined with testicle lumps or enlargement.
- Sexual problems, combined with testicle lumps or enlargement.

How to do a self testicular exam:

- A self exam is best done after or during a warm bath or shower, when skin is softest.
- Most testicle lumps are not cancerous, but any changes in size, shape, or weight should be checked by a doctor.
- Support the scrotum in the palm of the hand and become familiar with the size, shape, and weight of each testicle.
- Examine each testicle by rolling it between fingers and thumb. Press gently to feel for swelling, lumps, or changes in firmness.
- Each testicle has an epididymis at the top, which carries sperm to the penis. This may feel like a lump, but it is normal.
- Testicular cancer spreads through the body if left untreated. The farther testicular cancer spreads into the body, the more intense the treatment will be, and the less chance a guy has for survival.
- Learn more about testicular cancer at www.IansStory.org.

How testicular cancer spreads through the body:

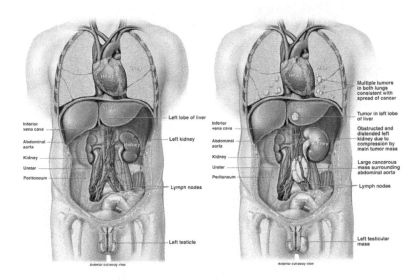

Above at left, is a normal body without cancer. The image on the right shows multiple cancerous lesions that have spread from the testicle to the abdomen, liver, and lungs.

Testicular cancer will spread in the body, first by invading the surrounding tissue. This spread creates a growing tumor mass in the testicle. Once the tumor is larger, cancer cells begin to break off and flow into the blood or the lymph system, where they travel to other parts of the body. Cancer cells then form other tumors by invading other organ tissues. The process is called metastasis, and you can't feel it happening any more than you can feel normal tissues growing. It is much easier to cure testicular cancer if it is treated before it reaches the point of metastasis.

References

University of Kansas Hospital and Medical Center - www.kumed.com
The Mayo Clinic - www.mayoclinic.com
Indiana University - www.indiana.edu
University of Maryland Medical Center - www.umm.edu
National Cancer Institute - www.cancer.gov

www.webmd.com
www.chemocare.com
www.medterms.com
www.hclfonline.com
www.checkemlads.com

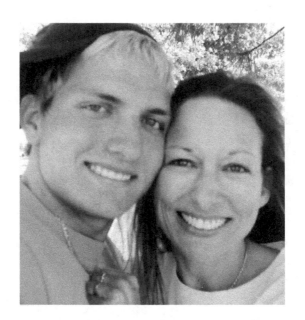

The author with her son in 2004

About the Author

Karen McWhirt is a freelance writer and Testicular Cancer Awareness advocate. From the year her son was diagnosed with the disease, Karen has been making endless efforts to continue teaching others about this most common, curable cancer of young men. Her son's main caretaker for the duration of his treatment, Karen saw elements of a cancer patient's life that most people never see. She shares Ian's poignant story to fulfill his wish that other young men would learn about the seriousness of testicular cancer and the importance of being proactive against the disease when it is in early stages, to avoid the fate that Ian suffered. Karen currently manages two websites for Testicular Cancer Awareness, volunteers at health fairs, and offers free public speaking, and free Testicular Cancer Awareness publications as her means of spreading awareness of testicular cancer. She has also published one music CD of Ian's music for Testicular Cancer Awareness.

Free Music CD - "Something To Remember"

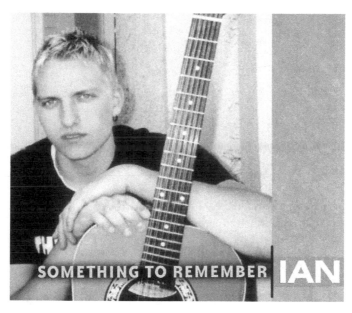

A collection of Ian's original music as written and performed live by Ian in a Kansas City radio station studio, with one bonus track, Ian's cover of "Love Song." Ian's original songs are about love, relationships, and moving on. His smooth vocals and melodic guitar chords are a compliment to any mood.

CD insert contains information about testicular cancer, its symptoms, and how to perform a TSE (testicular self-exam).

A great gift in the interest of Testicular Cancer Awareness for Young Men!

Receive one free music CD with purchase of this book. Offer good while CD supplies last. To request a free CD, please contact the author by e-mail from this website:

www.togetherwewillwin.net

CPSIA information can be obtained
at www.ICGtesting.com
Printed in the USA
BVHW07s1733111018
529897BV00001B/131/P

9 781432 748678